The History and Physical Examination Casebook

The History and Physical Examination Casebook

Diane L. Elliot, M.D.
Professor of Medicine
Department of Medicine
Division of General Medicine
Section of Health Promotion and Sports Medicine
Oregon Health Sciences University
Portland, Oregon

Linn Goldberg, M.D.
Professor of Medicine
Department of Medicine
Division of General Medicine;
Head, Section of Health Promotion and Sports Medicine
Oregon Health Sciences University
Portland, Oregon

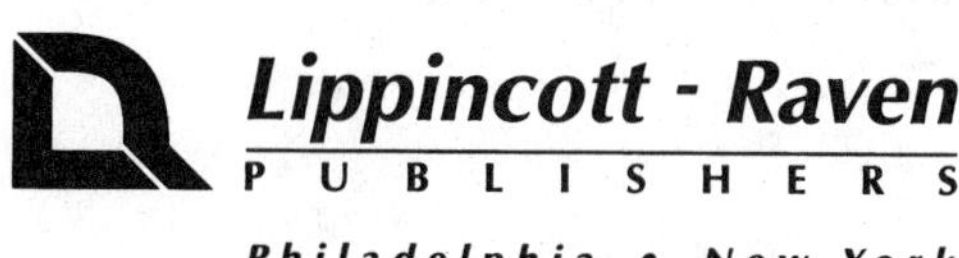
Lippincott - Raven
PUBLISHERS
Philadelphia • New York

Manufacturing Manager: Dennis Teston
Production Manager: Maxine Langweil
Production Editor: Kimberly Swan
Cover Designer: Karen Quigley
Indexer: Jayne Percy
Compositor: Compset, Inc.
Printer: Maple Press

Printed in the United States of America

9 8 7 6 5 4 3 2 1

Library of Congress Cataloging-in-Publication Data

Elliot, Diane L.
The history and physical examination casebook / Diane L. Elliot, Linn Goldberg.
p. cm.
Includes bibliographical references and index.
ISBN 0-316-23339-0
1. Medical history taking—Case studies. 2. Physical diagnosis—Case studies. I. Goldberg, Linn. II. Title.
[DNLM: 1. Medical History Taking. 2. Physical Examination. WB 290 E46h 1997]
RC65.E45 1997
616.07'51—dc21
DNLM/DLC
for Library of Congress 97-5555
CIP

Contents

Preface

"So, how do you put this case together?" is a question we have asked countless medical students and house officers. Interpreting a patient's medical history and physical findings, synthesizing information, and arriving at a working diagnosis are critical skills for physicians. As medical students move into their clerkship experiences, they are expected to reorder their disease-focused learning and apply it to patients presenting with undiagnosed problems—problems that often relate to several organ systems and the interaction of different illnesses. This book results from more than fifteen years of teaching physical diagnosis and helping students make the transition from disease-oriented pathophysiology and mechanical patient evaluation skills to assessment of patients.

Each chapter contains the following sections. The chapter **Objectives** are a listing of the key concepts covered in the chapter, including terms to understand, symptoms and signs of common illnesses (such as, aortic stenosis and temporal arteritis) and differential diagnosis of frequent presenting complaints, (for example, unintentional weight loss, back pain and lower extremity swelling). The list previews the chapter's contents and allows readers to self-assess their mastery of the material. The **Pertinent Points** section presents the critical elements of patient assessment for that chapter. They are a guide to specific questions and physical findings when evaluating patients with problems in that chapter's domain. The **Vignettes**, drawn from actual clinical cases, are edited accounts of patients whose illness exemplifies disorders in the chapter. The cases are designed to interest readers, encourage application of content, and provide a vicarious clinical experience that enhances retaining the content. The **Vignette Objectives** are learning points covered in that section of the chapter, and all are items that clinicians (including third year medical students) would be expected to know.

The **Content** focuses on information related to evaluating patients, such as how the history and physical examination are used to distinguish among diagnoses, what findings might be anticipated with particular disorders, and the sequence of findings as an illness progresses. The text assumes that readers are familiar with the "how to" of performing basic physical examination skills. We have included information concerning the reliability and utility of specific physical assessment maneuvers. Much of the material is organized into tables and algorithms to increase clarity and clinical application.

The **Vignette Follow-up** describes the patient's outcome and subsequent course. Each section of a chapter begins with one or more vignettes. An average of 12 patients are presented in each chapter. Following all the vignettes and content, chapters conclude with the **Objectives Review**, and with annotated **References**, concerning specific topics from that chapter. The review is a compilation of the chapter's **Vignette Objectives**, designed to promote self-assessment and review of material covered in the chapter.

This book may be used in several ways. Students may read its chapters coincident with their pathophysiology courses. The vignettes illustrate common disorders and demonstrate how patient assessment can define illnesses from the patient's complaint(s). In this way, the chapters illustrate the relevance of pathophysiology teaching and can increase a student's understanding and retention of course work. The book also can be read as students begin their clinical experiences. The casebook format makes interesting reading, and the information reviews important skills and concepts used in patient care.

This book can be a reference when evaluating patients. It is portable, and the chapter structure and index allow easy access to its content. For common disorders and patient complaints, the book outlines the relevant history and physical examination components and identifies the pertinent positive and negative findings to be identified. In addition, disorders are placed in context with other conditions with similar findings. Finally, the book is appropriate reading for clinicians at all levels of training and experience. The information is important for patient care, and the vignettes (as with all patient encounters) are interesting and illustrate the unique biologic variability of illnesses and how clinical manifestations are not as clear cut as a "classic presentation" suggests.

Acknowledgments

Our deepest gratitude goes to the patients who have allowed us the privilege of caring for them, learning from them, and sharing their stories and physical findings with others. We also want to thank the many individuals who have been our students. Their questions increase our understanding with each encounter. Their awe and excitement with patient assessment constantly renew our own interest in these enduring abilities.

1. Well Individuals and Special Situations

Objectives

List history and physical examination findings relating to the following issues:

- Screening physical examination
- Adolescent health care, including major health risks and confidentiality concerns
- Sports physical examination
- Falls and the elderly
- Advanced directives
- Risks for HIV infection
- Asymptomatic patients with HIV infection

Pertinent Points

History

Introduction: "small talk," calibration, set agenda
Chief complaint
Identify patient concerns and problems to address
Survey for other problems: ongoing medical problems? medications?
History of present illness (HPI)
- Time line, symptoms, PQRST (*p*alliate/*p*rovoke, *q*uality, location/*r*adiation, associated *s*ymptoms, tempo/*t*iming), affect on function/life-style, patient's attributes (what the patient thinks is going on and concerns about particular diagnoses)
- Pertinent positives that support and negatives that oppose diagnostic possibilities

Past medical history (PMHx)
- Childhood problems
- Medical illnesses
- Hospitalizations (medical, surgical, trauma, OB/GYN, psychiatric)
- Medications
- Allergy to medications
- Family history
- Habits: diet, smoking, alcohol, illicit drugs, exercise
- Sexual history
- HIV risk factors (sexual partners, including male-male contact, prostitutes, and those from high-risk groups; IV drug use; prior blood transfusion [1978–1985], and hemophiliacs receiving non–heat-treated concentrate [1978–1985]
- Immunizations (childhood, tetanus, Pneumovax, hepatitis A and B, influenza)
- Injury risk (seat belt, firearms, drinking-driving, helmet use)
- Abuse
- Occupational history (initial screening questions such as problems related to work, followed by more specific questions about exposure to chemicals, dust, noise, repeated musculoskeletal trauma, or infectious illnesses)

Review of systems
Social history/life-style

Physical Examination

(Modify on the basis of the patient's history and any conditions more prevalent in the patient's demographic group)

Inspection
- Nutritional state, height, weight
- Observe skin

Vital signs
- Blood pressure, heart rate

Integument
- Inspect skin, hair, nails

HEENT
- Inspect face and head
- Assess visual acuity, inspect fundi
- Test hearing
- Inspect oral cavity and pharynx
- Palpate neck for thyroid, cervical and supraclavicular adenopathy, carotid pulsations, and mass

Chest
- Auscultate lung fields

Cardiac
- Palpate point of maximal impulse (PMI)
- Auscultate precordium

Breasts
- Inspect and palpate (include axillary nodes)

Abdomen
- Percuss liver span
- Palpate for abdominal tenderness, liver edge, splenomegaly, and masses
- Digital rectal exam

Pelvic exam
- When indicated for Papanicolaou smear

Musculoskeletal
- Inspect for symmetry, deformities, and edema
- Palpate popliteal, dorsal pedal, and posterior tibial pulses

Neurological
- Mental status if more than 70 years old, confusion, neurologic complaint, or "a poor historian"
- cranial nerves: II (visual acuity), VII (symmetry of facial movement), VIII (hearing), XII (tongue movement)
- Inspect symmetry of muscle bulk and movements
- Observe gait

Vignette 1

Reliability: refers to the reproducibility or concordance between the findings of two examiners (interobserver reliability) or the findings from repeated examinations performed by the same observer (intraobserver reliability); this is an index of the degree of confidence and diagnostic certainty that can be placed in a finding; sources contributing to unreliability relate to the examiner, the patient, and the examination setting

Routine or screening physical examination: once advocated to be done annually for maintaining health and preventing illness; the utility of physical examination components has been critically assessed, and various health organizations have recommended the components of and the frequency with which these examinations should be performed (see Table 1-1).

AS is a second-year medical student who is visiting her parents during the winter break. While at home, two events occur that make AS wonder if what she has learned in medical school applies to the "real" world. First, she is unable to answer her mother's question about whether she needs a "complete" check-up and what procedures she should expect the physician to do. Then, while demonstrating her diagnostic equipment, AS cannot hear a murmur that her 16-year-old sister asks her to examine. Her sister's pediatrician noted a murmur years ago during a sports physical examination, and the sister wants to know if it is still present.

Vignette Objectives

1. What portions of the physical examination should be included in an adult, well-patient "screening" exam?
2. List factors that contribute to disagreement about physical examination findings and, for each, provide ways to increase exam reliability.

The Well-Patient Screening Examination

What Constitutes a Routine Exam?

Several excellent texts on physical examination are available (see the Preface, vii), and these books provide explicit instructions for performing physical examinations. However, most do not include recommendations for an expedient "screening examination," and physicians differ greatly on the exam procedures they usually perform. This variability among practitioners was demonstrated by a study in which similar new patients (trained by the investigators to present a consistent history) were evaluated by several different physicians. Despite comparable histories and patient characteristics, the interactions lasted from 5 to 60 minutes and providers performed from 16% to 89% of the potential physical examination components.

Some of the variability among practitioners may be due to changes in the recommendations for routine physical exams. The American Medical Association first endorsed periodic physical examinations in the early 1920s, and an annual check-up continued to be advocated into the 1970s. However, in recent years, specific physical examination maneuvers have been studied to define how useful they are for identifying illness. Table 1-1 lists physical examination components and the recommendations of four expert panels or reviewers with regard to whether each should be performed routinely. Only two examination procedures, (blood pressure measurement and clinical breast exam after 40 years of age), were recommended consistently.

Despite evidence that only a few exam features have been documented to be useful in detecting illness, physicians continue to perform examinations that include many features less useful in detecting illness. Luckmann and Melville found that more than 90% of family physicians think adults need to undergo periodic complete physical examinations, and more than 95% of these clinicians included the following components in their routine exams: weight and blood pressure measurement; mouth inspection; palpation of the lymph nodes and thyroid gland; abdominal examination; and auscultation of the lungs and heart. The observed discrepancy between what has been shown to be useful and what is done could be due to several factors: (1) habits are difficult to change; (2) practitioners do not believe or know current recommendations; (3) patients expect "complete" exams; and (4) the prior chance finding of an abnormality that affected patient care may cause a physician to continue to use that exam component(s).

An additional factor may be that physical examinations enhance physician-patient rapport in a way not appreciated by determining its utility for finding disease. This was substantiated by a study of physician-patient interactions, which showed that the time spent on physical assessment was positively related to patient satisfaction. Extrapolating from study of the medical interview, patient satisfaction is enhanced by maintaining patient comfort, avoiding patient embarrassment, and demonstrating facility with exam maneuvers.

Table 1-1. Recommended physical examination maneuvers

Maneuver	Canadian Task Force (1988, 1989)	U.S. Preventive Services Task Force (1989)	Oboler and LaForce (1989)	American Colleges of Physicians (1991)
Blood pressure	At least every 5 years and beginning at age 65 every 1 to 2 years	At least every 1 to 2 years and beginning at age 65 every year	At least every 1 to 2 years	At least every 1 to 2 years and annually if positive risk factors for coronary artery disease
Height and weight	Adolescents, women of low socioeconomic status, or those with unusual dietary habits	Each 1 to 3 years after age 40 and annually after age 65	Every 4 years	Not considered
Skin inspection	Annually after age 18 in those with excess sun exposure or dysplastic nevi	After age 18 if excess sun exposure, dysplastic nevi, or history of skin cancer	Evaluate for dysplastic nevi at initial visit; annually for high-risk patients	Not considered
Oral cavity	After age 65 and begin at age 18 if uses tobacco	After age 18 if uses tobacco or alcohol	Not recommended	Annual dental exam; mouth exam not recommended
Visual acuity	Not considered	Annually after age 65	Annually after age 60	Not considered
Hearing	After age 18 or if noise exposure	Annually after age 65 and begin at age 19 if noise exposure	Annually after age 60 by audioscope	Not considered
Auscultate carotids	Not recommended	Perform if (1) positive risks for or symptoms of atherosclerotic vascular disease, (2) every 1 to 3 years after age 40, and (3) annually after age 65	Not recommended	Not considered
Clinical breast examination	Annually after age 40 and after age 35 if family history of breast cancer	Annually after age 40 and after age 35 if family history of breast cancer	Annually after age 40 and after age 18 if family history of breast cancer	Annually after age 40 and after age 18 if family history of breast cancer
Chest and pulmonary exam	Not considered	Not considered	Not recommended	Not considered

Table 1-1. Recommended physical examination maneuvers *(continued)*

Maneuver	Canadian Task Force (1988, 1989)	U.S. Preventive Services Task Force (1989)	Oboler and LaForce (1989)	American Colleges of Physicians (1991)
Cardiac exam	Not considered	Not considered	Ausculate for valvular disease at initial visit and when age 60	Not considered
Abdominal exam* *Evaluation for hepatomegaly, splenomegaly, and ascites included in Chapter 7	Not considered	Not considered	Palpate for abdominal aortic aneurysm annually in men over age 60	Not considered
Stool for occult blood	Annually after age 40 if family history of colon cancer	Annually after age 40 if family history of colon cancer	Annually after age 50 and begin at age 40 if family history of colon cancer	Annually after age 50 and begin at age 40 if family history of colon cancer
Lymph nodes	Not considered	Not considered	Not recommended	Not considered
Musculoskeletal exam	Not considered	Not recommended	Back exam not recommended	Not considered
Bimanual pelvic examination and cervical cytology	Not considered	Cervical cytology every 1 to 3 years; routine pelvic exams not recommended	Cervical cytology if sexually active; after two negative annual cytologic exams, cervical cytology at least every 3 years; palpation of ovaries not recommended	Pelvic exam not considered; cervical cytology every 1 to 3 years
Digital prostate palpation	Not recommended	Not recommended	Not recommended	Not considered
Mental status	Not recommended	Not recommended	Not recommended	After age 65

How Reliable Are Physical Examination Findings?

Clinicians frequently disagree on their reported physical exam findings. This inconsistency is due to differences in the patient, examiner, and clinical setting (Table 1-2). Table 1-2 also lists ways to increase the **reliability** of examination findings. Bias can be minimized by asking a colleague, who is provided with minimal clinical information, to repeat portions of the exam. In addition, comparing findings with objective test results helps calibrate and refine an examiner's abilities. Similarly, repeated assessments of a patient over time acquaint clinicians with the potential variability in physical findings.

Table 1-2. Reliability of physical examination findings

Variables	Factors that decrease reliability	Methods to increase reliability
Patient	Biologic variation among people Effects of patient positioning Changes due to an illness's natural history and management	Examine many people to calibrate the range of normal variation Repeat assessments to evaluate the tempo of an illness and expected changes in a patient's findings
Examiner	Biologic variation in the senses Tendency to record inference rather than evidence Biased by prior experiences Incorrect use of diagnostic tools	Seek corroboration of key findings (repeating oneself and examination by others) Ask "blinded" (nonbiased) examiners to assess the patient Confirm key clinical findings with appropriate tests Report specific findings rather than inferences
Clinical setting	Disruptive examination environments (patient comfort and cooperation; setting's noise level and lighting) Malfunction or absence of examination equipment	Establish rapport before the examination Match environment to diagnostic task Use appropriate, well-functioning examination tools

Vignette Follow-up

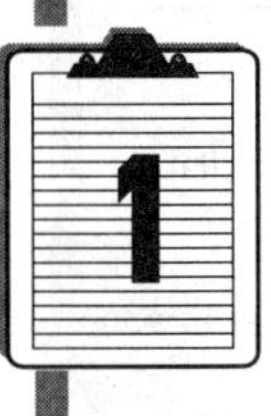

Once back at school, AS sends her mother the current screening recommendations and then calls her to clarify her understanding. In addition, AS reviews the section of her physical diagnosis text on cardiac assessment and concludes that her sister probably has a flow murmur. However, AS examined her sister sitting up in a noisy living room, rather than supine in a quiet office, and these factors may have contributed to her not hearing a murmur.

Vignette 2

Clinical breast examination: breast examination performed by a health care provider, as opposed to breast self-examination and mammography.

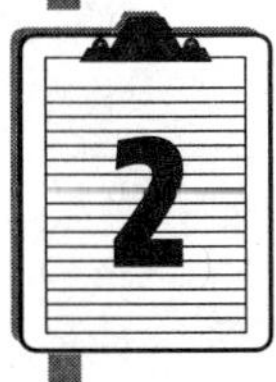

GLC is a 23-year-old woman with a clinic appointment as a new patient who needs a Pap smear. Her older sister had an abnormal Pap smear several years ago, and Ms. C is therefore somewhat apprehensive. Being new to the clinic, she is unsure about what is expected of her. The clinic aide escorts Ms. C to the exam room and asks her to change into a gown. Ms. C is not sure which way the gown closes, but guesses the opening goes in the front. After several minutes, the aide returns and instructs Ms. C to go to the bathroom, located down the clinic hallway, and "empty your bladder." The aide also tells Ms. C that her gown is on "backward." Ms. C adjusts her gown before leaving the room but still feels uncomfortable walking to the bathroom wearing only the gown. She waits several minutes for one of the bathrooms to become available and, after using it, returns to her assigned clinic room. She waits another 20 minutes before the resident physician appears.

The resident is late because of ward responsibilities, and the clinic nurse informs Dr. M that his patient is waiting as soon as he arrives in the clinic. A medical student, who is assisting in clinic, and Dr. M enter Ms. C's room and introduce themselves. The resident physician apologizes for being late and tells Ms. C that the pelvic exam will be done as quickly as possible. Her heels are placed in the metal stirrups, and with the medical student sitting at his side, the physician tells her to "spread your legs." This is followed by a rapid external genitalia exam that includes inspection of the labia, the urethral meatus, and the perineum. The resident inserts the double-blade metal speculum into the introitus to visualize the vaginal walls and cervix. A Pap smear is obtained, and the speculum is withdrawn. He then completes a bimanual and rectovaginal examination. No discussion takes place during the entire procedure, other than a few hushed words between the resident and medical student.

When the exam is completed, the resident tells Ms. C, who is still positioned with her feet in the stirrups, that the results will be mailed to her in a few days, and then he and the medical student leave the room. The aide helps the patient out of the stirrups and tells her she can dress and leave.

Vignette Objectives

1. List ways to decrease a woman's anxiety during a pelvic examination.
2. How does a woman's confidence in her ability to do breast self-examination relate to how likely she is to obtain a mammogram?

Breast, Pelvic, and Genitourinary Examinations

The breast, pelvic, and genitourinary examinations are most likely to cause a patient to feel embarrassed and vulnerable, and each requires special attention to patient comfort. Table 1-3 lists means to reduce a woman's anxiety during a pelvic examination. Women's preferences and physicians' practices vary concerning the presence of a chaperon during the pelvic examination. In general, younger women have a greater preference for a chaperon, and approximately half of women overall prefer to have a chaperon with a male examiner. Unlike

Table 1-3. Procedures that reduce patient anxiety during pelvic examination

Obtain the history before the patient disrobes
Elevate the head of the exam table to facilitate eye contact
Monitor patient comfort
Use an unhurried manner
Inform patient about findings

women's reaction to the pelvic examination, men's reactions to a genitourinary exam have not been well studied. When assessed, male adolescents have shown a preference not to have a chaperon present during the genitourinary examination.

The **breast examination** offers an opportunity to review exam technique with the woman and to emphasize the importance of mammography. Expressing the need for mammography is important, because the factors that most influence women to undergo mammography are a physician's personal recommendation and enthusiasm about its utility. Because women with more confidence in their breast self-exam abilities may think mammography is not needed, it is important to emphasize that both mammography and clinical or breast self-examination are useful. The use of one type of screening tool does not reduce the requirement for the other.

Vignette Follow-up

Ms. C receives a note from the clinic telling her that the Pap smear was normal. She is told to make another appointment in 2 years, but she chooses not to return to this clinic.

Vignette 3

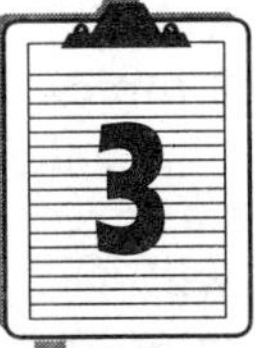

AV is 17 years old, and he comes with his mother to the clinic to have a precollege physical examination. They bring a form that needs to be completed. AV's parents have been patients for a couple of years, but previously AV has been seen only by a pediatrician. You know something about AV from interactions with his parents. He has done well in school and will be going out of state to a small private college.

Both AV and his mother are in the exam room, and she adds information to his answers to your questions. However, she spontaneously excuses herself when you announce the need to do a physical examination. Later the nurse enters the examination room and hands you a note that Mrs. V has written. In it she expresses her concern that AV may be using drugs and wonders if you could perform a urine drug screen without telling her son.

Vignette Objectives

1. What aspects of patient assessment are most useful when evaluating an adolescent?
2. What medical history questions relate to the leading cause of death among adolescents?

Adolescents: Health Risks and Sports Physical

"Routine" Examination of Adolescents

The well-patient, or "routine," evaluation of adolescents primarily focuses on the medical history (Table 1-4). Disease in this population is infrequent, and 80% of teenagers' deaths are due to unintentional injuries, homicide, or suicide. Motor vehicle and motorcycle accidents are the leading causes of the unintentional injuries. Adolescent deaths only represent a small fraction of the consequences of trauma. For every adolescent who dies as the result of some type of trauma, approximately 40 sustain injuries that necessitate hospitalization and another 1000 sustain injuries that are managed in the emergency room.

It is appropriate to talk with adolescents alone for at least part of the interview. Adolescents and their parents or guardians should understand that the physician's conversation with the teenager is confidential. Statements such as the following can be useful in encouraging an adolescent patient's trust:

> "I want my teenage patients to know that what they tell me is confidential. I will not repeat anything said, unless given permission. The exception is when, as with adults, a patient tells me something that suggests they might hurt themselves or others. But, parents often have questions about the visit. I'm going to tell them that they should ask you. So, you might want to think about what you would like to say to them."

This statement shows the physician's respect for an adolescent's desire for autonomy, acknowledges parents' interest in their child's health, and implies that parents and teens should talk about important health concerns.

Information about drug and alcohol use, sexuality, contraception, and sexually transmitted diseases is an important part of an adolescent's medical history. However, drug use and sexual history can be particularly difficult topics for adolescents to discuss, and young teenagers vary widely in their sexual knowledge and experience. Beginning with less intimate questions and asking about the habits of their friends facilitates an adolescent's comfort and willingness to disclose information about himself or herself. Potential questioning sequences are shown in Table 1-5, and additional history items are listed in Table 1-6. One means to remember each of the areas to cover is to use the mnemonic **HEADS** or **$HE^2A^3DS^2$**, as used at the Children's Hospital of Los Angeles. It consists of the following components:

- ***H*ome**
- ***E*ducation**
- ***E*ating**
- ***A*ctivities**
- ***A*mbitions**
- ***A*ffect**
- ***D*rugs** (including tobacco and alcohol)
- ***S*afety**
- ***S*uicide**

Table 1-4. Adolescent health care

History and physical examination component	Comment
Injury prevention	Seat belt, helmets, firearms, drinking and driving, smoke detectors
Tobacco, alcohol, and illicit drug use	When assessing illicit drug use, include anabolic steroids use and abuse of glue, paint, and other inhalants
Sexual behavior	Partner selection, condoms, STD prevention, unintended pregnancy, and contraception selection
Psychiatric disorders	Depression, suggested by drug use, social withdrawal, and decrement in school performance or personal hygiene; eating disorders
Height and weight	Serial observations monitor growth and development; obesity and eating disorders occur among adolescents
Blood pressure	Normal levels vary with age
Sexual maturation	Assess for appropriate maturation (see Chapter 9)
Skin	Assess high-risk group: increased exposure to sunlight or dysplastic nevi; evaluate for acne, warts, and other lesions
Visual acuity	Adolescents often show reduced acuity, with a value of less than 20/40 in 25%
Hearing	Perform at least once and more frequently if auditory trauma
Teeth and gums	Evaluate for caries
Cardiovascular	Evaluation for murmurs and clicks
Male genitourinary exam	Adolescents with a history of cryptorchidism, orchiopexy, or testicular atrophy are at increased risk for malignancy; sexual activity is indication for syphilis serology and cultures for *Chlamydia* and gonococci; homosexual youth also require hepatitis B screening, with vaccination of those not exposed
Pelvic examination	Exam indicated when sexually active, symptoms of severe menstrual disorders, pelvic pain, and vaginal discharge; sexual activity is indication for Pap smear and screening for gonococci, *Chlamydia,* and syphilis
Musculoskeletal	Evaluate for scoliosis

Table 1-5. Questioning strategy for adolescents

Topic	Sexual history	Drug use
Habits of others	"Are students at your school having sex?"	"What drugs do teens use at your school?"
Habits of friends	"Do your friends go on dates?" "How do they feel about having sex?"	"Have your friends tried drugs?" "How do you handle it when friends use drugs?"
Personal habits	"Are you sexually active now?"	"Have you used drugs?" "Teens frequently use tobacco and alcohol, but don't think of them as drugs. Have you used these?"

Table 1-6. Medical history discussion items for adolescents

Safety: seat belts, helmets, drunk driving, firearms, illicit substance use
School performance: favorite and least favorite classes, enjoyment, grades, disciplinary actions
Friends: relationships with members of same and opposite sex, number of close friends, qualities that are valued in friends
Home: family structure and relationships, occupation of parents, siblings, family arguments, running away
Personal interests: sports, hobbies, free-time activities, vocational plans
Emotional state: sadness, loneliness, depression, suicidal, eating disorders; any emotional problem should prompt asking about sexual and physical abuse
Concerns about sexuality: dating, intimacy and sexual activities, contraception and STDs; questions about changes in their bodies, menstruation, and "wet dreams"

Pre-participation Sports Physical Examination

A frequent reason for evaluating adolescents is to perform a "sports physical." As with other adolescent assessments, the history is the most important and revealing aspect of the interaction (Table 1-7). Suggested maneuvers to include in such an evaluation are listed in Table 1-7. Youth sports most prone to result in injury in boys are football and wrestling; the highest number of sports-related injuries among girls occur as the result of participating in softball and gymnastics.

Table 1-7. Pre-participation sports evaluation

History and physical examination component	Comments
Ask about current or past medical problems	Assess especially for symptoms that are cardiopulmonary (syncope, lightheadedness, chest pain), neurologic (seizures), and musculoskeletal (prior joint injury and current joint complaints)
Medications	Can be clue to chronic medical conditions; use of certain medications can result in altered exercise capacity
Surgery	Evaluate for loss of a paired organ
Drug use	Alcohol, tobacco, anabolic steroids, other performance-enhancing agents, weight control drugs (laxatives, diuretics), additional illicit drugs
Family history	Assess for sudden cardiac death and Marfan's syndrome
Menstrual history	Amenorrhea can be manifestation of an eating disorder and predispose to musculoskeletal injury
Prior sport injury	Identify areas for more detailed musculoskeletal exam; recent head trauma may preclude participation in contact sports
Height and weight	May add skin-fold measurement if concerned about evaluation and follow-up of underweight youth; may lead to additional counseling about appropriate weight and risks of dehydrating to "make weight" and/or eating disorders
Blood pressure	Normal levels vary with age
Cardiac	"Functional" or flow murmurs are common in younger adolescents; major concerns are hypertrophic cardiomyopathy and Marfan's syndrome
Musculoskeletal	Inspect for symmetry and scoliosis; range of motion of neck and upper extremities; lower extremities assessed with "duck-walk"; look for residual injury or conditions increasing injury risk (both may necessitate specific training activities)
Skin	Inspect for active infection

Vignette Follow-up

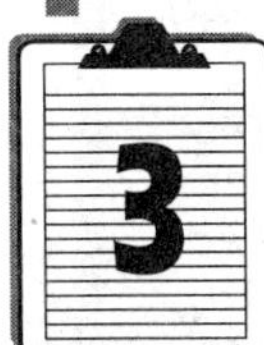

Areas of the medical history reviewed include AV's friends' and his sexual activity, as well as his family's structure, personal interests, career plans, personal substance abuse, automobile safety (including seat belt use and riding with intoxicated drivers), and firearm access. The confidentiality of the interaction is explained. AV denies drug use, other than some weekend experimentation with alcohol and cigarettes. His friends do not use drugs. Because he has an uncle who has major problems with substance abuse, AV believes that this has deterred him from using drugs. AV has a girl friend but has not been sexually active with her or other men or women. Risks for sexually transmitted diseases (STDs) and HIV are discussed, including condom use. Abstinence is presented as the only sure way to prevent pregnancy and the transmission of STDs.

AV's physical examination shows him to be a healthy-appearing young man, wearing Massimos and displaying three rings in his ear. He denies feelings of depression and displays a normal affective range and appropriate behavior during the interaction. His **blood pressure** is 110/70 mm Hg, with a **heart rate** of 110 beats/min (78 beats/min when checked later). His **height** is 68 inches, and his **weight** is 146 pounds. His **skin** shows a tattoo on his calf and mild acne over his face, but none on his back and chest. **Vision** is 20/20 in both eyes, and **hearing** is intact, as shown by assessment with an audioscope. His **mouth** exam shows a clear oropharynx and good dental hygiene. **Cardiac** exam shows a normal PMI; with auscultation, S_1 is normal and S_2 is physiologically split. His **genitourinary** exam reveals normal male genitalia, without skin lesions or abnormal scrotal mass, and his **maturation** is Tanner stage 5 (see Table 9-6, page 294). His **back** shows no scoliosis, and **joint** mobility of his shoulders, hips, knees, and ankles is normal.

Ms. V is told why surreptitious drug testing is not possible, and it is suggested that she might discuss her concerns in her son's presence. However, she decides not to mention it and explains that AV would only get angry and is already aware of her concerns.

Vignette 4

Advanced directives: explicit documentation of a person's choices concerning the use of "heroic" measures, including intubation and cardiopulmonary resuscitation; this also is referred to as a living will; the document can also name a person with "durable power of attorney for health care," who can "speak" for the incapacitated patient.

Activities of daily living (ADLs): systematic assessment of a person's ability to provide the basics of self-care (see Table 1-9); an acute decline in ADLs can indicate the presence of a new reversible disorder, such as a urinary tract infection or medication overdose.

Frail elderly: elderly people with the poorest health status, determined on the basis of low functional ability, the presence of several medical problems, or extreme age; elderly sometimes are classified into groups with different risks and health concerns, such as elderly versus frail elderly and young old versus old old.

Instrumental activities of daily living (IADLs): orderly evaluation of a person's ability to function independently; assesses ability to use the telephone, housekeeping (cleaning and laundry), shop, cook meals, take medications, manage personal finances, and use transportation (see Table 1-10); this evaluation provides information about safety and the need for additional resources.

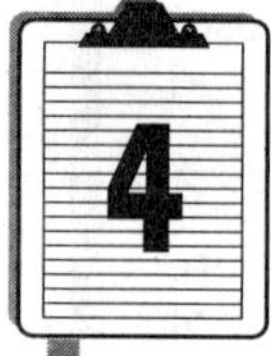

AG is a 91-year-old white woman who currently lives in a condominium. She has lived alone since her husband's death 46 years ago. Her son, who lives in the city, visits three times a week and does most of her shopping. There is a restaurant in her building that is open for "senior" meals. Mrs. G can feed and dress herself and occasionally takes the bus alone. She is independent and considers herself "very capable." Her current medical problems include hypothyroidism, treated with an appropriate replacement dose of levothyroxine, and mild degenerative arthritis of the hands.

She is a well-nourished, elderly woman, who is neatly groomed and pleasant. Vital signs reveal a **blood pressure** of 140/60 mm Hg and a **heart rate** of 76 beats/min. **HEENT:** her head is normocephalic and shows no evidence of trauma. Eye exam reveals a cataract in the left eye, and funduscopic evaluation reveals mild arteriovenous crossing changes. Visual acuity is not assessed. Ear examination reveals normal tympanic membranes, and her hearing appears normal, as assessed by determining her ability to hear a whisper. Mouth examination shows the patient to be wearing well-fitting dentures. Neck examination shows a normal-sized thyroid. **Cardiovascular** and **pulmonary** examination findings are normal.

Ms. G only wants her levothyroxine refilled, and she requests that she not have to return for a year. The physician orders a TSH level, writes a prescription for levothyroxine, and asks her to make a return appointment for a year later.

Vignette Objectives

1. What history and physical examination components are most helpful when evaluating elderly individuals?
2. What abnormal physical examination findings are more prevalent among older patients?
3. What features of the evaluation assess the risk of falls in an elderly patient?

Elderly Patients: ADLs and IADLs, Falls, Continence, Abuse, and Advance Directives

The medical interview and physical assessment of elderly patients may need to be modified to address changes brought about by the normal aging process and the altered prevalence of certain conditions (Table 1-8).

ADLs and IADLs

ADLs (Table 1-9) and **IADLs** (Table 1-10) are relevant to the elderly, and to any patient with a chronic debilitating condition. A simple way to view ADLs is to think of them as being comparable to the needs of a young child: toileting, feeding, bathing, and dressing. IADLs are activities that allow one to live alone, such as the ability to use the phone, cook, clean, manage finances, and use transportation. An acute decline in ADLs or IADLs may be the only clue to an underlying disorder, such as an otherwise asymptomatic urinary tract infection, silent cardiac ischemia, or adverse medication effects.

Falls

Falls are common among the elderly, with a prevalence of approximately 50% by 85 years of age. Falls usually stem from the combined effect of impairment in several systems (Table 1-11). Identifying a history of falls is worthwhile, because specific management (e.g., discontinuing certain drugs, buying new shoes, undergoing physical therapy for strength and gait training, removing throw rugs, and installing handrails) can then be implemented to reduce the risk of falls.

Continence

Approximately one third of elderly women have problems with incontinence, and half as many elderly men also experience incontinence. Incontinence causes embarrassment, reduces mobility, and impairs social interactions. The evaluation of people with incontinence is discussed in Chapter 5.

Elder Abuse

Result of epidemiologic studies indicate that 2% to 3% of those over 65 years old are abused. The risk is increased in those who (1) have cognitive impairment, (2) are living with relatives, or (3) have family members with substance abuse, mental illness, or prior antisocial behavior.

Table 1-8. Older patients

History and physical examination component	Comments
Medical interview	Anticipate a lengthy history; focus on current conditions and complaints; obtain prior records
Medication history	Include over-the-counter drugs; assess adherence to regimen and understanding of need for medications and any strategies used to promote adherence; polypharmacy is more than five medications, and the likelihood of medication problems increases markedly as the number of drugs increases; medications are most common cause of reversible mental status changes
Substance abuse	Alcohol abuse often goes unrecognized among the elderly; overuse of narcotics, sedatives, and anxiolytic agents also occurs; when suspected, confirm history through family and social contacts
Advance directives	Evaluate patient's choice concerning "heroic measures" (CPR and intubation) and whether patient understands and has completed advanced directives
Vital signs	Height loss can indicate spinal compression fractures due to osteoporosis; weight loss can be a sign of an underlying problem; although systolic pressure increases with aging (some consider 100 + age = normal systolic blood pressure in elderly), systolic hypertension is associated with increased cardiovascular morbidity; treatment of hypertension reduces that morbidity, and hypertension should not be ignored in the elderly; orthostatic blood pressure findings can be present in up to 25% of elderly people
Skin	Increased skin fragility, loss of skin turgor, seborrheic keratosis, and senile pigmented macules ("liver spots")
Visual acuity	Reduced upward gaze; approximately 10% of elderly are severely visually impaired; 30% have macular degeneration, which causes loss of central vision and is leading cause of blindness among the elderly; cataracts result in glare and sense of "looking through a screen"
Hearing	Hand-held audioscope has 90% sensitivity in detecting hearing defects in the elderly
Cardiac	Systolic ejection murmur of "aortic sclerosis" is common among the elderly; can be difficult to distinguish from calcific aortic stenosis, and echocardiogram may be needed to distinguish these two conditions
Breast	Breast cancer risk increases as women age; breast exam should not be omitted
Abdomen and genitourinary	Palpation for abdominal aortic aneurysm; Table 1-1 reviews recommendations for the stool occult-blood, digital prostate, and pelvic examinations
Extremities	Assess skin integrity, peripheral pulses, and joints for deformity
Mental status	Many studies document dementia often is missed; assess mental status early if history is tangential or if the patient is argumentative or a "poor historian," document mini–mental status; evaluate "spirits" and symptoms of depression
Neurologic examination	Decreased vibratory sense is frequent among elderly; assessment of strength and gait important for assessing risk for falls (see gait abnormalities Chapter 8); normal gait is shorter paced; evaluate functional ability (arise from chair, walk, turn around, walk back, pick up object from the floor)

Table 1-9. Activities of daily living index

For each area of functioning, check the description that applies.		
BATHING		
Able to get into and out of tub without help	Assisted with bathing only one part of the body, such as the back or a leg	Assisted with bathing more than one part of the body (or not bathed)
FEEDING		
Feeds self without assistance	Feeds self, except for help cutting meat or buttering bread	Assisted with feeding or fed through tubes or with IV fluids
DRESSING		
Gets clothes and dresses without assistance	Gets clothes and dresses without assistance, except for tying shoes	Assisted with getting clothes on or dressing
CONTINENCE		
Controls urination and bowel movement	Has occasional accidents	Assisted with control of urination or bowel movement, catheter use, or incontinence
TOILETING		
Goes to bathroom, cleans self, and arranges clothes without assistance (may use walker or wheelchair for support; and at night, can use bedpan or commode)	Assisted with going to bathroom, cleaning self, or arranging clothes	Does not go to bathroom to eliminate
TRANSFER		
Moves in and out of bed and chair without assistance	Moves in and out of bed or chair with assistance	Does not get out of bed

Advanced Directives

Approximately 30% of elderly people state that they do not want cardiopulmonary resuscitation (CPR), and that percentage increases with age. Although most say they would like to discuss the issue with their physician, less than 15% are given that opportunity. It is important to ask a patient about his or her wishes in this regard, because physicians, nurses, and families, even when they "know" the patient well, cannot predict a patient's decision about CPR.

These discussions are much easier to hold during a clinic visit than during an acute illness. Discussing them during a clinic visit also allows the patient time to think about the issues, talk with family members, and plan advanced directives. Sample questions to begin the discussion may include: "If you become very ill, how should your family be involved in your care?", "If you had a terminal illness, how would you want it to be handled?", and "Would you want us to try to resuscitate you if your heart stopped beating?"

Table 1-10. Instrumental activities of daily living scale

For each ability, identify the category that best describes the patient.

TELEPHONE				
Operates telephone; looks up and dials numbers	Answers telephone but does not dial	Dials a few well-known numbers	Does not use telephone	
SHOPPING				
Does all shopping independently	Shops independently for small purchases	Accompanied on any shopping trip	Unable to shop	
COOKING				
Plans, prepares, and serves own meals	Prepares meals if supplied with ingredients	Heats and serves prepared meals or prepares meals but does not maintain adequate diet	Meals must be prepared and served	
HOUSEKEEPING				
Maintains house alone or with occasional assistance	Performs light daily tasks, such as dish washing and bed making	Performs light daily tasks but cannot maintain acceptable level of cleanliness	Needs help with all home maintenance tasks	Does not participate in any housekeeping tasks
LAUNDRY				
Does personal laundry completely	Launders small items	All laundry done by others		
TRANSPORTATION				
Travels independently on public transportation or drives own car	Arranges own travel by taxi, but does not otherwise use public transportation	Travels on public transportation when accompanied by another	Travels only by taxi or car with assistance.	Does not travel
MEDICATIONS				
Takes own medications in correct dose at correct times	Takes own medications, if prepared in advance	Not capable of dispensing own medications		
FINANCES				
Manages financial matters (such as writes checks, pays rent, and does banking)	Manages day-to-day items but needs help with major purchases	Incapable of handling money		

Table 1-11. Falls

History and physical examination component	Comments
History of present illness	Circumstances surrounding the fall; the history and assessment can be similar to that of people with syncope (see Table 3-11, Chapter 3); assess for impairment of sensorimotor systems (such as vision, balance, proprioception, and peripheral sensation)
Home environment	Hazards include poor lighting, stairs, throw rugs, and the bathroom arrangement; adaptive devices, such as railings for stairs, elevated toilet seats, bath and shower mats and chairs, and grab rails and side bars for the bathtub are useful; assess for proximity of help in an emergency
Inspection	Evaluate potential for being abused; assess for signs of trauma and level of hygiene
Vital signs	Arrhythmia, orthostatic hypotension (near-syncope can be manifested as a fall)
HEENT	Visual impairment, cervical spine range of motion (can suggest limitations in ability to see and presence of cervical myelopathy)
Extremities	Arthritis and joint deformities, evidence of peripheral vascular disease
Neurologic	Mental status, muscle strength, tremor, gait, reflexes

Vignette Follow-up

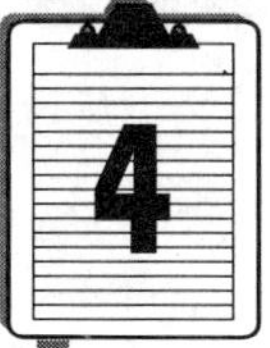

AG returns to the clinic 6 weeks later with her 65-year-old son. She fell while showering in the bathtub and was unable to get out of the tub. Because no one heard her intermittent yells for help, she sat in the tub for more than 18 hours. Her son discovered her the following day, when he came to deliver her groceries. He took Ms. G to an emergency room, where she was given intravenous hydration for several hours and then discharged to her son's care. She has been admitted to a nursing home that offers assisted living. Her new apartment has been checked for hazards, and adaptive equipment has been installed. She has also been provided with an emergency call device that she can wear.

Vignette 5

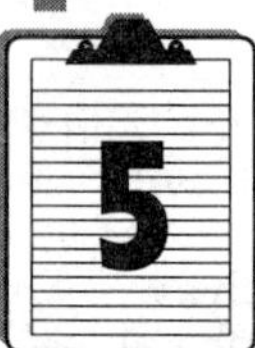

TR is a 32-year-old high school teacher who relates that he has been found to be HIV positive by anonymous testing. He is concerned about seeking medical care and how it may affect his future employability and ability to obtain health insurance. He played 3 years of single-A baseball after college graduation and believes he acquired the infection during that interval. During that time, he had several women sexual partners, including prostitutes. He denies other risk factors for HIV infection. Currently he feels well, but it was the identification of prominent sports figures as being HIV positive that prompted his obtaining anonymous testing. He has not revealed the test results to anyone else. He is married and has two children. He teaches science and coaches baseball. Mr. R had been seen in the office twice previously, but HIV risks were not assessed at either visit.

His **height** is 73 inches and **weight** 187 pounds (84 kg) (unchanged from when seen 4 months ago). He appears healthy, with a **blood pressure** of 125/85 mm Hg and **heart rate** of 68 beats/min. His **skin** is normal, without suspicious lesions. **HEENT:** his visual acuity is 20/20 bilaterally, his pupils are equal and reactive to light, and his fundi appear normal. His oropharynx is clear, without evidence of candidiasis or hairy leukoplakia. His neck has no palpable adenopathy (nodes also are not palpable in his axilla and groin). **Chest:** clear to auscultation. **Cardiac:** normal PMI, normal S_1, and physiologically split S_2. **Abdomen:** liver 9 cm to percussion span in the midclavicular line. His spleen is not palpable, and no mass or tenderness is present. His **genitalia** are normal. **Digital rectal exam** findings are normal, with a normal-sized prostate and occult-blood–negative stool. His **extremities** show no edema. His **mental status** is normal, as assessed by the mini–mental status examination (30 of 30 points). **Cranial nerves** II through XII are intact. **Peripheral sensation** is normal to light touch and vibratory testing. **Strength** is normal and symmetrical, and **reflexes** are symmetrical at 1+ to 2+, with downgoing toes.

Vignette Objective

1. What components of the history and physical examination are most important when evaluating an asymptomatic person who is HIV positive?

Patients with Asymptomatic HIV Infections: Detection and Assessment

Assessing HIV risk factors should be a routine component of most medical interviews. However, practitioners often fail to do this and detect only a third of those at increased risk. Evaluating the risk for HIV infection can be done at several points in the medical interview. If the history of the present illness does not trigger a discussion of HIV risk, it can be evaluated during discussion of other health behaviors and habits, such as smoking, alcohol, and seat belt use, or it can be an addendum to the sexual history. Table 1-12 lists questions that can be asked to evaluate HIV risk.

More than 50% of people known to be HIV positive are asymptomatic. Tables 1-13 and 1-14 outline the history and physical examination components especially important for these patients. In addition, when people are found to be HIV positive, their contacts should be notified. Safe sex practices need to be reviewed and the patient informed of community resources available for the education and support of people with HIV. Safe sex practices include body massage, hugging, mutual masturbation, and closed-mouth kissing. Latex con-

Table 1-12. HIV risk assessment questions

I try to ask all patients whether they have had any experiences that would increase their risk for HIV infection. Have you engaged in any behaviors that would put you at risk? (Many patients know the risks for HIV infection, and some will have undergone prior HIV testing.)
Many people have undergone HIV testing or are concerned that they might be at risk for HIV infection. Is this true for you?
Are you single? Do you have a partner? Are you married? Is your partner a man or woman? Because it affects your risk for certain conditions, have you been sexually active with men, women, or both?
Do you practice safe sex (use condoms)?
About how many sexual partners have you had in the past 10 years?
Have you had male-male sexual contact or sexual contact with a prostitute or others from high-risk groups?
Do you have a history of IV drug use?
Have you received blood transfusions (prior to 1985)?
Do you have a history of sexually transmitted disease or hepatitis B?

Table 1-13. Asymptomatic HIV-infected people

History component	Comments
When was infection probably acquired?	Relates to disease progression and expected stage of illness
Prior infections: STDs, chickenpox, hepatitis, tuberculosis (PPD status)	These infections indicate potential problems and need for specific prophylaxis
Immunizations	Helps identify those considered for hepatitis B and Pneumovax immunizations
Medications, including adjuvant and unconventional therapies	Adjuvant therapy use is common
Travel habits	Identifies risk for certain infections
Sexual practices	Safe sex practices, notification of partners
Mental health	Depression and anxiety are common
Review of systems: energy loss, weight loss, skin or vision changes, cough, prior abnormal Pap smear	Specific symptoms can indicate early manifestations of illness; cervical dysplasia can progress rapidly
Social and economic support	Identification of problems allows referral to appropriate resources, if needed

Table 1-14. Asymptomatic HIV-infected people

Examination component	Comments
Height and weight	Weight loss, or "wasting," is a sign of disease progression; a greater than 10% weight loss can be a component of an AIDS-defining illness
Skin	Seborrheic dermatitis (eyebrows, cheeks, ears, and anterior chest); molluscum contagiosum (pox virus); KS (initial macular phase, becoming violaceous nodule; also can have appearance of hemangioma, ecchymosis, or cellulitis); herpesvirus infection ("cold sore," genital herpes)
HEENT	CMV retinitis appears as white-yellow necrosis and red hemorrhage ("cottage cheese and catsup"); oral candidiasis; 20% of asymptomatic patients have hairy leukoplakia of lateral and dorsal surfaces of tongue; KS lesions of gingiva and hard palate
Chest	Pulmonary findings can stem from infection and less frequently from neoplastic disorders (as with KS); infections can include bacterial pneumonia, PCP, mycobacterial infections, and CMV pneumonitis
Abdomen	Splenomegaly can be associated with generalized adenopathy; mycobacterial infection can cause hepatomegaly and splenomegaly; perirectal lesions
Genitourinary	Rapid progression of cervical dysplasia can necessitate Pap smear each 6 months; recurrent *Candida* vaginitis common; perirectal condyloma; herpes simplex virus ulceration
Lymph nodes	Adenopathy can be manifestation of HIV infection or indicate malignancy or regional infection
Extremities	Hyperalgesic pseudothrombophlebitis (painful calf associated with swelling and erythema)
Mental status	Depression and anxiety common, cognitive dysfunction can occur with disease progression
Neurologic	Peripheral neuropathy can be manifestation of illness and its treatment; myopathy can be manifestation of HIV or be due to treatment

KS = Kaposi's sarcoma; CMV = cytomegalovirus; PCP = *Pneumococcus carinii* pneumonia;

doms with monoxynol-9–containing spermicide can be used to decrease HIV transmission, but a concern about their use is that the rate of condom failure may be over 10%. HIV-positive people should not share razors, toothbrushes, tweezers, or other items that may be contaminated with blood.

HIV can affect every organ system. Several patients with such HIV-associated problems are described in other chapters (see Index). Tables 1-13 and 1-14 list additional concerns applicable to the evaluation of asymptomatic people with HIV-infection.

Vignette Follow-up

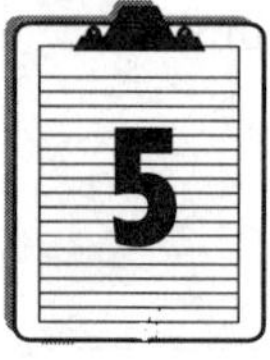

TR is questioned concerning prior travel and infectious illnesses. He takes no medications and denies tobacco, alcohol, and other drug use. Since his marriage 5 years ago, his only sexual partner has been his wife. She uses oral contraceptives, and they have not used condoms. A detailed review of systems does not disclose any abnormalities. TR appears anxious but denies depression or despondency. He has planned how he would tell his wife about the diagnosis.

The current visit has been scheduled as a routine follow-up, and time limitations confine the interaction to the history, physical examination, the plan for laboratory evaluation, and immediate concerns about his wife, children, and job. He is scheduled to return in 2 days to have a PPD (purified protein derivative) read and offers to bring his wife with him for that visit. (Subsequent evaluation shows that Mrs. R is HIV negative.)

Objectives Review

1. What portions of the physical examination should be included in an adult, well-patient "screening" exam?
2. List factors that contribute to disagreement about physical examination findings and for each, provide ways to increase exam reliability.
3. List ways to decrease a woman's anxiety during a pelvic examination.
4. How does a woman's confidence in her ability to do breast self-examination relate to how likely she is to obtain a mammogram?
5. What aspects of patient assessment are most useful when evaluating an adolescent?
6. What medical history questions relate to the leading cause of death among adolescents?
7. What history and physical examination components are most helpful when evaluating elderly individuals?
8. What abnormal physical examination findings are more prevalent among older patients?
9. What features of the evaluation assess the risk of falls in an elderly patient?
10. What components of the history and physical examination are most important when evaluating an asymptomatic person who is HIV positive?

Suggested Reading

Alpert EJ. Violence in intimate relationships and the practicing internist: new "disease" or new agenda? *Ann Intern Med* 1995;123:774–81.
Obtaining a history about abuse is appropriate in any patient seen in a primary care setting, but it is especially appropriate in women who come for emergency room care or who are injured; abuse is associated with chronic abdominal/pelvic pain, chronic headaches, drug abuse, and psychiatric diagnoses; the author presents a strategy for the clinical evaluation of such women and the management of abuse.

American Medical Association. *Policy compendium on confidential health services for adolescents* (JE Gans, ed). Chicago: AMA, 1993.
Available from Department of Adolescent Health, AMA, 515 North State St, Chicago, IL 60610; 312-464-5570.

Canadian Task Forces on the Periodic Health Examination. The periodic health examination: 2; 1987 update. *Can Med Assoc J* 1988;138:619–28.

After evaluating the scientific evidence, this task force made recommendations about appropriate health maintenance procedures; information is presented on both the quality of the evidence and the strength of the recommendations; this update includes a discussion of teen pregnancy, endometrial cancer, and postmenopausal osteoporosis.

Carney PA, Dietrich AJ, Freeman DH Jr, Mott LA. The period health examination provided to asymptomatic older women: an assessment using standardized patients. *Ann Intern Med* 1993;119:129–35.

These researchers trained standardized patients to present consistent histories and found practitioners varied widely in the exam components they performed.

Department of Clinical Epidemiology and Biostatistics, McMaster University. Clinical disagreement: I. How often it occurs and why. *Can Med Assoc J* 1980;123:499–504; Clinical disagreement: II. How to avoid it and how to learn from one's mistakes. *Can Med Assoc J* 1980;123:613–17.

These two articles contain information about why clinical disagreement occurs and strategies to prevent or minimize its occurrence.

Eddy DM, ed. *Common screening tests.* Philadelphia: American College of Physicians, 1991.

American College of Physicians recommendations for the screening physical examination.

English A. Treating adolescents. *Med Clin North Am* 1990;74:1097–112.

The author is a JD at the National Center for Youth Law; she discusses issues concerning consent, "mature minors," contraceptive services, pregnancy care, and abortion.

Fields SD. Special considerations in the physical exam of older patients. *Geriatrics* 1991;46:39–44.

The author discusses the changes that can occur during normal aging, including gait disorders, incontinence, visual loss, and deafness.

Frame PS. The complete annual physical examination refuses to die. *J Fam Pract* 1995;40:543–5.

This is an editorial that accompanied the Luckman and Melville article concerning family physicians' periodic physical examination practices.

Ginsburg KR, Slap GB, Cnaan A. Adolescents' perceptions of factors affecting their decisions to seek health care. *JAMA* 1995;273:1913–8.

These researchers concluded that adolescents value infection control procedures, such as hand washing, the demonstration of respect for their confidentiality, and the use of effective interpersonal skills.

Gomez JG, Landry GL, Bernhardt DT. Critical evaluation of the 2-minute orthopedic screening examination. *Am J Dis Child* 1993;147:1109–13.

The history is the most important aspect of the "sports physical"; this brief musculoskeletal exam (symmetrical appearance, joint range of motion, scoliosis, dynamic function of the lower extremities, stand on toes, and walk like a duck) showed a sensitivity of approximately 50% at detecting orthopedic problems.

Hayward RSA, Steinberg EP, Ford DE, Roizen MF, Roach KW. Preventive care guidelines: 1991. *Ann Intern Med* 1991;114:758–83.

The authors compare guidelines issued by the American College of Physicians, the Canadian Task Force, and the U.S. Preventive Services Task Force.

Johnson JD, Meischke H. Factors associated with adoption of mammography screening: results of a cross-sectional and longitudinal study. *J Women's Health* 1994;3:97–105.

A physician's recommendation to have a mammogram was the most important predictor of a woman obtaining a mammogram; surprisingly, women confident in their ability to do a self-exam are less likely to have mammography, which emphasizes the need to inform women of the additive benefits of the test.

Lachs MS, Feinstein AR, Cooney LM Jr, et al. A simple procedure for general screening for functional disability in elderly patients. *Ann Intern Med* 1990;112:699–706.
The authors propose an initial simple screen for problems, with more extensive evaluation if needed; mobility and extremity function are assessed by having elderly patients touch the back of the head, rise from a chair, walk 10 feet, and return to the chair.

Lachs MS, Pillemer K. Abuse and neglect of elderly persons. *N Engl J Med* 1995;332: 437–43.
The authors present a brief review and tabulate risk factors and physical findings that indicate abuse; they also propose an algorithm for responding to suspected abuse.

Luckmann R, Melville SK. Periodic health evaluation of adults: a survey of family physicians. *J Fam Pract* 1995;40:547–54.
The authors surveyed New England family physicians and found that more than 90% supported the need for periodic physical exams; more than 95% included the following in their routine examinations: weight, blood pressure, the palpation of nodes, mouth inspection, palpation of thyroid, auscultation of heart and lungs, palpation of abdomen, and evaluation of extremities.

MacKenzie RG. Approach to the adolescent in the clinical setting. *Med Clin North Am* 1990;74:1085–94.
Two thirds of this article constitutes a review of the physical, psychological, and intrapersonal changes that occur during adolescence; the author also discusses how to interview adolescents and cites use of the HE^2A^3DS *mnemonic.*

Mitchell TL, Tornelli JL, Fisher TD, Blackwell TA, Moorman JR. Yield of the screening review of systems: a study on a general medical service. *J Gen Intern Med* 1992;7:393–7.
The cost-effectiveness of the review of systems was found to be equivalent to that of other accepted screening procedures, yielding a new diagnosis for approximately 5% of patients.

Mulrow CD, Lichtenstein MJ. Screening for hearing impairment in the elderly. *J Gen Intern Med* 1991;6:249–58.
The authors critically review data and advocate screening using an audioscope and brief questionnaire about hearing.

Newman LS. Occupational illness. *N Engl J Med* 1995;333:1128–34.
The author reviews the occupational history, using an initial quick survey to reveal work-related problems and then detailed questioning, if needed; a useful list of information sources concerning occupational illnesses also is presented.

Oboler SK, LaForce FM. The periodic physical examination in asymptomatic adults. *Ann Intern Med* 1989;110:214–26.
The authors critically review the evidence for the efficacy of different maneuvers; those that hold up to scrutiny are tabulated.

Penn MA, Bourguet CC. Patients' attitudes regarding chaperons during physical examinations. *J Fam Pract* 1992;35:639–43.
The results of studies, such as this one, depend on the population of women studied and the women's prior experiences; it is difficult to generalize findings, making it important to ask patients about their preferences; overall, younger women were more likely to want a chaperon with a male examiner.

Scheitel SM, Fleming KC, Chutka DS, Evans JM. Geriatric health maintenance. *Mayo Clin Proc* 1996;71:289–02.

Recommendations concerning components of the physical assessment listed in Table 1-1 do not specify the effects of aging on the conclusions; the authors review data for the elderly to determine the utility of screening physical exam maneuvers, diagnostic studies, immunization, and aspirin and estrogen replacement therapy; they provide a bottom-line recommendation for each.

Sox HC Jr. Preventive health services in adults. *N Engl J Med* 1994;330:1589–95.
This succinct review article includes a listing of appropriate "screening" procedures, and the author compares recommendations from the American College of Physicians, Canadian Task Force, and U.S. Preventive Services Task Force.

Tinetti ME. Performance-oriented assessment of mobility problems in elderly patients. *J Am Geriat Soc* 1986;34:119–26.
The author provides tables of specific actions that assess balance and gait; use of performance criteria allows more precise identification of problems, some of which can be addressed therapeutically.

Uhlmann RF, Pearlman RA. Perceived quality of life and preferences for life-sustaining treatment in older adults. *Arch Intern Med* 1991;151:495–7.
Physicians generally underestimate a patient's own perception about the quality of his or her life; impressions of health care providers and families cannot be substituted for finding out from a competent patient their wishes concerning CPR; families' and physicians' predictions regarding patients' wishes for resuscitation did not prove to be accurate.

U.S. Preventative Services Task Force Guide to Clinical Preventive Services, 2nd ed. Baltimore, Williams & Wilkins, 1996.
The first edition was published in 1989; in the second edition, the 169 interventions described in the first edition are updated and seven chapters are added; six laminated cards are included, with recommendations for different age groups.

Ward J, Sanson-Fisher R. Prevalence and detection of HIV risk behavior in primary care: implications for clinical preventive services. *Am J Prev Med* 1995;11:224–30.
The study documented that physicians do not judge a person's risk for HIV infection accurately; physicians identified less than half of those at risk for HIV infection.

White JC, Levinson W. Lesbian health care. What a primary care physician needs to know. *West J Med* 1995;162:463–6.
The authors briefly present unique issues related to obtaining a history in lesbians and specific disease concerns and psychosocial issues that pertain to them.

2. Head, Ears, Eyes, Nose, and Throat Problems

Objectives

List history and physical examination findings for the following problems:

- Amaurosis fugax
- Bell's palsy
- Blepharitis
- Cavernous sinus thrombosis
- Central retinal artery occlusion
- Conjunctivitis
- Hearing loss
- Iritis
- Neck mass
- Optic neuritis
- Otitis externa
- Otitis media
- Pharyngitis
- Ramsay Hunt syndrome
- Red eye
- Sialolithiasis
- Sinusitis
- Uveitis
- Visual loss

Pertinent Points

History

Any trouble with your vision? Last eye examination?
Any trouble hearing? Tinnitus? Ear pain?
Any trouble with your nose or sinuses?
Any sores in your mouth? Toothaches?
Any swellings or lumps in your neck?
For those with sudden visual loss:
- Onset
- Description of visual deficit
- Associated symptoms: pain, photophobia, tearing, discharge, preceding flashing lights
- Trauma
- Scintillating scotoma, history of migraine headache
- Myopia
- Medical illnesses (such as hypertension, diabetes, atrial fibrillation, multiple sclerosis)
- Tongue or jaw claudication
- Headache
- Scalp tenderness
- Malaise
- Weight loss

For those with a "red" eye:
- Onset
- Associated symptoms: itching, pain, photophobia, tearing, or discharge (watery, purulent)
- Contacts with similar complaint
- Seasonal
- Trauma
- Exposure to chemicals or ultraviolet light
- Contact lens use
- Medical illnesses (e.g., tuberculosis, toxoplasmosis, syphilis, ankylosing spondylitis, inflammatory bowel disease, sarcoidosis)

For those with a progressive hearing loss:
- Onset
- Unilateral versus bilateral
- Otitis media or "plugged" ears
- Medication exposure (aspirin, furosemide, aminoglycosides)
- Acoustic trauma
- Vertigo
- Family history of deafness

For those with suspected sinusitis:
- Preceding allergic rhinitis or upper respiratory tract infection
- Purulent discharge
- Facial or dental pain
- Headache
- Effect of position
- Prior "sinusitis" (similarity of symptoms, how was diagnosis established, treatment)

For those with pharyngitis:
- Fever, coryza, cough
- Exposure to viral illness, streptococcal infections, or mononucleosis
- Prior rheumatic fever
- Diabetes or other condition reducing immunity

For those with isolated facial weakness:
- Onset
- Associated symptoms (dysesthesia, changes in taste, hearing loss, vertigo)
- Trauma
- Viral prodrome
- Medical illnesses (e.g., diabetes, cerebrovascular disease, malignancy)

For those with a neck mass:
- Onset, progression, other masses
- Pain, fever
- Pharyngitis, facial infection
- Smoking
- Exposure to cats

Physical Examination

Vital signs
- Blood pressure, heart rate, respiratory rate

Inspection
- Nutritional state

Head

Inspect head and facies (asymmetry, temporal wasting) and scalp (distribution and texture of hair)
Palpate temporal arteries (tenderness or beading)

Eyes

Inspect brows, lids, lashes (xanthelasma, ptosis, proptosis), conjunctiva, sclera), iris
Test visual acuity
Assess extraocular movement (EOM) in the six cardinal directions, conjugate eye movement, nystagmus, lid lag
Assess pupil size, shape, consensual and direct response to light and accommodation
Test visual fields by confrontation
Inspect cornea (arcus senilis, Kayser-Fleischer ring of Wilson's disease)
Examine lens
Examine fundi: vessels (hypertensive changes, emboli), optic disk (sharpness of borders, cup size, color, edema), retina (hemorrhages, exudates, abnormal pigmentation, scars), macula

Ears

Inspect auricle
Test hearing
Inspect canal and tympanic membrane (TM) (canal patency, cerumen, and TM mobility)
Perform Rinne and Weber tests

Nose and sinuses

Inspect septum (deviation, perforation), turbinates, mucosa (erythema, discharge)
Palpate maxillary and frontal sinuses
Transilluminate maxillary and frontal sinuses

Mouth

Inspect tongue (atrophy, glossitis, ulceration), palate, gingival and buccal mucosa, dentition, oropharynx; palpate any lesions for induration
Palpate temporomandibular joint during jaw motion

Cranial nerves

I (olfactory)—Usually not tested; when performed each nostril is tested separately
II (optic)—Visual acuity, visual fields, afferent limb pupillary response
III (oculomotor), IV (trochlear), VI (abducens)—EOMs, efferent limb pupillary response
V (trigeminal)—Sensation in its three branches, afferent corneal reflex, muscles of mastication
VII (facial)—Facial muscles, taste in anterior two thirds of tongue
VIII (vestibuloauditory)—Hearing, balance (vestibular)
IX (glossopharyngeal)—Gag (motor response), palate elevation
X (vagus)—Laryngeal function, gag (sensation)
XI (spinal accessory)—Sternocleidomastoid, trapezius
XII (hypoglossal)—Tongue movement

Neck

Palpate thyroid; size, symmetry, nodules, tenderness
Palpate and auscultate carotids
Palpate for adenopathy: anterior cervical (high, middle, and low), posterior cervical, occipital, supraclavicular, submental, submandibular, and anterior midline (define size, location, tenderness, consistency, and mobility)
Palpate for neck masses (location, size, erythema, tenderness, firmness, associated skin findings and adenopathy, movement with tongue protrusion)
Assess tracheal position and movement

Vignette 1

Afferent defect: normally, pupillary constriction is similar for both eyes when a light is shone into either eye; an afferent defect is demonstrated by shining a light into the uninvolved eye, which should cause both pupils to constrict, but when the light is shone into the affected eye, that eye's pupil dilates; a decrease in receptor density (as occurs after optic neuritis) can preserve acuity but cause a deficit in afferent input.

Amaurosis fugax: transient and painless monocular visual loss; often described as a "shade coming down"; it usually is due to microemboli resulting from atherosclerotic disease; cholesterol emboli (Hollenhorst plaques) sometimes can be seen in retinal arteries on funduscopic exam.

Anisocoria: unequal pupillary size. 20% of normal individuals have mild anisocoria, but each pupil responds briskly and symmetrically.

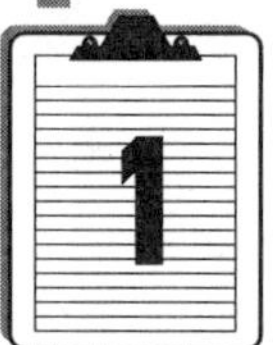

SS is an 86-year-old retired college professor who is active despite several medical problems. Two days ago he suffered visual loss in his right eye. The event was not preceded by eye pain or symptoms of amaurosis. He specifically denies jaw claudication, headache, scalp tenderness, and proximal muscle soreness. Mr. S's chronic problems include stable coronary artery disease, gout, and degenerative joint disease, which has necessitated bilateral total hip replacements and causes chronic low back pain.

Physical examination reveals a **blood pressure** of 155/90 mm Hg and a **heart rate** of 74 beats/min, which is regular. **HEENT:** lids and lashes are normal; visual acuity (with correction) is 20/300 in the right eye and 20/50 in the left. Pupils are 3 mm and reactive bilaterally, but a right afferent defect is demonstrable; conjunctivae and sclerae are normal; intraocular pressure is 22 mm Hg in the right and 17 mm Hg in the left. The right retina appears normal, but the right optic nerve head shows prominent edema. Arterial narrowing is present, but no other vessel abnormalities are seen. **Chest:** clear to auscultation. **Cardiac:** carotids were 2+ and equal, without bruit; no jugular venous distention; the point of maximal impulse (PMI) is not palpable; S_1 and S_2 are normal; S_4 is present. **Abdomen:** soft, without organomegaly; no bruit or aortic enlargement. **Extremities:** no edema, full active range of motion; muscles are nontender. **Neurologic:** reflexes 2+ and symmetrical; strength, dexterity, and rapid movements are symmetrical and normal; the only deficit is associated with cranial nerve II.

Vignette Objective

1. List the diagnoses to be considered in a patient presenting with an acute visual loss and the history and physical examination findings typifying each diagnosis.

Ophthalmologic Disorders

Acute Blindness

Acute visual loss is a medical emergency that requires evaluation by an ophthalmologist. Conditions that cause acute visual loss are listed in Table 2-1. The evaluation of these patients requires documentation of the visual impairment (visual fields and acuity). People can perceive a visual field cut as a loss of vision in one eye, and monocular problems must be distinguished from a deficit affecting both eyes (such as an homonymous hemianopia, in which the same half of the visual field is lost in both eyes, or bitemporal hemianopsia, in which the temporal fields of both eyes are affected (Fig. 2-1). If both eyes are affected, this usually indicates a problem at or distal to the optic chiasm, rather than a

Table 2-1. Acute monocular blindness

Condition	Findings
Retinal detachment	Associated with extreme myopia and head or eye trauma; often preceded by floaters or flashing lights; painless; detachment can be visible on funduscopic exam
Central retinal vein occlusion	No prodrome; painless; funduscopic exam shows edema, hemorrhages, and dilated veins ("squashed tomato"); associated with hypertension, diabetes, blood dyscrasias, and glaucoma
Central retinal artery occlusion	Acute onset; painless; history of thromboembolic disease, atrial fibrillation, or carotid disease; pale optic disk, bloodless arteries, and cherry red spot in the macula; occasionally, gently palpating eye can dislodge clot and restore arterial flow
Acute (narrow-angle or angle-closure) glaucoma	Painful, red eye or brow; sudden onset, which can coincide with pupil dilatation that occurs when the person enters a dark room; poorly reactive, midposition pupil; corneal edema can blur vision; shallow anterior chamber and markedly increased intraocular pressure; immediate therapy is 2% pilocarpine drops to constrict the pupil, while waiting for emergency ophthalmologic consultation
Ischemic optic neuropathy	Develops acutely or over several days; within 24 hours, disk becomes pale or edematous; extent of visual loss can vary; afferent pupil defect; associated with temporal arteritis (often affects elderly women; symptoms such as headache, jaw claudication, or polymyalgia rheumatica; elevated erythrocyte sedimentation rate); disorder also can be due to atherosclerotic disease
Optic neuritis	Visual loss occurs over hours to days; central scotoma; if anterior optic nerve affected, pain occurs with eye movement; causes papillitis, which can be mistaken for papilledema (but with loss of vision); in approximately half of patients with idiopathic optic neuritis multiple sclerosis will develop

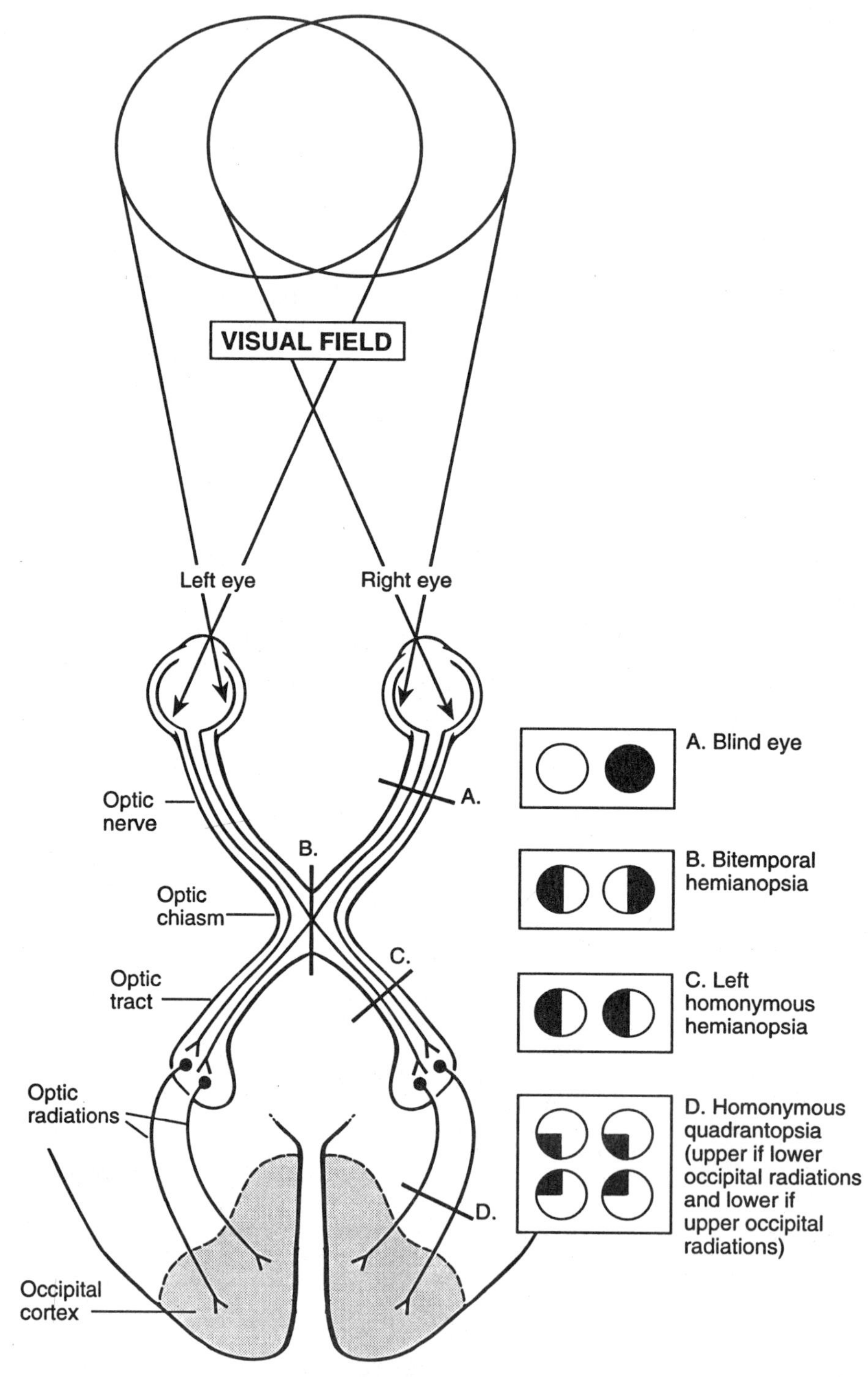

Figure 2-1. The visual fields and optic pathways. Also shown are the field cuts produced by lesions at particular locations along these paths.

problem affecting the globe or optic nerve. No afferent defect is present if both eyes are similarly affected.

The etiology of gradually progressive visual loss differs from that of acute visual loss and varies with the patient's age. Diabetes is the most common cause of non-acute progressive visual loss among people aged 20 to 60 years old. Macular degeneration is the leading cause in people older than 60.

Temporal Arteritis

Temporal arteritis (TA) (also called *giant cell arteritis*) is primarily an illness of the elderly, with women affected more often than men and caucasians more than the members of other racial groups. A granulomatous inflammation of the larger extracranial arteries leads to the disorder's symptoms and signs. The manifestations of temporal arteritis are listed in Table 2-2. Most patients have a markedly elevated sedimentation rate, but no laboratory tests are diagnostic.

Visual loss is a severe complication of temporal arteritis, which is caused either by ischemia of the optic nerve (ischemic optic neuritis) or by central retinal artery occlusion. Central retinal artery occlusion results in a more sudden and profound loss of vision; on inspection, the retinal arteries appear bloodless and narrowed. Optic nerve ischemia causes a more gradual vision loss in which the optic disk margins can be blurred but the vessels do not have a bloodless appearance. The blindness that results from TA often is irreversible, and because of this potential, empiric treatment with corticosteroids must be initiated while the patient is being assessed and before the diagnosis is established. Although optic nerve ischemia can be caused by TA, most cases are due to atherosclerotic disease involving the migration of small emboli to these vessels.

Polymyalgia rheumatica (PMR) is a disorder that affects the same patient group as that affected by TA. Both disorders can coexist, and approximately 10% of patients with PMR also have TA. PMR is characterized by the development of severe pain in the shoulders and pelvic girdle. Although patients may complain of weakness, the limitation is due to pain. Because PMR often occurs in association with TA, they may both be manifestations of a similar inflamma-

Table 2-2. Temporal arteritis

History and physical examination	Findings (reported prevalence in selected series)
Age of onset	Rare before age 50
Sex	Women > men
Race	Caucasians > African-Americans and Asians
Associated symptoms	Headache (60%), jaw claudication (30%), malaise or weight loss (40%), depression (25%), diplopia, sudden-onset blindness
Palpation of scalp and temporal arteries	Temporal artery or scalp tenderness (55%)
Eye	Scotoma or unilateral loss of vision (ischemic optic neuropathy or central retinal artery occlusion), nonconjugate gaze due to palsy of cranial nerves III, IV, or VI

tory process. Therefore all patients with PMR should be carefully evaluated for findings of TA. Some experts believe that all patients with PMR should undergo temporal artery biopsy to evaluate for that possibility.

Vignette Follow-up

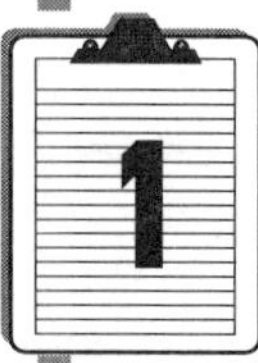

TA is a concern as a cause of Mr. S's ischemic optic neuritis, and a sedimentation rate is obtained, which is 41 mm/hr (slightly elevated). Because of the elevated sedimentation rate, the patient is begun immediately on a high-dose regimen of prednisone. Temporal artery biopsy is negative for arteritis, and the prednisone therapy is discontinued. Mr. S's ischemic optic neuritis is thought to be due to atherosclerotic disease.

Vignettes 2 and 3

Blepharitis: infection or inflammation of the eyelid margins.

Chalazion: pea-sized cyst in a meibomian gland (sebaceous gland); the glands are located deep in the lid and can be seen protruding when the lid is everted.

Chemosis: conjunctival edema.

Hordeolum: red, tender mass caused by infection of a superficial hair follicle gland; the infecting organism is usually *Staphylococcus aureus;* also called a **stye.**

Pinguecula: fatty, fibrous growth under the conjunctiva on the medial sclera; from the Latin word for "fat"; related to wind and dust exposure: when it extends over the iris, it can obstruct vision and is called a **pterygium.**

Uveitis: inflammation of the uveal tract, which includes the iris (causing **iritis**), ciliary body, and choroid plexus.

RE is a 48-year-old man who comes to the clinic complaining of pain in his right eye of 3 days' duration. He describes a constant ache in his eye, accompanied by tearing and photophobia. He thinks that perhaps he has gotten "something in my eye," but repeated washing of the eye has not helped. His eye has been red, but he has not noted any "mattering." His wife, child, and co-workers have been well, and no one has "pink eye."

Physical examination abnormalities are limited to those revealed by the **ophthalmologic** examination. His **visual acuity,** as determined by using a near vision card, is 20/50 in the right eye, 20/30 in the left eye, and 20/30 for both eyes. His **lids** and **lashes** are normal, and no foreign body is seen when the lids are everted. The **conjunctiva** of his right eye is injected. Both **pupils** are round and reactive to light, with the right 2 mm and the left 4 mm in diameter. **Fundi** examination reveals normal disks, vessels, and retina.

RG is a 43-year-old man who comes to clinic because of a "headache" and a "goose egg on my forehead." He has noted that the left side of his forehead

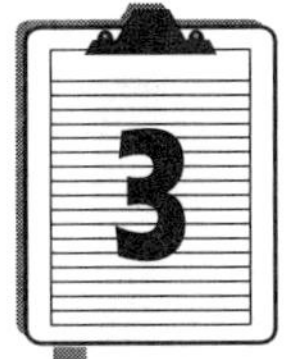

has been painful for 2 days. His symptoms are unrelieved by acetaminophen, and he seeks care because of forehead redness and swelling. Mr. G's general health is good, and he usually does not get headaches. He is gay, and in a stable relationship; a HIV antibody test done 14 months ago was negative.

Physical examination reveals a healthy-appearing man whose **blood pressure** is 135/80 mm Hg and **heart rate** is 68 beats/min. General physical examination findings are normal, and the only abnormal finding on **HEENT** exam is a small "abrasion" at his scalp line that is surrounded by dermal erythema. (When questioned about the area, the patient says that he thinks he may have traumatized himself with a sharp comb.) Sensation over his face is normal, and there is no sinus tenderness.

Mr. G is thought to have cellulitis and is begun on dicloxacillin therapy. However, the erythema and discomfort persist. Because of concern that the cellulitis is extending from a sinusitis, he is seen by an ENT physician and undergoes a sinus computed tomographic series, which is normal. The ENT physician also is concerned about periorbital cellulitis and hospitalizes the patient for 24 hours so that he can receive parenteral antibiotics, after which he is discharged on a regimen of oral antibiotics. However, the patient's discomfort continues and he returns to the clinic.

Vignette Objectives

1. What information from a patient's history and physical examination would mandate an emergency ophthalmologic consultation?
2. How can the history and physical examination assist in the evaluation of a patient with a red eye?
3. Explain the pathogenesis and list the complications of periorbital cellulitis.

"Red Eye"

The differential diagnosis for a red eye includes conjunctivitis, corneal injury, keratitis, anterior uveitis or iritis, scleritis and, acute-angle closure glaucoma (Table 2-3). Findings that indicate a condition requiring emergency ophthalmologic intervention are: (1) reduced visual acuity (assessed using corrected vision), (2) visual field loss, (3) photophobia, (4) severe pain, and (5) abnormal pupillary response. In the absence of these findings, a patient probably has bacterial, viral, or allergic conjunctivitis, which together are the most common causes of a red eye.

Corneal abrasions are the second most common cause of a red eye. Eversion of the lids to locate a foreign body should be a routine measure when assessing people with a painful or inflamed eye. Corneal damage sometimes can be observed with oblique illumination, but the instillation of fluorescein dye, followed by inspection of the eye using a penlight with a cobalt blue filter, can illuminate corneal defects. Contact lens users can have corneal ulcerations, which can become infected with *Pseudomonas* or *Acanthamoeba,* especially if

Table 2-3. Red eye

Condition	Findings
Allergic conjunctivitis	Bilateral; itchy eyes; watery discharge; often seasonal; can be nonseasonal and due to sensitivity to contact lenses or cosmetics
Infectious conjunctivitis	"Mattering," purulent discharge; lids crusted closed in A.M.; foreign body sensation; minimal eye pain; exposure to others with conjunctivitis ("pink eye"); no effect on vision; normal pupillary response; unilateral or bilateral; epidemic viral keratoconjunctivitis can be associated with fever, pharyngitis, and preauricular adenopathy
Herpes conjunctivitis (varicella-zoster or simplex)	Vesicles of shingles in V_1 distribution; cornea especially at risk if vesicles on nose; simplex associated with "cold sores"; corneal herpetic dendrite seen with fluorescein exam
Cornea trauma	History of trauma or ultraviolet light exposure (welding, tanning lamp, sunlight); exquisitely painful; vision can be impaired if central cornea affected; foreign body under lid will cause multiple vertical corneal abrasions; ultraviolet light exposures result in multiple punctate lesions ("starry night")
Anterior uveitis or iritis (choroid plexus, ciliary body, and iris)	Photophobia, aching pain; ciliary blush (erythema concentrated around iris); decreased visual acuity; pupil may be slightly constricted; consider whether there is an associated infection (TB, toxoplasmosis, syphilis) or rheumatic illness (sarcoid, ankylosing spondylitis, Reiter's syndrome, inflammatory bowel disease)
Acute angle closure glaucoma	Sudden onset of eye or brow ache, nausea; decreased vision (due to corneal edema); pupil mid-position and nonreactive; shallow anterior chamber; marked increase in intraocular pressure; ophthalmologic emergency

they use tap water as a contact lens solution. A corneal ulcer constitutes an ophthalmologic emergency, requiring urgent evaluation. Iritis can result in eye pain, and pupillary constriction increases the discomfort. This can be detected by asking the patient to close the affected eye and shining a light into the nonaffected eye. Consensual pupillary constriction in the closed eye is not painful in the presence of conjunctivitis but is in the presence of iritis.

Periorbital and Orbital Cellulitis

The location of a cellulitis surrounding the eye indicates both its origin and its potential for intracranial extension. Cellulitis can involve the preseptal space and be anterior to the eyelid's septum (i.e., periorbital). It often results from bacterial infection of the lashes (hordeolum). The findings of cellulitis are present in the setting of periorbital infections (erythema, warmth, edema, and tenderness), but orbital pressure and eye motion do not cause pain. "Orbital" cellulitis often is an extension of sinusitis. It involves structures deep to the lid's septum, including the retroorbital structures. Because the infection extends to the orbit, it can result in proptosis and pain with eye movement. Infection can extend intracranially and result in cavernous sinus thrombosis.

Eye In Systemic Illness

Many diseases have ophthalmologic manifestations. Specific findings are discussed in the respective chapters covering these entities. The selected signs of different types of illnesses are summarized in Table 2-4.

Ear Disorders

Hearing can be evaluated by determining a patient's ability to hear a whisper or watch tick but is best assessed with an audioscope. The Rinne and Weber tests are used to distinguish conductive from sensorineural hearing loss (Table 2-5). Formal audiometry provides more reliable information about the cause of a hearing loss. Sensorineural loss ("nerve deafness") often is accompanied by tinnitus. The common causes of progressive hearing loss and the associated findings are listed in Table 2-6.

Table 2-4. Eye and systemic illnesses

Condition	Comments
Diabetes	Most frequent cause of blindness in the U.S. for those <60 years old; dot-and-blood hemorrhages (microaneurysms); cotton wool spots (retinal infarcts); neovascularization and vitreous hemorrhages (see also stages of retinopathy Chapter 9)
Hypertension	Arteriolar narrowing and arteriovenous compression (arteriovenous nicking or crossing changes); flame hemorrhages; papilledema (see also progression changes Chapter 3)
Graves' disease (hyperthyroidism)	"Stare," lid retraction, and lid lag (von Graefe's sign) (can occur with hyperthyroidism of any cause); chemosis, proptosis, limitation of extraocular movements, compression of optic nerve (signs Graves' ophthalmopathy)
Connective tissue/autoimmune illnesses	Sjögren's syndrome (dry eyes or keratoconjunctivitis sicca; Schirmer's test quantitates tearing using strips of filter paper); temporal arteritis (ischemic optic neuropathy, retinal artery occlusion); sarcoidosis (uveitis); systemic lupus erythematosus (retinal infarcts cause cotton wool exudates or cytoid bodies); spondyloarthropathies (uveitis); myasthenia gravis (diplopia); rheumatoid arthritis (episcleritis and scleritis)
Hematologic problems	Anemia associated with pale conjunctiva (see Chapter 6 discussion of its sensitivity and specificity); polycythemia (dilated retinal veins); sickle cell disease (retinal hemorrhages and neovascularization)
Infectious illnesses	Leptospirosis (bulbar and palpebral conjunctivitis); endocarditis (Roth's spots); HIV illness (cytomegalovirus retinitis)

Vignette Follow-ups

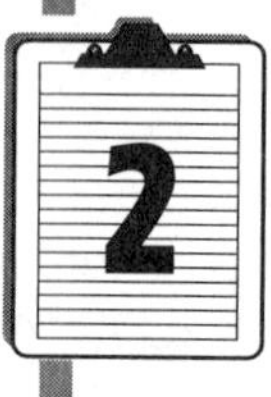

Mr. E is seen that day by an ophthalmologist, who finds inflammatory cells in the anterior chamber on slit-lamp examination, a finding consistent with uveitis. Forty percent of the cases of uveitis are associated with a systemic illness, and the most frequent of these are ankylosing spondylitis, Reiter's syndrome, and Sjögren's syndrome. Most coexisting conditions are detected by history and physical examination, and Mr. E has no findings to suggest these conditions. He is treated with topical steroids to decrease the inflammation and homatropine to dilate the pupil and prevent the formation of synechiae (adhesions) from the iris to the lens. The iritis resolves, and Mr. E remains healthy.

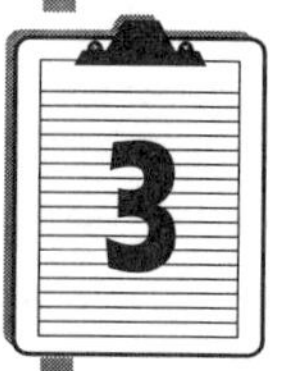

Seven days after the appearance of the initial symptoms, Mr. G is seen again, and at this time, vesicles in a V_1 distribution have formed. Because of this V_1 distribution (with one vesicle on his nose), corneal involvement is a concern but an ophthalmologist consultant finds no evidence of ocular involvement. Mr. G is given oral acyclovir and the condition resolves over several days. Mr. G undergoes repeat anonymous HIV antibody testing after the onset of this problem, and results are negative.

Herpes zoster in a V_1 distribution can have eye manifestations, especially if lesions extend to the nasal bridge. In general, most episodes of zoster ("shingles") are idiopathic. However, it can be associated with states of immunosuppression (such as a lymphoma and after chemotherapy or infection with HIV).

Vignette 4

Presbycusis: sensorineural hearing loss that occurs with aging.
Cholesteatoma: growth of epithelium in the middle ear in the form of a keratin-containing cyst; often a consequence of tympanic membrane (TM) perforation or chronic TM retraction; can result in conductive hearing loss.
Tinnitus: a ringing or rushing sound that seems to originate in the ear or ears.

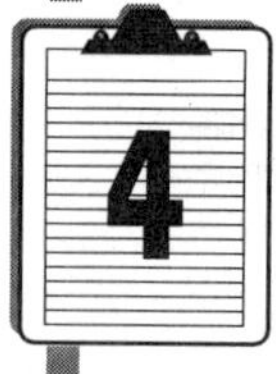

RG is a 43-year-old woman who feels her "hearing is worse." She relates a history of bilateral tinnitus of many years' duration and a progressive, bilateral hearing loss occurring over the past 4 months or so. She is in good health, has no significant medical history, and takes no medications. Her only prior ear problem is bilateral otitis media that was a complication of influenza about 10 years ago. She has no significant history of noise exposure, and she has no family history of deafness, renal disease, or mental retardation. Her parents and two siblings are alive and well.

General physical examination findings are normal. Of the **HEENT** findings relevant to her complaint, the **nasal mucosa** appears normal and the **nasopharynx** and **oropharynx** are clear. Both **tympanic membranes** are normal in appearance and mobility. An audiogram is obtained.

Vignette Objective

1. What history and physical examination findings are of particular relevance to a patient complaining of decreased hearing?

Table 2-5. Conductive versus sensorineural deafness

	Unilateral hearing loss	
Test	Sensorineural	Conductive
Rinne* (mastoid bone and air conduction)	Air > bone in both ears	Bone > air in "bad" ear
Weber* (bone conduction from the midline)	Louder in "good" ear	Louder in "bad" ear (not masked by competing conducted sound)

*Normal response is air > bone, and Weber heard the same in both ears; use 256-Hz tuning fork.

Table 2-6. Hearing loss

Origin/etiology	Findings
CONDUCTIVE (EXTERNAL EAR AND CANAL, TYMPANIC MEMBRANE, MIDDLE EAR CONTENTS)	
External canal	Obstruction with cerumen, foreign body, inflammation, and debris of external otitis
Tympanic membrane	Impaired movement due to perforation or scar tissue
Middle ear and its contents	Effusions (eustachian tube dysfunction or obstruction due to adenoids, tumor); otitis media; cholesteatoma; otosclerosis (inherited as autosomal dominant trait with variable penetrance, overall prevalence approximately 0.5%, women > men, onset in early adulthood, occasionally combined with sensorineural loss due to cochlear involvement); tumor of jugular bulb (glomus jugulare) associated with pulsating tinnitus, red mass behind tympanic membrane
SENSORINEURAL (COCHLEA, ACOUSTIC NERVE, AND CENTRAL AUDITORY PATHWAYS)	
Congenital	Most cases are either genetic or due to problem in utero
Ototoxins	Aminoglycosides, furosemide, aspirin, erythromycin
Infection	Mumps, measles, adenoviruses, meningitis, congenital syphilis
Acoustic trauma	Prolonged exposure to excessive noise
Vascular	Brainstem involvement can cause central or retrochochlear deafness
Acoustic neuroma	Associated tinnitus and vertigo; unilateral; as the neuroma extends, also can affect cranial nerves V, VI, VII, IX, and X; similar findings can result from a meningioma of the cerebellopontine angle
Meniere's disease	Usually unilateral; 20% of cases bilateral; episodic vertigo and tinnitus lasting a few days; low-frequency hearing loss
Presbycusis	Begins with loss of high tones and speech discrimination; progresses to lower frequencies; affects 30% of U.S. population over 70 years old
Syndromes of hereditary deafness with other abnormalities	Alport's disease (1% of cases of genetic deafness, onset in adolescence, associated with glomerulonephritis); Waardenburg's syndrome (1% of cases of congenital deafness, white forelock, heterochromia of iris [different-colored eyes], autosomal dominant trait); Usher's syndrome (3% to 10% of cases of congenital deafness; retinitis pigmentosa and visual problems develop in late childhood); Alström's syndrome (retinitis pigmentosa, diabetes, obesity, and deafness); Jervall's disease (autosomal dominant trait, prolonged QT interval, arrhythmias, deafness)

Vignette Follow-up

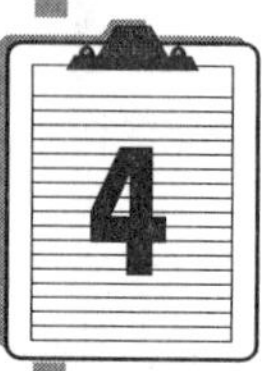

The audiograms show bilateral, high-frequency sensorineural hearing loss. There is no asymmetry or evidence of a conductive loss or retrocochlear disease. It is thought that Ms. G's hearing loss is most likely due to presbycusis or a hereditary disorder. She is being observed for symptoms and followed with serial audiograms.

Vignette 5

Cavernous sinus thrombosis: extension of an infection from the angular vein (drains the central face) or retroorbital structures to the cavernous sinus can cause thrombophlebitis; this is associated with a deep headache, eyelid edema, and paralysis of nerves traversing the sinus (cranial nerves III, IV, or VI); this is a life-threatening emergency, with a mortality approaching 50%.

Otitis media: disorders of the middle ear; can be classified further as acute (usually infectious, with a dull or erythematous, outwardly bulging TM) or chronic (such as serous otitis, with fluid or "bubbles" behind the TM).

Otitis externa: disorders of the external auditory canal; can be due to infections or allergic dermatitis.

JR is a 15-year-old high school student who has an intractable headache and has experienced visual loss. She first complained of a frontal headache and ear pain almost 2 weeks ago. A local physician examined her, diagnosed sinusitis and otitis media, and prescribed oral ampicillin. Two days later, she complained of increasing headache and nausea, and her physician called in a prescription for acetaminophen with codeine to the local pharmacy. For the next several days, JR continued to complain of photophobia and sustained headache, despite taking the antibiotics as prescribed. JR has no significant medical history, other than occasional "strep" throat infections. No one at home has been ill. She takes no medications.

Physical examination reveals an uncomfortable-appearing adolescent who is holding her forehead in her right hand and trying to avoid looking up at the light. Her oral **temperature** is 38.5°C, her **blood pressure** is 150/78 mm Hg, and her **heart rate** is 92 beats/min. **HEENT:** periorbital swelling is present bilaterally, with associated frontal sinus tenderness. **Extraocular movement** testing shows a palsy of the right superior oblique muscle (cranial nerve IV). **Visual field** testing is attempted, and it appears that only gross central vision remains. **Funduscopic** exam reveals the existence of bilateral papilledema and retinal hemorrhages. Her **nose** and **mouth** show no lesions. The TMs of both **ears** are erythematous. Her **neck** is supple, and there is no rigidity in response to flexion, extension, or rotation. She had no mastoid tenderness. **Chest:** clear to auscultation. **Cardiac:** no jugular venous distention; PMI is normal; S_1 and S_2 are normal, with physiologic splitting of S_2. **Abdomen:** soft; bowel sounds are present and no organomegaly or masses are found. **Neurologic** examination shows involvement of cranial nerves II, III, IV, and VI; others are intact (cranial nerve I is not tested). No pathologic reflexes are present, and deep tendon reflexes are 2+ and symmetrical.

Vignette Objectives

1. List causes of ear pain and the physical findings of otitis media.
2. List the history and physical examination findings indicative of sinusitis.
3. List complications of otitis and sinusitis.

Otitis

Otitis Media

Acute otitis media is a common problem. Patients with the disorder complain of ear pain and often have an associated upper respiratory tract infection. Symptoms also can include fever, hearing loss, tinnitus, and vertigo. The TM is erythematous, with loss of its landmarks. As middle ear pressure increases, the TM loses its mobility and can bulge outward. Occasionally, bullae are seen on the TM ("bullous myringitis"), which can be indicative of an infection with *Mycoplasma pneumoniae* or other atypical organisms. Otitis media is associated with several complications, including hearing loss, vertigo resulting from labyrinthitis, and mastoiditis. In rare cases, the temporal bone can become infected.

Complaints of acutely decreased hearing (described as "plugged ears" or a sensation of "water in the ears") do not necessarily indicate the existence of a middle ear infection, because eustachian tube dysfunction, without infection, can cause a sterile middle ear effusion or "serous otitis." In serous otitis, however, the TM is retracted and fluid can be seen behind it. In addition, ear pain (otalgia) can be referred from disorders in other locations, such as dental problems, and temporomandibular joint arthritis, pharyngitis, glossopharyngeal neuralgia, thyroiditis, and, rarely, angina.

Otitis Externa

Otitis externa is an inflammation of the external ear canal and skin of the auricle. The inflammation can be due to eczema, contact dermatitis, infection, trauma, or foreign bodies. Bacterial infection, as with most skin infections, often is due to *S. aureus* and *Streptococcus* species. Because *Pseudomonas* organisms can colonize the canal, this bacteria also can be a cause of external otitis. Swimmers often have stagnant water in their external canals, which predisposes to infection ("swimmer's ear"). In addition, an otitis externa can be an extension of a middle ear infection. If the canal is occluded as the result of edema and the TM cannot be visualized, it can be difficult to determine whether an otitis media is present. In such situations, empiric treatment for both disorders is appropriate.

"Malignant" otitis externa is a rapidly advancing infection of the external canal, usually occurring in patients with compromised immunity, such as poorly controlled diabetes mellitus. Because of the contiguity of the central nervous system structures and the aggressive nature of the infection, the condition is an emergency usually requiring treatment with parenteral antibiotics.

Sinusitis

Obstructed sinus ostia, resulting from an upper respiratory tract infection or allergic rhinitis, predispose to the development of sinus infections. Rarely, sinusitis is due to the extension of a tooth infection. Findings characteristic of sinusitis are listed in Table 2-7. Complications of sinusitis include extension of the infection into contiguous structures, resulting in such conditions as orbital cellulitis, osteomyelitis, cavernous sinus thrombosis, meningitis, and brain abscess. Superior orbital fissure syndrome can result from sphenoid sinusitis and cause lateral rectus palsy, possible involvement of cranial nerves III and IV, proptosis, and severe pain.

Vignette Follow-up

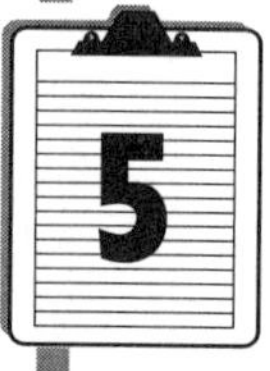

JR has septic thrombosis of her intracranial venous sinuses, secondary to her sinusitis and otitis. Increased intracranial pressure has developed as the result of superior sagittal sinus occlusion. Broad-spectrum antimicrobial therapy is begun, and her condition gradually improves. Tragically, Ms. R has been legally blind since leaving the hospital 14 months ago. A claim for malpractice is pending.

Table 2-7. Sinusitis

History and physical examination	Findings (reported prevalence in selected series)
Symptoms preceding the current complaints	Upper respiratory tract infection or allergic rhinitis
Head, facial, or dental pain?	Aching over involved sinus (60%); pain increased by bending over; headache (60%); tooth pain (20%)
Change in smell	Decreased smell (40%)
Palpation of sinuses	Sinus tenderness (30%)
Inspection of nasal mucosa	Unilateral purulent nasal discharge (70%)
Sinus transillumination	Opacification of maxillary or frontal sinus (70%)

Vignette 6

Pharyngitis: pain due to inflammation of the oropharynx or nasopharynx. The discomfort often worsens with swallowing.
Odynophagia: pain or discomfort on swallowing. It can be associated with dysphagia (difficulty in swallowing).
Rhinorrhea: nonbloody nasal discharge.

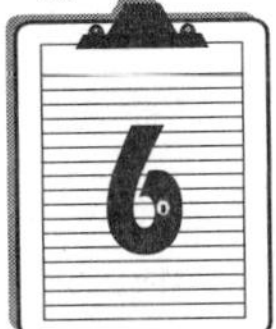

SG is a 16 year old who comes to the clinic because of a "sore throat." She also has experienced malaise, headache, and a low-grade fever for the past 2 days. Her mother is worried about mononucleosis. SG has no other complaints, and her general health has been good. She denies sexual activity or drug use.

Physical examination findings are significant for an oral **temperature** of 38.3°C (101°F). Her **blood pressure** is 90/60 mm Hg and **heart rate** is 88 beats/min. **HEENT:** anicteric, clear conjunctiva, and findings from a **funduscopic examination** are normal. Her **oropharynx** shows erythema without palatal petechiae, and there is an exudate over moderately enlarged tonsils. Her **tympanic membranes** are clear, with normal landmarks. Her **trachea** is midline and movable, with normal crepitance. She has tender **bilateral anterior cervical adenopathy** but no posterior cervical adenopathy. **Chest:** clear to auscultation. **Cardiac:** normal S_1 and physiologically split S_2; no additional sounds are heard. **Abdomen:** nontender, with no hepatosplenomegaly or masses.

Vignette Objectives

1. How does the history and physical examination help identify the cause of pharyngitis and indicate whether a throat culture is needed?
2. What are the acute complications of bacterial pharyngitis, streptococcal infections, and infectious mononucleosis?

Pharyngitis

Complaints of a "sore throat" usually refer to pharyngeal discomfort (pharyngitis) that is worsened by swallowing (odynophagia). This common problem usually is caused by a viral infection. Although less common, streptococcal infections are a concern because of their potential to lead to rheumatic fever or poststreptococcal glomerulonephritis.

The history and physical examination help prioritize potential causes. By stratifying the risks, a management plan can be selected, ranging from symptomatic treatment alone (salt-water gargles and acetaminophen treatment) to empiric antibiotic treatment. Several strategies are available to estimate a patient's likelihood of having a streptococcal infection. One method is to score one point each for (1) the presence of tonsillar (not pharyngeal) exudate, (2) the presence of swollen, tender anterior cervical nodes, (3) a fever of 38.3°C (101°F) or more, and (4) lack of cough. The likelihood of "strep throat" increases with the number of points (Table 2-8). Throat culture can be reserved for patients more likely

Table 2-8. Stratifying risk for a streptococcal pharyngitis

Points	Probability of streptococcal infection	Management
0	0–2%	Symptomatic treatment
1	1%–6%	
2	4%–18%	Throat swab (for rapid streptococcal test* or throat culture)
3	11%–40%	
4	25%–60%	Treat without throat swab

*Sensitivity 80%, specificity 90%.

to have infection. Other factors that increase risk include a documented streptococcal exposure, a history of acute rheumatic fever, an immunocompromised state, and diabetes mellitus. In addition, the incidence, and therefore the likelihood, of streptococcal infection is greater in the winter and spring.

Infectious mononucleosis accounts for less than 10% of patients with pharyngitis, and most of these people have a self-limited illness, similar to other types of viral pharyngitis. Mononucleosis usually occurs in the second decade of life. A unique manifestation in patients with mononucleosis is that treatment with ampicillin (often given to treat a presumed "strep" infection) causes a morbilliform rash. Other findings associated with infectious mononucleosis include an exudative pharyngitis (approximately 50% of patients), posterior cervical adenopathy (90% of patients), and petechiae on the palate.

Finding a positive heterophile antibody, along with a lymphocytosis of more than 50%, confirms the diagnosis. Transient splenomegaly can occur in patients with infectious mononucleosis, and spontaneous splenic rupture is an uncommon, but potentially fatal, complication. Even in the absence of palpable splenomegaly, patients with mononucleosis are advised to avoid engaging in contact sports and other activities that could result in splenic rupture.

Complications of pharyngitis can occur as a result of the infection's extension to form a peritonsillar ("quinsy") or retropharyngeal abscess. The former is identified by the finding of marked pharyngeal asymmetry, resulting from the unilateral abscess. Retropharyngeal abscesses are rare in adults, and normal tracheal movement and crepitance are additional evidence against that diagnosis.

Vignette Follow-up

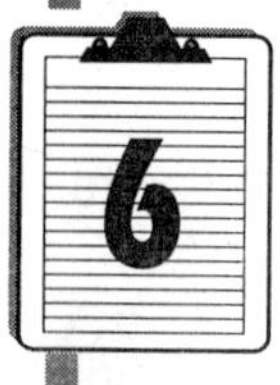

A rapid strep test result is positive and SG is treated with oral penicillin VK (250 mg qid for 10 days).

Vignette 7

Cheilosis: dryness, inflammation, and cracking of the angle of the mouth; also called *angular stomatitis.*

Gingivitis: inflammatory process confined to the gingiva; an early stage of periodontitis.

Periodontitis: inflammation involving the gingiva, alveolar bone, and periodontal ligament.

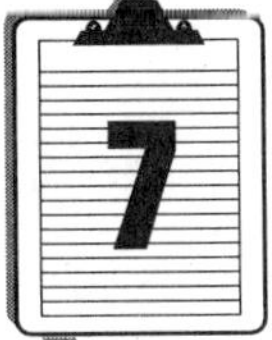

CD is a 20 year-old man who has noticed a white area on the inside of his left cheek. He thought it would go away and has used a nystatin solution for the past 2 weeks. However, over the past few days, the area has become sore. He has no history of mouth trauma or oral problems. He has been otherwise well. He plays baseball on a college team and has been using chewing tobacco daily, a practice he started in junior high school at age 14. He usually places the chewing tobacco on the left side of his mouth between his left cheek and mandibular gingiva. His alcohol use is confined to several beers on the weekend.

Physical examination reveals a well-developed, athletic-appearing man who is in no distress. His **blood pressure** is 110/70 mm Hg, and he has a regular **heart rate** of 68 beats/min. **HEENT:** the only abnormality noted during his **mouth exam,** is a 2-cm ulcerated, nontender, firm, white plaque with surrounding erythema on his left bucca mucosa. His tongue is normal, and his teeth are in good repair. No cervical, submandibular, submental, or supraclavicular nodes are present. The remaining findings from CD's physical examination are normal.

Vignette Objectives

1. List the causes of painful and painless oral lesions, and the features of each.
2. What are the causes of pigmented oral lesions?

Oral Lesions

The tongue is susceptible to "glossitis," which is evidenced by erythema and loss of papillae. It is a nonspecific finding suggestive of nutritional deficiencies, such as those of niacin, thiamine, iron, or vitamin B_{12}. Tongue enlargement also can reflect several problems, for example, acromegaly, myxedema, and amyloidosis. Different types of oral lesions are listed in Table 2-9. Inspection of the tongue's ventral surface is especially important, because that is the location of approximately 80% of oral malignant tumors.

Table 2-9. Oral lesions

Condition	Findings
Aphthous ulcer ("canker sore")	Painful, shallow ulcer; normally 2 to 4 mm in diameter; white with erythematous border, lasts 1 to 2 weeks
Syphilitic chancre	Lips or tongue, painless ulcer; manifestation of primary syphilis; occurs approximately 3 weeks after exposure
Herpes simplex ("cold sore" or "fever blisters")	Initial infection can cause a diffuse gingivostomatitis; recurrences usually appear on the lip's border; painful; lasts 1 to 2 weeks; precipitated by trauma, fever, sun exposure
Leukoplakia	White, flat dysplastic epithelium; associated with alcohol and tobacco use; approximately 5% undergo malignant transformation
Squamous cell carcinoma	80% on the floor of mouth on underside (ventral surface) of the tongue; can appear as white lesion; usually firm, ulcerated, painless; often in an area of leukoplakia; history of tobacco and alcohol use
Coxsackie ("herpangina")	Childhood illness associated with fever and small punctate lesions of palate
Pemphigus vulgaris and pemphigoid	>80% of patients with pemphigus have oral lesions, which appear as bullae on a noninflamed base; oral manifestations can precede skin lesions by several weeks; oral lesions occur in >90% of patients with pemphigoid; the disorders are distinguished by results of biopsy
Trauma	Should heal in 1 to 2 weeks; if lesion persists longer than 2 weeks, biopsy indicated
Oral candidiasis ("thrush")	White pseudomembranes or coating over an erythematous mucosa; associated with broad-spectrum antibiotic use, AIDS, suppressed cellular immunity
Pigmented lesions	1. Peutz-Jeghers syndrome: brown macules on buccal mucosa; lesions also on lips and nose, surrounding eyes and on hands; associated with potentially malignant intestinal polyps 2. Heavy metal exposure, especially lead and mercury: thin, blue-black line at gingival margin of teeth 3. Addison's disease: dark pigment, mainly on buccal mucosa; can be associated with skin pigmentation, including palmar creases and any scars formed subsequent to disease onset 4. Melanin pigmentation: varied color, often due to racial pigmentation; similar pigmentation can be seen with smoking

Vignette Follow-up

A biopsy specimen of the white, indurated, and ulcerated lesion is obtained, which shows leukoplakia. CD undergoes surgical removal of this precancerous lesion. He stops all tobacco use.

Vignette 8

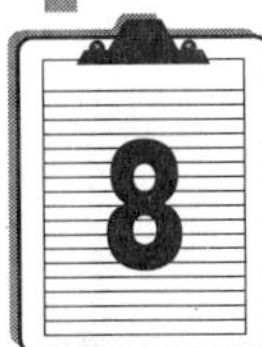

PE is a 52-year-old man who comes to the clinic because of the sudden onset of right facial weakness. He has suffered no preceding trauma or viral illness, and he is well, other than being obese and having an elevated cholesterol level. He reports that his face felt "funny" the day before, and he awoke this morning with facial weakness and inability to close his right eye. He denies prior neurologic problems, and his current symptoms are limited to the face.

Physical examination reveals a man with obvious facial asymmetry, with drooping of his right face and a reduced blink in the right eye. His **blood pressure** is 136/84 mm Hg, with a **heart rate** of 78 beats/min. Physical examination findings include a **height** of 70 inches (1.75 cm), with a **weight** of 243 pounds (109 kg). Both **TMs** and external auditory canals are clear, and **hearing** is intact, as tested by whisper and watch tick. **Cardiovascular** examination findings are normal, with full pulses and no bruits. On **neurologic evaluation**, he has weakness of the right **seventh cranial nerve,** including weakness of his forehead. The remaining cranial nerves are intact. Reflexes, motor strength, fine motor movement, and sensory examination findings are normal.

Vignette Objective

1. Explain how facial paralysis due to cranial nerve VII involvement (a peripheral palsy) differs from that due to a central deficit.

Facial Paralysis

Cranial nerve VII innervates the muscles of facial expression, and its sensory fibers supply taste to the anterior two thirds of the tongue. Facial paralysis can be either central (upper motor neuron) or peripheral (brainstem and seventh cranial nerve) in origin. Because both cortical motor strips influencing the forehead innervate both brainstem nuclei, the forehead is spared when there are central lesions. In addition, because structures are associated closely in the cortical motor strip, central facial weakness usually is accompanied by weakness of the upper extremity.

Most facial weakness is idiopathic (i.e., Bell's palsy). The etiology is unknown, but the disorder may be due to a viral infection or nerve ischemia. Weakness usually is greatest 2 days after the onset of the initial symptoms. Eighty percent of people with Bell's palsy recover completely, although crossed reinnervation can result in misconnections, such as those resulting in gustatory tearing. Ramsay Hunt syndrome, the second most common cause of a peripheral seventh cranial nerve palsy, is due to zoster infection of the geniculate ganglion. In this latter disorder, the peripheral seventh cranial nerve palsy is accompanied by ear pain and vesicles on the TM and auditory canal.

Vignette Follow-up

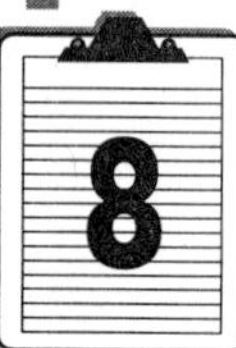

PE is thought to have Bell's palsy. He is started on a high-dose regimen of corticosteroids, with the dose slowly tapered over several weeks. To prevent corneal drying, he wears a patch over his right eye at night. His facial paralysis resolves over 4 weeks, and he is found to be doing well 4 months after resolution of the symptoms.

Vignettes 9 and 10

Ranula: minor buccal salivary gland retention cyst
Trismus: pain with jaw opening
Virchow's node: the left supraclavicular node drains the abdomen, and adenopathy in that location can be a sign of intraabdominal malignancy

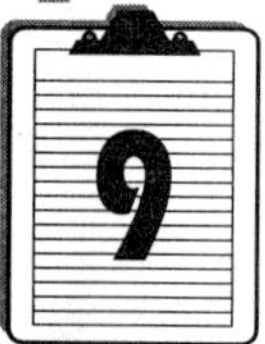

FP is a 37-year-old woman who reports feeling a lump "just under the right-side of my jaw, down in my neck." She first noticed the lump after she experienced discomfort, deep to her tongue, while she was eating a "midnight snack of fresh pineapple." Although the lump seemed smaller in the morning, she felt more pain when she began eating a bagel for breakfast. The pain has increased as the lump has become larger. Before this event, she has felt well, without a recent history of sore throat, fever, cough, or dental problems. She believes she had mumps as a child. Her family history is positive for a father who died from non-Hodgkins lymphoma, and she is concerned about having cancer.

Physical examination reveals an anxious woman who continues to touch her right submandibular region while she recounts her history. Her **blood pressure** is 124/74 mm Hg, her **heart rate** is 88 beats/min, and **temperature** is 37°C. **HEENT** examination reveals a 2.5 × 2.5–cm, mildly tender, firm, rounded submandibular mass just proximal to the angle of her jaw. Mouth findings and mucous membranes are normal. Gloved palpation of the right sublingual area confirms the existence of a submandibular, rounded mass. Her neck is free of lymphadenopathy or thyromegaly. Carotid upstrokes are normal, without bruit. The remainder of the findings from her physical examination, which includes palpation for **lymph nodes** (cervical, preauricular, supraclavicular, axillary, and inguinal) and **percussion for liver size and splenomegaly,** are normal.

MG is a 36-year-old woman who has noticed a "bulge" on the right side of her neck. The area is not tender, and no local redness or heat is associated with the swelling. She has not had fevers or chills, weight loss, anorexia, or other systemic symptoms, and she does not complain of cough, hoarseness, or increased sputum production. She is married, exercises daily, and takes no medications. Ms. G's husband is concerned about the possibility of an infection or cancer.

Physical examination reveals a healthy-appearing woman. Her **blood pressure** is 110/70 mm Hg, with a **heart rate** of 62 beats/min. **HEENT:** her **head** is normocephalic, without any skin lesions or foci of infection. Her **mouth** and **throat** are clear, and there is no posterior pharyngeal drainage. There are no facial masses or swelling. Her **neck** shows a swelling on its right lateral aspect deep to the sternomastoid muscle that protrudes to the anterior triangle. The mass is fluctuant, but attempts to transilluminate the area are unsuccessful. There is no thyromegaly or **thyroid** mass. No **lymph nodes** are palpable, and this includes the cervical, submandibular, submental, occipital, supraclavicular, and axillary nodes. Her **chest** is clear to auscultation, and **cardiac** examination findings are unremarkable. **Abdominal** examination reveals a scaphoid abdomen without hepatomegaly, splenomegaly, or mass. Bowel sounds are normal. The remainder of the findings from the examination, including evaluation of **cranial nerves** II through XII, are normal.

Vignette Objectives

1. List the common causes of a nontender neck mass.
2. How do the medical history and physical examination findings differentiate among the causes of a neck mass?

Neck Mass

There are many causes of neck swelling (Table 2-10). When describing a neck mass, it often is practical to separate these swellings into midline and lateral masses. The lateral neck can be divided by the sternocleidomastoid muscle to the anterior and posterior triangle. In addition, palpation can assist determining whether a neck mass is superficial, such as with lipomas and sebaceous cysts, or is deep to the underlying cervical fascia.

Midline masses can be thyroglossal duct cysts, dermoids, and thyroid abnormalities. A thyroglossal cyst elevates when the tongue protrudes. The thyroid gland does not move with swallowing. Branchial cleft cysts are lateral swellings that arise deep to the sternomastoid fascia. These cysts are nontender and fluctuant, and they normally occur in patients younger than 40 years of age. Because they arise deep to the sternocleidomastoid fascia, they do not transilluminate. A cervical rib can present as a firm mass in the supraclavicular fossa.

Lymph nodes of the neck are located in five places. The anterior cervical nodes drain the mouth, nasopharynx, larynx, and thyroid gland, and cervical lymph node enlargement can cause a lateral neck mass. The submandibular nodes drain the lip and anterior tongue. The left supraclavicular nodes drain the abdomen, and their enlargement, called a *Virchow's node,* often is a sentinel sign of an intraabdominal malignant tumor.

Salivary glands can enlarge as the result of retained secretions, duct obstruction, local inflammation, or malignancy (Table 2-11). The three major salivary glands (parotid, submandibular, and sublingual) vary in their susceptibility to

Table 2-10. Neck mass

Condition	Findings
Thyroglossal duct cyst	Usually develops before age 20; localized in midline along the path of thyroid gland migration; painless until becomes infected; moves upward when tongue is protruded
Thyroid nodule	Nodule, acute hemorrhage into thyroid cyst
Dermoid	Smooth midline mass, usual onset in twenties
Salivary gland enlargement due to infection, duct obstruction, or malignancy	Infection (usually with *S. aureus*) causes tenderness; possibly a purulent drainage from the gland's duct; painful swelling that increases when salivation increases; 80% of cases are submandibular, due to that gland's more viscous secretions; approximately 40% of stones are visible on radiograph
Lymphadenitis	Tender node(s), usually with acute enlargement; associated with viral upper respiratory tract infections or bacterial cellulitis; rarely cat scratch disease
Toxoplasmosis	Mononucleosis-like illness; mildly tender posterior cervical adenopathy; history of exposure to undercooked meat or to cats
Tuberculous adenopathy (scrofula)	Posterior cervical node, nontender; nonmycobacterial form usually submandibular and not associated with pulmonary disease
Malignant adenopathy	Nontender, firm to hard, slowly enlarging; metastatic squamous cell carcincoma of head and neck, which often is associated with alcohol and tobacco use; lymphoma; thyroid malignant tumor
Branchial cleft cyst	Painless mass; located in anterior to upper third of the sternocleidomastoid muscle; soft, fluid filled
Jugular vein thrombosis	Rare complication of pharyngitis that results in swollen neck and septic pulmonary emboli (Lamer's syndrome)

Table 2-11. Salivary gland enlargement

Condition	Findings
Suppurative parotiditis	Acutely inflamed or infected gland; usually occurs in elderly, debilitated people; associated with dehydration and partial duct obstruction; usually due to *S. aureus* or gram-negative organisms; radiographs useful to exclude a stone causing obstruction; can localize to abscess and require drainage
Viral parotiditis	Usually due to mumps; bilateral in 75% of cases; can be associated with aseptic meningitis (10%) and orchitis (25% of postpubertal males) and oophoritis (5% of women); other viral causes include Coxsackie A, influenza, ECHO, and Epstein-Barr virus
Sialolithiasis	Painful swelling that increases when salivation increases; 80% of cases are submandibular, due to that gland's more viscous secretions; approximately 40% of stones are visible on radiograph
Sjögren's syndrome	60% of patients have parotid enlargement; low gland secretion rate and xerostomia predispose to infection
Malignant tumor	Slowly growing, firm, nontender mass; approximately 50% are benign pleomorphic adenomas
Bulimia	Parotid gland enlargement is thought to be due to protein and other nutrient deficiencies; other stigmata include loss of tooth enamel and knuckle calluses (from self-induced vomiting)
Alcoholic liver disease	Parotid gland enlargement is thought to be due to protein malnutrition

different problems. Mumps, the most common salivary gland infection, usually affects only the parotid glands. This gland is palpable behind the mandibular ramus, and its duct (Stensen's), which opens opposite the upper second molar, can be felt when palpating over the contracted masseter muscle. Parotid gland inflammation causes trismus, leading to the name "mumps," from *mompen,* the Danish word for 'mumbling.'

The sublingual and submandibular salivary glands are most susceptible to stone disease because of the more viscous nature of their secretions. Sarcoidosis can affect the lacrimal glands as well as the parotid and other salivary glands, but the swelling is not tender. Likewise, malignant tumors of the salivary glands develop slowly and are nonpainful. The minor salivary glands in the buccal mucosa also can become obstructed, resulting in a soft, translucent retention cyst, or ranula (so called because of its resemblance to the belly of a little frog).

Vignette Follow-ups

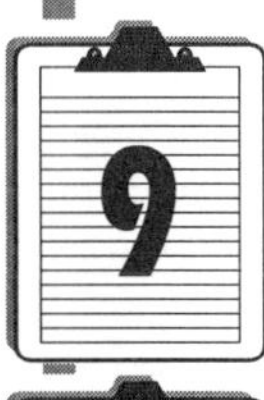

FP is found to have a small salivary duct stone. The swelling, which occurred with eating, indicates that it was due to increased salivary flow. Because there is some reduction in gland size between eating, this indicates the gland is not totally obstructed. A calculus is identified on a radiograph, and oral surgery is needed to remove the stone.

MG undergoes diagnostic ultrasound imaging, which reveals a cystic structure with characteristics most compatible with those of a branchial cleft cyst. A moderate amount of "debris" is noted in the cystic fluid. She is started empirically on a regimen of an oral second-generation cephalosporin, and the mass resolves over the following 2 weeks. Ms. G is offered surgery but prefers continued conservative treatment. Five years later, the mass has not recurred.

Objectives Review

1. List the diagnoses to be considered in a patient presenting with an acute visual loss and the history and physical examination findings typifying each diagnosis.
2. What information from a patient's history and physical examination would mandate an emergency ophthalmologic consultation?
3. How can the history and physical examination assist in the evaluation of a patient with a red eye?
4. Explain the pathogenesis and list the complications of periorbital cellulitis.
5. What history and physical examination findings are of particular relevance to a patient complaining of decreased hearing?

6. How does the history and physical examination help identify the cause of pharyngitis and indicate whether a throat culture is needed?
7. What are the acute complications of bacterial pharyngitis and infectious mononucleosis?
8. List causes of ear pain and the physical findings of otitis media.
9. List the history and physical examination findings indicative of sinusitis.
10. List complications of otitis and sinusitis.
11. List the causes of painful and painless oral lesions, and the features of each.
12. What are the causes of pigmented oral lesions?
13. Explain how facial paralysis due to cranial nerve VII involvement (a peripheral palsy) differs from that due to a central deficit.
14. List the common causes of a nontender neck mass.
15. How do the medical history and physical examination findings differentiate among the causes of a neck mass?

Suggested Reading

Baum JL. Ocular infections. *N Engl J Med* 1978;299:28–32.
A brief review that includes a discussion of keratoconjunctivitis, infected corneal ulcers, endophthalmitis, and uveitis; this and several other references are from a New England Journal of Medicine Current Concepts in Ophthalmology series.

Busse WW. Chronic rhinitis. *Postgrad Med* 1983;73:325–35.
The author presents a framework for distinguishing among and treating allergic rhinitis, nasal polyps, prolonged medication use (rhinitis medicamentosa), and vasomotor rhinitis.

Nadol JB, Jr. Hearing loss. *N Engl J Med* 1993;329:1092–102.
Almost a third of those over age 65 have significant hearing loss; the author reviews the anatomy and physiology of hearing and the common causes of hearing loss.

Patz A. Retinal vascular diseases. *N Engl J Med* 1978;298:1451–4.
The author covers the effects of diabetes and the pathophysiology of retinal vein and artery occlusion.

Quigley HA. Open-angle glaucoma. *N Engl J Med* 1993;328:1097–106.
The author discusses the epidemiology and pathogenesis of and treatment options for open-angle glaucoma.

Reuler JB, Lucas LM, Kumar KL. Sinusitis. *West J Med* 1995;163:40–8.
These general internists present a concise review from the perspective of primary care providers.

Rose DE. Noise and hearing loss. *Postgrad Med* 1981;70:119–29.
This review is helpful, especially regarding the appropriate use and interpretation of audiograms.

Rosenbaum JT. Uveitis. *Arch Intern Med* 1989;149:1173–6.
Forty percent of those with uveitis have a systemic illness; the most common associated illnesses are Reiter's syndrome, ankylosing spondylitis, Sjögren's syndrome, and sarcoidosis.

Sanchez-Menegay C, Hudes ES, Cummings SR. Patient expectations and satisfaction with medical care for upper respiratory infections. *J Gen Intern Med* 1992;7:432–4.
The degree of a patient's satisfaction was found to relate to the provider's interest in the patient and the reassurance and advice given, rather than to the specific diagnosis rendered.

Thoft RA. Corneal disease. *N Engl J Med* 1978;298:1239–41.
The author briefly reviews the nutritional causes (worldwide, the most common cause of blindness) as well as the infectious, inflammatory, and traumatic causes of corneal disease.

Williams JW Jr, Simel DL. Does this patient have sinusitis? Diagnosing acute sinusitis by history and physical examination. *JAMA* 1993;270:1242–6.
From the Rational Clinical Examination series; factors predictive of sinusitis include maxillary tooth pain, poor response to decongestants, colored nasal discharge, and changes in the way the sinus transilluminates (the last is only useful when transillumination is done properly, which can be difficult and takes practice).

3 Cardiovascular Problems

Objectives

List history and physical examination findings for the following problems:

- Angina
- Aortic dissection
- Aortic stenosis
- Cardiac tamponade
- Chronic venous insufficiency
- Claudication
- Congestive heart failure
- Endocarditis
- Flow or innocent murmur
- Hypertrophic cardiomyopathy (asymmetrical septal hypertrophy or idiopathic hypertrophic subaorticstenosis [IHSS])
- Mitral regurgitation
- Mitral valve prolapse
- Myocardial infarction
- Pericarditis
- Peripheral arterial occlusive disease
- Pulmonary edema
- Syncope
- Unstable angina

Pertinent Points

History

Any problems with your heart?
Any history of chest pain?
- Location, radiation
- Severity (scale of 1 to 10)
- Quality of pain (sharp, dull, squeezing)
- Duration
- Frequency
- Change in pattern
- Provoked by exercise, anxiety, or meals
- What do you do when having pain?
- Relieved by rest, nitroglycerin, or antacids
- Associated symptoms (nausea, shortness of breath, diaphoresis)
- Cardiac risk factors (hypertension, diabetes, smoking tobacco, lipid levels, family history)
- Related to chest movement or respiration
- Symptoms of gastroesophageal reflux

Ever told about a heart murmur?
- When, by whom?
- History of rheumatic fever (carditis, arthritis, chorea)
- Prior evaluation for murmur
- Using endocarditis prophylaxis before dental procedures

Any spells of light-headedness or fainting?
- Onset, frequency
- Duration of symptoms
- Prodromal palpitations, nausea, perioral tingling
- Related to position change
- Residua immediately after the symptoms

Problems with palpitations?
- Duration
- Pattern of the beats
- Frequency
- Related to anxiety, use of stimulants, caffeine, drug use, alcohol, or tobacco
- Associated symptoms

For those with congestive heart failure (CHF):
- Onset, etiology
- Weight gain
- Leg swelling
- Dyspnea on exertion (quantify limitations)
- Orthopnea
- Paroxysmal nocturnal dyspnea
- Salt intake
- Medication adherence
- New medications

Physical Examination

Vital signs
- Blood pressure in both arms, heart rate
- Orthostatic change, respiratory rate

Neck veins
- Elevation (jugular venous pressure [JVP])
- Waveform
- Movement with respiration
- Hepatojugular reflex

Carotid arteries
- Upstroke, contour, volume
- Bruits

Point of maximal impulse (PMI)
- Location
- Size
- Duration

Cardiac auscultation
- Heart sounds of valve closure (S_1 mitral and tricuspid; S_2 aortic and pulmonic)
- Murmur
- Gallop (S_3, S_4), other sounds
- Rub

Pulmonary percussion and auscultation
- Dullness to percussion
- Rales, wheezes

Abdominal examination
- Abdominal bruits
- Hepatomegaly
- Aorta width

Extremities
- Dermal appendages
- Cyanosis
- Clubbing
- Peripheral pulses
- Bruits
- Edema

Vignette 1

Hypotension: a systolic blood pressure that is less than 90 mm Hg; however, a patient whose usual blood pressure is higher than normal can have "relative hypotension" at a systolic pressure of greater than 90 mm Hg.
Orthostatics: measuring the pulse and blood pressure supine and upright assesses a patient's intravascular volume status; when the intravascular volume is depleted, changing from supine to upright causes the heart rate to increase and blood pressure to drop.
Pulsus paradoxus: an accentuation of the 10 mm Hg or less reduction in systolic pressure that occurs with inspiration. Pulsus paradoxus can be caused by cardiac tamponade, reactive airway disease, and, less frequently, constrictive pericarditis.
Shock: hypotension associated with inadequate tissue perfusion.

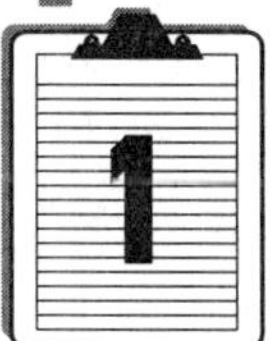

You are watching your 14-year-old son's junior high football team practice. They have been practicing for 90 minutes in full gear on a hot August afternoon. One of the boys is tackled and receives a hard blow to the abdomen with the tackler's helmet. The coach sees you on the sidelines and asks you to assess the player, who now feels "dizzy." You get your stethoscope and blood pressure cuff from the car and assess the player.

Vignette Objectives

1. What are the symptoms of orthostatic hypotension?
2. What is the sequence of pulse and blood pressure changes that occur with increasing intravascular volume depletion?
3. How do normal blood pressure values vary with age?

Hypotension

As a rule of thumb, a blood pressure of less than 90 mm Hg (for an adult) is considered hypotension. Hypotension can lead to shock, a condition characterized by inadequate tissue perfusion. Shock can be classified into the categories listed in Table 3-1. Establishing a person's usual resting blood pressure allows interpretation of their current level. Many young, healthy people have systolic blood pressures that are normally 90 mm Hg, whereas a systolic pressure of 120 mm Hg in a 70-year-old woman whose usual systolic pressure is 160 mm Hg indicates the existence of significant hypotension.

Orthostatic Hypotension

The upright posture accentuates any intravascular volume depletion and can result in hypotension. This typically leads to a feeling of "graying-out," due to

Table 3-1. Categories of problems causing hypotension

General category	Specific conditions	Findings
Cardiogenic "pump failure"	1. Tachyarrhythmias or bradyarrhythmias 2. Obstruction to cardiac outflow (valvular and perivalvular) 3. Myocardial dysfunction 4. Cardiac tamponade 5. Massive pulmonary embolism	*History:* chest pain dyspnea. *Physical signs:* elevated jugular pressure; cool, clammy skin (due to decreased perfusion); CHF (rales, S_3, peripheral edema); tamponade (Kussmaul's sign, distant-sounding heart sounds)
Hypovolemic (acute blood loss, dehydration, or autonomic insufficiency)	1. Hemorrhage 2. Dehydration (nausea, diarrhea, burns, peritonitis, pancreatitis) 3. Relative hypovolemia due to automonic neuropathy	*History:* trauma, vomiting, diarrhea or blood loss, diabetes or other neuropathy. *Physical signs:* orthostatic changes in vital signs; inadequate heart rate increase with standing or absent heart rate change with respiration suggests autonomic neuropathy
Septic (vasodilatation)	Gram-negative sepsis or other overwhelming infection	*Physical signs:* fever, flushed warm skin; findings of the cause for sepsis (e.g., pneumonia or pyelonephritis); can be orthostatic changes if vasodilatation is causing hypovolemia

reduced perfusion of the central nervous system. One can simulate the symptoms by squatting for a few minutes, then standing quickly. This maneuver pools blood in the lower extremities; on standing, blood return to the heart is reduced, causing a lower cardiac output and blood pressure. It takes several seconds for the autonomic nervous system to respond and normalize blood pressure. Assessing supine and upright pulse and blood pressure (measuring "orthostatics"), is a diagnostic test of intravascular volume status. When the intravascular volume is depleted, the pulse and blood pressure changes can quantify the amount of volume depletion (Table 3-2). Sitting upright can cause light-headedness or near syncope if the intravascular volume is severely decreased. However, a palpable systolic pressure usually can be obtained quickly to gauge the orthostatic changes.

Blood pressure can take several minutes to reequilibrate after a person moves from a supine to upright position. Therefore, to accurately interpret blood pressure, it should be measured immediately after a position change and then again 3 minutes later. A decrease in blood pressure, without an increase in heart rate, is suggestive of an autonomic insufficiency, such as can occur in the settings of diabetes, other neuropathies, and parkinsonism.

Other Information Gained from the Blood Pressure

Besides its importance in the diagnosis of hypertension and the assessment of intravascular volume, blood pressure measurement is important in the identifi-

Table 3-2. Vital signs and intravascular volume

	Supine		Standing		
Intravascular volume	Heart rate	Blood pressure	Heart rate	Blood pressure	Other findings
Normal	Normal	Normal	No change	No change	—
Early volume depletion (15% decrease)	Normal	Normal	Increase of 10–15 beats/min	No change	Usually no symptoms
Moderate volume depletion (25% decrease)	Increase of 10–15 beats/min	Normal	Increase of 15–25 beats/min	Decrease of 10–15 mm Hg	Light-headed when upright
Severe volume depletion (35% decrease)	Increase of >15 beats/min	Decrease of 10–15 mm Hg	Increase of >20 beats/min	Decrease of >15 mm Hg	Thirst, light-headed, skin pale and cool

cation of arterial narrowing and obstruction (such as a coarctation of the aorta and peripheral vascular disease) and cardiac tamponade.

Blood pressure differences between the left and right arm or between the upper and lower extremities can indicate a vascular obstruction or narrowing. For example, differences between the arm blood pressures can result from stenosis of a subclavian artery or a dissecting aneurysm of the aortic arch that affects the great vessels. In young adults with hypertension, lower extremity pressures that are less than the arm pressures can indicate the presence of coarctation of the aorta. A difference in pressure between the upper and lower extremities among older adults usually indicates the existence of peripheral vascular disease.

Pulsus paradoxus is defined as an inspiratory decrease in the systolic pressure of more than 10 mm Hg. The name is actually a misnomer, in that it is not paradoxical but an accentuation of the normal decrease in the systolic pressure that occurs with inspiration. It is assessed by measuring the systolic pressure when it is only audible during exhalation, then slowly lowering the pressure until it is heard through a respiratory cycle. Assessing for pulsus paradoxus is critical for diagnosing cardiac tamponade; it also can be a manifestation of reactive airway disease and, less frequently, of constrictive pericarditis.

Blood Pressure in Children

Normal blood pressures in children and adolescents are lower than those in adults. Table 3-3 lists the normal values for children of different ages.

Table 3-3. Normal vital signs for children of different ages

Age	Heart rate (beats/min)	Systolic pressure (mm Hg)*	Diastolic pressure (mm Hg)*	Severe hypertension (mm Hg)
Premature	140	45	25	—
Newborn	125	60	35	>105/–
1 month	120	80	45	>105/–
6 months	120	90	60	>110/–
12 months	120	95	65	>115/80
2–3 years	110	100	65	>125/85
4–5 years	100	100	65	>125/85
6–8 years	90	100	60	>130/85
9–12 years	80	110	60	>135/90
≥13 years	70	115	60	>145/95

*90% of normal values within ±15 mm Hg.

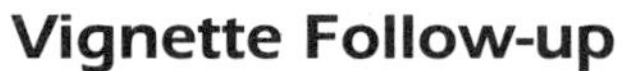

Vignette Follow-up

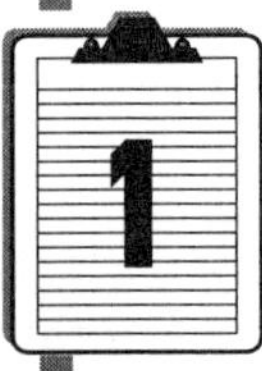

The player has a **heart rate** of 80 beats/min when supine, which increases to 100 beats/min on standing; his **blood pressure** does not change with the position change. The youth tells you that the helmet blow was to the lower abdomen. On examination, his **abdomen** is found to be soft and nontender, with normal bowel sounds. Your impression is that the blood pressure decrease is due to dehydration, not intraabdominal bleeding caused by splenic rupture or liver contusion. His dehydration probably results from the heat, sweating to regulate body temperature, and inadequate volume replacement. The young player's symptoms resolve, and his vital signs normalize with oral fluid intake.

Vignette 2

Emergent hypertension: elevated blood pressure accompanied by a condition, such as unstable angina, congestive heart failure, or acute renal failure, that would be ameliorated by blood pressure reduction.

Hypertension: systolic pressure of more than 140 mm Hg and diastolic pressure of more than 90 mm Hg. A "high normal" blood pressure is a systolic pressure of 130 to 139 mm Hg or a diastolic pressure of 85 to 89 mm Hg.

Malignant hypertension: markedly elevated blood pressure associated with papilledema, proteinuria, hematuria, and a microangiopathic hemolytic anemia.

Osler's maneuver: performed by observing whether the radial artery remains palpable when a blood pressure cuff is inflated above the patient's systolic pressure. The finding of a palpable radial artery may indicate the existence of pseudohypertension; however, others have found that the specificity of Osler's maneuver is low.

Pseudohypertension: a cuff blood pressure reading that is falsely elevated above the measured intraarterial pressure.

You are examining a 56-year-old man for a "sprained" ankle. You have not seen the patient for several years because he has felt well and does not like to visit physicians. The patient has not had his blood pressure measured for at least 3 years. His **blood pressure** today is 190/110 mm Hg. He is in minimal distress as the result of his sprained ankle, has taken no medications, and has no other complaints.

Vignette Objectives

1. What evidence of long-standing hypertension can be detected during a physical examination?
2. What findings from the history and physical examination help determine the appropriate management for hypertension?

Hypertension

Most of the 50-million people in the United States with an elevated blood pressure have mild hypertension, that is, a diastolic pressure between 90 and 105 mm Hg. Hypertension is generally asymptomatic. The history and physical examination are directed at identifying consequences of an elevated blood pressure (end-organ damage) and seeking causes of the hypertension. More than 95% of cases of hypertension are "essential"; that is, there is no known cause. Secondary hypertension can result from drug use (e.g., sympathomimetic agents or nonsteroidal antiinflammatory drugs [NSAIDs], alcohol withdrawal), chronic renal failure, renal artery stenosis, endocrine disorders (e.g., Cushing's syndrome, hyperaldosteronism, pheochromocytoma), or aortic coarctation. Despite the low yield, a consideration of causes is important during an initial evaluation of a patient with hypertension or when previously well controlled hypertension has become difficult to treat.

Both the duration and degree of the blood pressure elevation determine whether any sequelae have resulted from hypertension. The existence of such sequelae and any acute problems affect the urgency of blood pressure management. Life-threatening problems indicating the need for emergent treatment include unstable angina, congestive heart failure, and acute renal failure. Even in the absence of symptoms, a systolic blood pressure that is 210 mm Hg or more and a diastolic pressure that is 120 mm Hg or more require immediate treatment. These management decisions are based on many factors, and general categories and guidelines are presented in Tables 3-4 and 3-5. "Malignant" hypertension is characterized by confusion, papilledema (hypertensive encephalopathy), proteinuria and hematuria, and a microangiopathic hemolytic anemia. Although malignant hypertension can be confused with a cerebrovascular event, focal neurologic deficits are unusual in malignant hypertension.

Table 3-4. Hypertension: mode of presentation and findings

Presentation	Symptoms	Physical examination
Symptomless	None	Elevated blood pressure is the only abnormality
Symptomless, but long-standing	None	Narrowing of retinal arterioles; S_4, sustained PMI (due to cardiac hypertrophy)
"Emergent," symptomatic	Dyspnea, orthopnea, peripheral edema (symptoms of CHF); chest pain (cardiac ischemia); tearing chest pain, can radiate to posterior neck or back (aortic dissection); headache, asymmetrical neurologic findings (CNS hemorrhage)	Narrowing of retinal arterioles, arteriovenous crossing changes; $S_4 \pm S_3$, laterally displaced, sustained PMI (cardiac hypertrophy and dilitation), elevated jugular venous pressure, rales, dependent edema; asymmetry in blood pressures or pulses (aortic dissection)
"Malignant" hypertension	Severe headache, confusion, blurred vision	Blood pressure usually markedly increased (diastolic, >120 mm Hg), papilledema and retinal hemorrhages or exudates, abnormal mental status

Table 3-5. Recommendations for follow-up of an initial blood pressure measurement

Systolic blood pressure (mm Hg)	Diastolic blood pressure (mm Hg)	Initial management
≥210	≥120	Assess for manifestations of malignant hypertension, evaluate complications, initate treatment, and consider hospitalization
180–209	110–119	Evaluate for findings of cardiac, renal, and other end-organ damage; initiate treatment and obtain follow-up within 1 week
160–179	100–109	Probable hypertension; assess for signs of long-standing hypertension; confirm with at least two additional blood pressure assessments within 4 weeks
140–159	90–99	Possible hypertension; assess for signs of long-standing hypertension and evaluate and treat within 8 weeks; consider life-style changes*
130–139	85–89	Consider life-style changes* to lower blood pressure and recheck blood pressure in 6 months to 1 year

*Life-style changes are the suggested initial therapy for mild hypertension. These include weight loss, limiting alcohol intake, sodium restriction, dietary modifications, and exercise.
Source: Modified from the fifth report of the Joint National Committee on Detection, Evaluation and Treatment of High Blood Pressure (JNC V), 1993; 153(2):154–83.

Pseudohypertension is the name applied to an intraarterial pressure that is lower than the indirectly assessed cuff blood pressure. This is occasionally found in elderly people and is probably due to the patient's stiff blood vessels, which require additional pressure to be compressed. Some have found a palpable radial artery, revealed by performance of **Osler's maneuver**, indicates the existence of pseudohypertension, but others have found the specificity of Osler's maneuver to be low.

Vignette Follow-up

The patient's history and physical examination findings are normal, except for the elevated blood pressure and swollen ankle. Repeat blood pressure, measured after 15 minutes of rest, is 180/105 mm Hg. Laboratory studies are performed to assess the patient's renal function and cardiac risk factors. The patient is asked to return the following morning for repeat blood pressure measurement and further consideration of initiating therapy for hypertension.

Vignette 3

Angina pectoris: chest pain caused by myocardial ischemia.
Aortic dissection: disruption of the arterial wall, with creation of a false vascular lumen.
Unstable angina: an angina pattern showing an increase in the frequency, duration, or severity of attacks or a decrease in the amount of exertion causing pain or in the promptness of relief with nitroglycerin; its presence is an indication for the institution of specific emergent management; also called *crescendo* or *accelerated angina.*

EJ is a 62-year-old widow in good health. You are seeing her in the clinic because of concern about "chest pain." One week ago she experienced 6/10 (moderate) anterior chest discomfort. The pain was localized from her sternum to left chest but did not radiate to her neck, jaw, or arms. The pain was not accompanied by other symptoms, such as sweating, shortness of breath, anxiety, nausea, or palpitations. It began while she was standing at the kitchen sink. She was concerned that it might be "heart trouble," so she sat down at the kitchen table. The pain slowly resolved after approximately 45 minutes. She is physically active, swims twice a week, and has not had any previous chest discomfort.

Vignette Objectives

1. What aspects of the history are important in predicting the cause of a patient's chest pain?
2. What questions would you ask to assess cardiac risk factors?

Chest Pain

Causes of Chest Pain

Chest pain is a frequent complaint, and it is one of the few conditions for which you may hospitalize a patient, with a normal physical examination, on the basis of the history alone. Two aspects of the patient's story are used to assess whether the chest pain is angina pectoris: the patient's risk factors for coronary artery disease and the patient's description of the pain.

There are six major risk factors for coronary disease: (1) male sex, (2) family history of early atherosclerotic vascular disease, (3) diabetes, (4) a high LDL cholesterol or low HDL cholesterol level, (5) hypertension, and (6) tobacco use. Although male sex is a risk factor, after menopause, women (who are not receiving estrogen replacement therapy) have a risk that approaches that of men. And, overall, more American women than men die from cardiovascular disease. Estrogen replacement therapy appears to decrease the risk of cardiovascular disease among estrogen-deficient women. Other independent risk factors include a sedentary life-style, age, and possibly obesity and hypertriglyceridemia. The greater the number of risk factors, the higher the probability the pain is cardiac in origin.

A mnemonic to use when obtaining a description of any pain is **PQRST,** which stands for **P**rovoke and **P**alliation of pain, **Q**uality (intensity and character), **R**adiation and location, **S**ymptoms which are associated with the pain, and the pain's **T**iming (onset, duration, and frequency). Data from many people with chest pain have been used to identify certain clinical features that predict the existence of angina or ischemic chest pain. These are age greater than 60 years, smoking, pain upon exertion, pain necessitating stopping activity, and pain that is relieved within 3 minutes of the administration of nitroglycerin.

Many problems can cause chest pain. The differential diagnosis can be organized using one of several strategies; for example, it can be organized by anatomic structures or by disease processes (e.g., infections, malignant, vascular, immunologic). Causes of chest pain are organized by anatomic structures in Table 3-6.

Besides prioritizing the causes of a patient's chest pain, it is also important to consider life-threatening conditions, even ones with a low probability. Three life-threatening intrathoracic disorders cause chest pain: myoacardial infarction, aortic dissections, and pulmonary embolus (Table 3-7). Distinguishing a myocardial infarction from aortic dissection can be difficult, however. Both have similar risk factors, and the symptoms can overlap. In addition, both can coexist if the coronary ostia are disrupted by the dissection. The chest radiograph can be evaluated for signs of mediastinal widening, and if needed, a

Table 3-6. Causes of chest pain

Anatomic system	Cause of pain
Cardiac	Coronary artery disease, aortic valvular disease, pulmonary hypertension, pericarditis
Vascular	Aortic dissection
Pulmonary	Pulmonary embolism, pneumonia, pleuritis
Musculoskeletal	Costochondritis, muscular spasm, rib or vertebral fracture
Neural	Herpes zoster, cervical radiculopathy
Gastrointestinal	Esophageal spasm, esophagitis, peptic ulcer disease, pancreatitis, cholecystitis
Emotional	Anxiety, hyperventilation, depression

Table 3-7. Life-threatening causes of chest pain

Diagnosis	History	Physical examination
Myocardial infarction	Cardiac risk factors: smoking, hypertension, diabetes, ↓HDL, ↑LDL, male sex, family history Severe retrosternal pressure, prolonged >10 min.; associated nausea, diaphoresis, dyspnea; prior angina	Stigmata of atherosclerotic vascular disease, bruits
Aortic dissection (prevalence of findings varies depending on site of dissection)	History of hypertension; Marfan's syndrome Acute severe pain, pain maximal at onset, anterior chest or interscapular, can be "tearing" sensation	2/3 aortic regurgitation, pulse deficit
Pulmonary embolus	Factors predisposing to thrombotic disease: bed rest, malignant tumor, vascular trauma, surgery Pleuritic chest pain, dyspnea, hemoptysis	Can have asymmetrical leg swelling and pain, but exam neither sensitive nor specific for deep venous thrombosis; other than tachycardia, physical examination findings can be normal

chest computed tomographic scan or transesophageal echocardiogram can be obtained to exclude an aortic dissection.

Vignette Follow-up

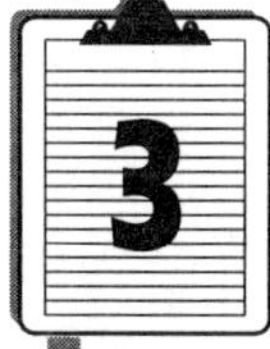

The patient's only cardiac risk factor is a history of cigarette smoking (she quit 6 months ago). A 12-lead electrocardiogram and chest radiograph are normal. A graded exercise electrocardiogram test also is normal. Her symptoms do not recur, and she is thought to have non–cardiac-related chest pain of undetermined etiology.

Vignette 4

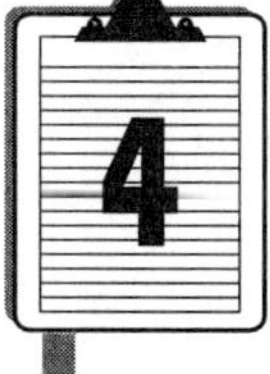

RW is a 67-year-old man who is in your office for evaluation of "chest pain." He is known to have atherosclerotic peripheral vascular disease and underwent a femoropopliteal bypass 4 years ago. The patient tells you that he had a "positive" stress test 2 years ago, when seen by another physician for evaluation and treatment of chest pain. He was given nitroglycerin to use as needed. However, he has only rarely (less than once per month) experienced exertional chest pain, until the past 10 days. His prior episodes have been completely relieved by rest or sublingual nitroglycerin. In the past 10 days, he has been experiencing two to three episodes of chest pain each day. Although the pain continues to be relieved by sublingual nitroglycerin, it is now provoked by minimal exertion (such as walking to the bathroom) and has occurred at rest.

Vignette Objective

1. Chest pain due to angina or cardiac ischemia can be classified as new onset, stable, unstable, or as a myocardial infarction. What questions can help in characterizing these types of anginal pains?

Angina Pectoris

Table 3-8 presents a categorization of angina. It is a simplification of what often is a difficult clinical distinction. This classification can be thought of as a con-

Table 3-8. Types of angina pectoris

Type of angina	Chest pain history	Management
New-onset	Severe and often described as squeezing or pressure; can be a "discomfort," not identified as "pain" Exertional Lasting less than 15 minutes Retrosternal and can radiate to the neck, jaw, or left arm Can be associated with shortness of breath, diaphoresis, nausea, and feelings of anxiety or impending doom Usually occurs in patients with cardiac risk factors	Short- or long-acting nitrates, beta-blockers, calcium antagonists, aspirin; consider an exercise test to stratify the degree of cardiac risk
Stable	Pain description as with "new onset" Fixed pattern, reproduced by a certain amount of exertion Relieved by rest or nitroglycerin Functional class based on the degree of limitation due to chest pain (see Table 3-12 for functional classification)	Management as for new-onset; monitor for disease progression
Unstable	Change in frequency, duration, severity, amount of exertion that causes pain or less prompt relief with nitroglycerin New-onset angina (especially when at rest or with minimal exertion)	Admit to hospital and "rule out" myocardial infarction; medical management (aspirin, nitrates, beta-blockers, heparin); consider urgent coronary angiography
Prolonged angina	Symptoms lasting more than 15 minutes, can be initial episode of angina	If no ECG changes, managed as unstable angina; if ECG changes, managed as acute myocardial infarction until diagnosis excluded

tinuum of increasing symptoms severity, ultimately leading to a myocardial infarction. More than 80% of patients with myocardial infarction experience chest pain, but only about a quarter of the people describe "classic" anginal pain. The clinical distinction is often difficult, but it is important because it has a direct bearing on the prognosis and management rendered and relates directly to the pathophysiology involved.

Acute Myocardial Infarction

The mnemonic to remember when assessing a patient suffering an acute myocardial infarction is HEART, with each letter referring to an important aspect of management, as follows:

H: Do you understand the patient's **h**emodynamics? Low blood pressure can be due to left ventricular failure or inadequate left ventricular preload (e.g., hypovolemia or a right ventricular infarct). When the hemodynamics are unclear, invasive hemodynamic monitoring may be needed.

E: **E**motion and pain control are important.

A: **A**rrhythmias of various types, such as brady- and tachyarrhythmias are associated with a myocardial infarction; their occurrence depends on the location and extent of the infarct.

R: The **r**atio of the myocardial oxygen supply to myocardial demand needs to be optimized. Supply-side factors are oxygenation, hematocrit, and perfusion (e.g., perfusion is augmented by dilating myocardial vessels). Demand can be reduced by slowing the heart rate, lowering the blood pressure, reducing inotropy, and decreasing myocardial wall stress (by decreasing cardiac dilatation).

T: Patients should be considered for receipt of **t**hrombolytic therapy, heparin and aspirin.

Complications of a myocardial infarction causing hypotension or cardiac decompensation and the associated findings are given in Table 3-9.

Vignette Follow-up

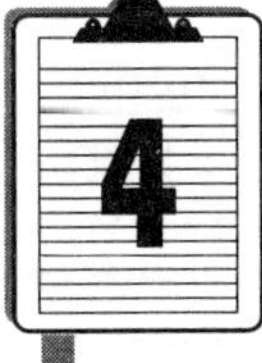

RW is admitted to the hospital and treated for unstable angina. He is begun on a regimen of aspirin, beta-blockers, and nitrates but continues to have pain. A heparin infusion is added, and he undergoes urgent cardiac catheterization and angiography early the next morning, followed by coronary artery bypass graft surgery for three-vessel disease later that day. He does well, and after 2 months in a cardiac rehabilitation program, he is back to playing golf.

Vignette 5

Ankle brachial index: ratio of ankle pressure (measured with a regular cuff just above the ankle) divided by the upper extremity pressure. This ratio is usually greater than 1.0. A value of 0.5 to 0.9 can be associated with claudication, and levels less than 0.5 often are associated with pain at rest.

Claudication: exercise increases the muscles' oxygen requirements; when perfusion is limited, exertion can result in pain due to muscular ischemia.

IL is an 85-year-old woman who is complaining of left calf and foot pain. For 2 months she has noted pain in these areas while walking, and for the last 2 weeks the pain has been present at rest. Her general health is good, and she rarely sees a physician. Her only medication is calcium supplements, and she has smoked half a pack of cigarettes per day for over sixty years.

Physical examination reveals a spry elderly woman. Her **blood pressure** is 170/80 mm Hg in both arms, and **heart rate** is 78 beats/min. Examination findings are normal, other than the **vascular** and **skin** assessments. A superficial 1.5-cm ulcer is present over the left lateral malleolus. Her systolic pressures (in mm Hg) are as follows:

Location	*Right*	*Left*
Brachial	172	170
Upper thigh	240	166
Above knee	212	168
Below knee	160	72
Dorsal pedal	142	34
Posterior tibial	120	0

Vignette Objective

1. List the findings characteristic of peripheral arterial occlusive disease and define the ankle brachial index.

Peripheral Vascular Disease

Peripheral artery narrowing reduces blood flow to the extremities. During exertion, the blood flow limitation results in symptoms of claudication, as muscular ischemia is manifested as pain. Depending on the location of the narrowing, the pain can be in the calf, thigh, or buttock; more proximal aortoiliac disease can result in impotence and gluteal claudication (Leriche's syndrome).

The physical examination can indicate the existence of peripheral arterial disease by showing decreased or absent pulses and audible bruits. Bruits usually are indicative of arterial narrowing. Care is required when performing auscultation, because even slight pressure from the stethoscope can cause a bruit. In addition, the dorsalis pedis pulse is absent in approximately 10% of normal people. By comparing the lower extremity blood pressure to that in the upper

Table 3-9. Complications of myocardial infarction

Problem	History and physical examination findings
Hypotension due to left ventricular failure (survival 20% in this subgroup patients)	Large infarction, elevated jugular venous pressure (JVP), pulmonary congestion with rales ± wheezes
Hypotension due to right ventricular infarction	Inferior infarction (present in approximately half of patients with inferior MIs), elevated JVP, clear lungs
Ruptured papillary muscle	3 to 10 days after MI; apical systolic murmur and LV failure; hemodynamic consequences depend on extent of muscle damage
Ruptured ventricular septum	1 to 2 weeks after anteroseptal MI, acute LV failure and harsh systolic murmur at left lower sternal border
Cardiac rupture	5 days to 2 weeks after MI: recurrent chest pain, hypotension, and death
Pulmonary embolus	Reduced incidence with use of minidose subcutaneous heparin and anticoagulant therapy; chest pain, dyspnea (see Chapter 4 for discussion pulmonary emboli)

MI = myocardial infarction.

extremities (the ankle brachial index), the degree of vascular insufficiency can be gauged, and it is more reliable than grading the pulses from 0 (absent) to 4+ (bounding). Normally the systolic pressure is slightly higher in the lower extremities (measured at either the popliteal or dorsalis pedis artery). The ankle brachial index is the ratio of ankle pressure (measured with a regular cuff just above the ankle) divided by the upper extremity pressure. This ratio is usually greater than 1.0. A value of 0.5 to 0.9 can be associated with claudication, and levels less than 0.5 often result in resting pain.

In addition to pulse and pressure changes, peripheral artery disease causes skin perfusion to be decreased, resulting in cool and dry skin, brittle and thick nails, and loss of dermal appendages (hairs). The distribution of the changes reflects the relative blood flow. If perfusion is severely reduced, ulceration and gangrene can occur.

When an extremity affected by arterial insufficiency is elevated, it is usually pale. However, such limbs also can be pale when horizontal. When an ischemic limb is made dependent, the time to return of skin perfusion is delayed more than the usual 10 seconds. With continued dependency, the limb can demonstrate rubor, which is a consequence of the cyanosis and vasodilatation stemming from local ischemia.

Peripheral venous disease also is manifested by abnormalities in the extremities. However, unlike arterial insufficiency, venous disease results in increased venous pressure, stasis edema, and venous ulcerations. The differences between arterial and venous disease are summarized in Table 3-10.

Acute arterial occlusion can occur in the setting of chronic peripheral artery disease or develop acutely as the result of an embolus. Acute restriction of blood flow results in the "4 Ps" of an extremity, that is, pale, pulseless, paralyzed, and extremely painful.

Table 3-10. Comparison of peripheral arterial and venous disease

	Arterial occlusive disease	Chronic venous insufficiency
Etiology	Risks for atherosclerosis: smoking, hyperlipidemia, diabetes, hypertension; Thromboangiitis obliterans (Buerger's disease), associated with smoking in younger men	Trauma, prior thrombophlebitis, family history; incompetent deep vein valves
Symptoms	Claudication progressing to pain at rest; other symptoms of atherosclerotic disease, such as angina or history of myocardial infarction	History of varicosities or deep venous thrombosis or recurrent phlebitis; achy legs, relieved with leg elevation, leg swelling
Signs	Reduced or absent pulses, bruits, absent hair, pale cool skin; thromboangiitis obliterans associated with migratory thrombophlebitis and higher incidence of ulcers of fingers	Normal arterial findings, varicosities, dependent brawny edema, skin pigmentation due to hemosiderin from chronic microhemorrhages, recurrent cellulitis, ulceration

Vignette Follow-up

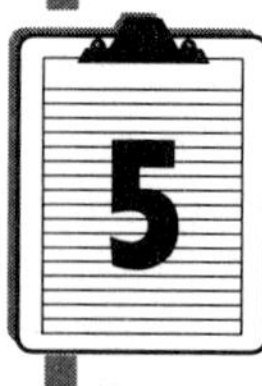

IL undergoes a left femoropopliteal (below the knee) bypass grafting using a reverse saphenous vein graft. She tolerates the procedure well and is able to discontinue smoking.

Vignette 6

Syncope: transient loss of consciousness.

Vasovagal syncope: typically provoked by noxious, painful, or other unpleasant stimuli, it results in increased vagal tone and slowed heart rate. Prodromal symptoms prior to syncope include light-headedness or graying-out, nausea, salivation, and diaphoresis; symptoms can progress to loss of consciousness.

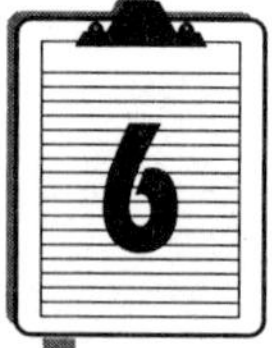

RG is a 79-year-old man who has experienced two episodes of syncope during the past month. He reports that each time he has fainted suddenly without a prodrome of chest pain, palpitations, shortness of breath, or light-headedness. The last episode occurred while he ate breakfast, and his face landed in the cereal bowl. He awakens after a few seconds. Immediately after the episode, he has no weakness, difficulty speaking, visual disturbances, or cardiac complaints. His wife has observed the latest "spell" and confirms the history. He reports that he had a myocardial infarction 12 years ago. However, he has had no heart problems since that time. His **vital signs, cardiac examination** and **neurologic** findings are normal.

Vignette Objective

1. How would a patient's history and physical examination findings distinguish among the causes of syncope?

Syncope

Prospective evaluations of patients with transient loss of consciousness, or syncope, have shown that the history and physical examination provide the most important diagnostic clues to the cause. Approximately 25% of the diagnoses are determined on the basis of the history, with an additional 10% determined on the basis of the physical examination findings. Features related to the causes of syncope are listed in Table 3-11. Immediate questions to be asked concern the patient's activity and position just prior to fainting. Syncope resulting from cardiac problems rarely occur when a person is recumbent. Vasovagal episodes normally are preceded by a symptom complex consisting of sweating, lightheadedness, and abdominal queasiness. Seizures often are characterized by postictal confusion (see Chapter 8 for further discussion).

As already noted, vasovagal syncope typically is provoked by something noxious. The central nervous system hypoperfusion is corrected when the patient is supine or is positioned with the head lower than heart. Typically the

Table 3-11. Differentiating causes of syncope

	Vasovagal syncope	Seizure	Cardiac syncope
Onset	Often preceded by nausea, weakness, and diaphoresis	Brief aura or sudden onset without warning	Sudden onset or preceded by chest pain, palpitations, or other cardiac symptoms; history cardiac disease
Typical setting	Noxious, painful stimuli or emotional upset	Sometimes precipitated by blinking lights or monotonous music	Valvular outflow obstruction can be exertional; dynamic outflow obstruction usually occurs immediately after exertion
Occurrence	Only when upright	Any position	Any position
Physical findings	Pallor, diaphoresis, bradycardia	Repetitive jerking movements, gross tonic-clonic movements (major motor seizure), tongue bites, incontinence	Pallor; if due to arrhythmia, pulse rate and rhythm will be helpful; cardiac findings if due to valvular disease
Findings after syncope or seizure	Rapid recovery; symptoms can recur on standing	"Postictal" confusion; can have residual neurologic abnormalities (such as asymmetrical reflexes or a Todd's paralysis)	Recovery can be rapid or prolonged, depending on duration hypoperfusion

person recovers quickly, without any neurologic symptoms or abnormal physical findings.

Cardiac disorders can reduce cerebral blood flow. They include tachyarrhythmias and bradyarrhythmias, obstruction to cardiac outflow, decreased cardiac filling (as occurs with hypovolemia or massive pulmonary embolus), or a combination of these problems. Finally, metabolic problems (e.g., hypoglycemia, hyperglycemia, hypoxemia, and drug ingestion) can alter brain function and also cause loss of consciousness.

Palpitations

"Palpitations" are a symptom that may indicate an arrhythmia. However, palpitations also are a common complaint of normal, healthy people. When obtaining a history from a patient complaining of palpitations, four aspects are especially important: (1) a history of known cardiac disease; (2) characterization of the rhythm (e.g., can the patient tap out the rhythm?); (3) establishment of any provoking stimuli (e.g., exercise, coffee, anxiety, alcohol, and medication); and (4) associated symptoms (e.g., chest discomfort, light-headed feeling, and shortness of breath).

Vignette Follow-up

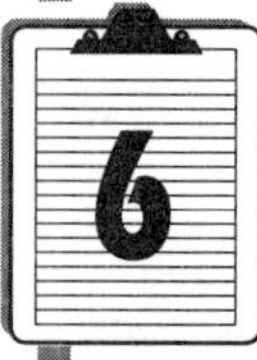

An event monitor captures a 4-second sinus node pause which is associated with the occurrence of the symptoms. Because of his cardiac syncope, RG receives a pacemaker.

Vignette 7

Dyspnea on exertion: shortness of breath or an abnormally uncomfortable awareness of breathing brought on by exercise.

Orthopnea: difficulty breathing when supine. An upright or semirecumbent position lowers the diaphragm and decreases venous return to the heart by allowing blood to pool in the lower extremities.

Paroxysmal nocturnal dyspnea: an hour or two after going to bed, fluid from the lower extremities slowly shifts to the intravascular space and results in pulmonary congestion. The person awakens with shortness of breath and sits or stands to decrease venous return and relieve the symptoms.

SW is a 72-year-old woman who returns to the clinic because of bilateral "leg swelling." The patient has a 20-year history of hypertension. Before this visit, she has had no chest pain or palpitations, and no record of heart disease. During the past 2 months, she slowly has gained 14 pounds (6.3 kg) and dyspnea on exertion, orthopnea, and swollen legs have developed.

Physical examination reveals a pleasant, talkative woman who **weighs** 148 pounds (67 kg) (up 13 pounds [5.85 kg] from the last visit 7 weeks ago), **blood pressure** is 160/100 mm Hg in both arms, **pulse** is 104 beats/min and irregularly irregular, **temperature** is 37.1°C orally, and **respirations** are 20 breaths/min. **HEENT:** corneal arcus and arteriolar narrowing are noted on funduscopic examination. Her neck is supple without thyromegaly or adenopathy. **Chest:** decreased breath sounds in the right base and bibasilar rales. **Cardiac:** jugular venous distention to the angle of her jaw when sitting at 90 degrees; her PMI is laterally displaced to the anterior axillary line and 2.5 cm in diameter; an S_3 is palpable; S_1 is variable in intensity; S_2 is normal; and an S_3 is audible; a 2/6 systolic murmur is present at the apex, with radiation to the axilla; peripheral pulses are all present and symmetrical without bruits. **Abdomen:** obese with normal bowel sounds; liver span is 11 cm to percussion, with the hepatic edge just palpable and mildly tender; no masses are palpable; and stool is occult-blood negative. **Extremities:** 3+ pitting edema extending up to her knees bilaterally; no venous cords are palpable. **Mental status:** she is alert and oriented, with normal cognitive function. **Reflexes:** 2+ and symmetrical, with normal **tone** and **strength** bilaterally.

Vignette Objectives

1. What are the symptoms of CHF?
2. What questions would you ask to clarify the cause of new-onset CHF and define the cause of an exacerbation of chronic CHF?
3. What are the physical examination findings associated with CHF?

Congestive Heart Failure

Symptoms

Several symptoms are typical of CHF, but none are specific to the disorder. Dyspnea is one such symptom, but patients describe dyspnea in a variety of ways. For example, they may say "I'm short of breath," "I cannot catch my breath," or "My chest feels tight." Dyspnea on exertion is the earliest symptom of left ventricular failure, and the circumstances of its occurrence provide information about the severity of CHF. As heart failure progresses, dyspnea occurs with less exertion and patients with severe CHF can have dyspnea at rest. The disability of patients with CHF can be quantified using a functional classification such as the New York Heart Association functional classification (Table 3-12).

Table 3-12. New York Heart Association functional classification

Class	Description
I	Patients with disease but usual physical activity does not cause undue fatigue, palpitations, dyspnea, or anginal pain.
II	Patients with disease who are comfortable at rest. Cardiac symptoms slightly limit physical activity.
III	Patients with disease who have moderate limitations, so that the usual activities, (e.g., making a bed or showering without stopping), result in fatigue, palpitation, dyspnea, or anginal pain.
IV	Patients with disease who are not able to carry on any physical activity without discomfort. Symptoms of congestive heart failure or angina may be present at rest.

As noted earlier, paroxysmal nocturnal dyspnea (PND) usually occurs an hour or two after a patient has gone to bed and fallen asleep. As the person sleeps in the recumbent position, fluid from the lower extremities slowly shifts to the intravascular space, resulting in increased intravascular volume, a higher pulmonary capillary pressure, and pulmonary edema. The patient awakens feeling short of breath and anxious. To obtain relief, he or she sits up in bed or on the side of the bed, with the feet hanging down, resulting in decreased venous return. He or she may open a window "to get more air." In mild cases, relief is obtained in a few minutes. In more severe attacks, respiratory distress can persist for an hour or two. After breathing returns to normal, the patient may have undisturbed sleep for the rest of the night or may sleep in a recliner all night for fear of the symptoms recurring. Orthopnea is another form of dyspnea. Patients with orthopnea sleep propped up on pillows or in a reclining chair to prevent respiratory distress. The sitting position relieves dyspnea by lowering the diaphragm and decreasing venous return to the heart, allowing blood to pool in the lower extremities.

Acute pulmonary edema is due to the sudden development of pulmonary congestion. When left ventricular end diastolic pressure increases above normal, a fluid transudate enters the alveoli from the pulmonary capillaries. During an episode of pulmonary edema, a patient either sits upright or stands, causing blood to be redistributed to the legs, and cardiac filling is reduced. Affected patients are often anxious, agitated, pale, and diaphoretic. Their respiratory rate is rapid, and they may develop a cough or wheezing ("cardiac asthma"). Rales and wheezes are heard on pulmonary examination, and their sputum may be pink, frothy, or blood streaked.

General fatigue, weakness, and a feeling of heaviness in the limbs are related to poor perfusion of the skeletal muscles resulting from the reduced cardiac output associated with CHF. Nocturia is a symptom that occurs early in CHF. It results from suppression of urine formation during the day, because the limited cardiac output is directed away from the kidneys while the patient is upright and active. This pattern is reversed at night, when the cardiac output is distributed less to the periphery and more to visceral organs. Congestive hepatomegaly can produce anorexia and a dull ache or a feeling of heaviness in the right upper quadrant or epigastrium. Impairment of memory, headache, confusion, nightmares, and occasionally disorientation can occur in elderly patients with advanced heart failure and reduced cerebral perfusion.

Signs

The physical examination findings associated with CHF often are categorized as either right sided (caused by an elevated right ventricular [RV] end-diastolic pressure) or left sided (resulting from an elevated left ventricular [LV] end-diastolic pressure), or as due to low cardiac output.

"Pure" right-sided CHF can be due to pulmonary disease and hypoxia (cor pulmonale), RV myocardial infarction, and pericardial disease. However, isolated right-sided CHF is infrequent, because the most common cause of RV failure is LV failure. Therefore the two usually coexist. With long-standing left sided CHF, the pulmonary lymphatics enlarge to accommodate the high volume of fluid transudate. Accordingly, chronic biventricular heart failure is unaccompanied by pulmonary edema, despite the elevated LV end-diastolic pressure. The "right-sided" findings of CHF are an elevated jugular venous pressure and hepatomegaly resulting from liver congestion.

Left-sided CHF results in pulmonary congestion, and the findings include rales (especially in the bases or dependent regions), bronchospasm, wheezes, and right-sided or bilateral pleural effusion. On physical examination, LV enlargement usually is detectable, resulting in a PMI that is laterally displaced, sustained, or dyskinetic. When a patient is examined in the left-lateral position, a PMI of greater than 3 cm in diameter or more than 10 cm from the midsternal line (when supine) are sensitive tests for left ventricular enlargement. An S_3 often can be heard at the apex. LV dilatation can be associated with a mitral regurgitation murmur. Dependent edema affecting the lower extremities and the presacral area when the patient is supine also reflects an elevated central venous pressure and decreased renal perfusion, with increased sodium reabsorption.

A hepatojugular reflex can be elicited in patients with CHF. To elicit it, the liver is gently compressed for 20 seconds, which causes blood to be released from the hepatic sinusoids into the inferior vena cava, which elevates the jugular venous pressure. The normal response is a transient, brief increase in jugular venous pressure, but in CHF the elevation persists for as long as the liver is compressed.

Etiologies of New (or Worsening) Congestive Heart Failure

Establishing the cause of an exacerbation of chronic CHF is as important as determining the cause of new heart failure. Potential considerations include a superimposed new cardiac disorder (e.g., a recent myocardial infarction or arrhythmia), increased cardiac demands, (e.g., anemia, infection, or hyperthyroidism), increased sodium intake, nonadherence to medications, progression of the underlying disease, and new drugs (e.g., NSAIDs, beta-blockers, or verapamil). Possible causes of CHF are organized by anatomic structures in Table 3-13 and presented using a mnemonic in Table 3-14.

Table 3-13. Anatomic approach to causes of congestive heart failure

Structures outside of the chest
- Endocrinopathies (thyroid, pheochromocytoma)
- Anemia

Vascular
- Hypertension: systemic or pulmonary
- Pulmonary emboli

Pericardial
- Effusion
- Constriction

Coronary
- Ischemic cardiomyopathy
- Inflammatory arteritis

Myocardial
- Cardiomyopathies
- Conducting system disease
- Infiltrative problems (hemochromatosis, amyloid)

Valvular
- Stenosis
- Regurgitation

Table 3-14. Causes of congestive heart failure (SAVE MY HTS mneumonic)

Systemic problems: anemia, endocrinopathies
Arrhythmias
Valvular disease
Endocarditis
Myocardial muscle disease: infiltrative, inflammatory, hereditary
Y
High blood pressure
Thrombosis of coronary vessels (coronary artery disease)
Surface or pericardial disease

Vignette Follow-up

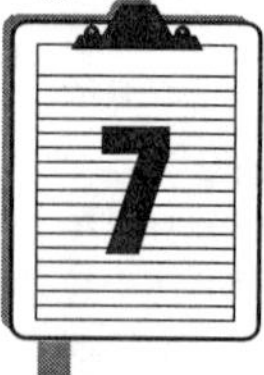

SW is treated with digoxin to decrease her rapid atrial fibrillation rate, and intravenous furosemide, to reduce intravascular volume. Treatment with an angiotensin-converting enzyme inhibitor is initiated to reduce her blood pressure and decrease afterload. Because of the potential for embolic events, SW is anticoagulated with warfarin. Three weeks later, she is in New York Heart Association functional class II and able to do light housework without suffering dyspnea.

Vignettes 8, 9, and 10

Systolic ejection murmur: murmur characterized by a pattern of increasing then decreasing intensity; usually an aortic or pulmonic outflow murmur.

Holosystolic murmur: murmur that remains the same in intensity throughout systole; often best heard at the cardiac apex and due to mitral regurgitation.

You have signed up to help with pre-participation physical examinations for your local university athletes. Two students (HB and DD) are of particular concern to you:

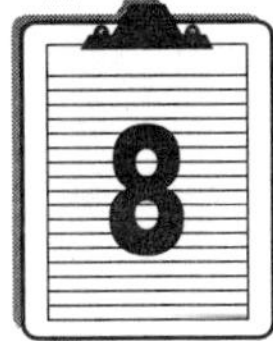

HB is an 18-year-old woman on the basketball team. She has no history, symptoms, or signs of cardiac disease, and she has been playing volleyball since age 9. There also is no family history of heart disease or sudden death, and all family members tend to be tall and slender, as she is. Her **height** is 73 inches (1.8 m), her **weight** is 158 pounds (71 kg), her **blood pressure** is 108/60 mm Hg, and her **pulse** is 78 beats/min. **HEENT:** eye exam findings are normal; her oropharynx is clear, and she has a high arched palate; her neck is supple without thyromegaly. Her **chest** is clear to auscultation. **Cardiac:** no jugular venous distention; the PMI is normal in size and just lateral to the midclavicular line: S_1 is normal; S_2 is physiologically split; and a midsystolic click is audible but without systolic or diastolic murmurs. **Abdomen:** soft without organomegaly, masses, or bruits. **Extremities:** long, slender limbs, without edema or clubbing.

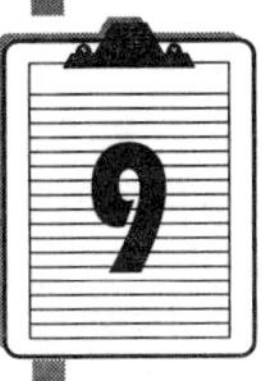

DD is a 19-year-old baseball player with no history of cardiac symptoms. His family history is negative for atherosclerotic vascular disease, although he does report a paternal uncle who died suddenly in his 40s of an "unknown" cardiac disease. The physical examination reveals a healthy, muscular man. His **blood pressure** is 118/82 mm Hg, and his **heart rate** is 56 beats/min. Abnormal findings are confined to the **cardiac** examination. There is no jugular venous distention. The PMI is normally positioned and sustained. S_1 is normal, and S_2 is narrowly split. A 2/6 systolic ejection murmur is present at the left sternal border; no S_3, S_4, or diastolic murmurs are heard.

ET is a 60-year-old woman who has been admitted from the emergency room after an episode of syncope. On the day of admission, while in church, she felt a "tingling" in her forehead. This was followed by a sudden loss of consciousness, and she awoke after about 5 minutes. At that time, her mental status was normal, and she had no focal neurologic complaints. Paramedics were called, and they brought her to the emergency room. Additional questioning discloses that about 2 months ago, she had a "gray-out" spell, without a prodrome or loss of consciousness. She has had a known heart murmur since age 40, but she has not been evaluated further nor told she had a "heart problem." She maintains a vigorous life-style and has no history of chest pain, palpitations, or shortness of breath.

Physical examination reveals a slightly obese woman in no distress. Her **blood pressure** is 148/92 mm Hg in both arms. Her **heart rate** is regular at 74 beats/min. **HEENT:** normal fundi; no thyromegaly, and carotids are grade 2+

bilaterally with transmitted murmurs. **Chest:** clear to auscultation. **Cardiac:** sustained but nondisplaced PMI; carotid upstroke is normal; S_1 is normal; a 3/6 midpeaking systolic ejection murmur and an S_4 are heard; no diastolic murmur is appreciated. **Extremities:** no edema, and pulses are full and symmetrical. **Neurologic** examination findings are normal.

Vignette Objectives

1. What features are used to decide whether a murmur is originating from the aortic or mitral valve?
2. What are the characteristics that distinguish among an innocent flow murmur, and the murmurs of aortic stenosis, asymmetrical septal hypertrophy, and an atrial septal defect?
3. What features of the history and physical examination indicate that a systolic ejection murmur represents hemodynamically significant aortic stenosis?

Murmurs

Every type of murmur can be described in terms of its location, pattern, intensity, timing, radiation, and changes with maneuvers. Determining a murmur's origin is facilitated by an understanding of the types of murmurs and the cardiac findings characteristic of the particular cardiac abnormality.

Systolic murmurs can be caused either by blood being ejected out through the pulmonary artery or aorta (ejection murmurs) or by blood traveling back through the mitral or tricuspid valve into the left and right atrium (regurgitant murmurs). The distinguishing features of systolic murmurs are listed in Table 3-15. Certain causes of systolic murmurs require additional consideration, however. The most common cause of sudden death in young athletes is hypertrophic cardiomyopathy, or asymmetrical septal hypertrophy (sometimes also referred to as *idiopathic hypertrophic subaortic stenosis* [IHSS]). This disorder is inherited as an autosomal dominant trait, and many affected people have a family history of the problem. The cardiomyopathy results in increased ventricular mass, usually associated with asymmetrical hypertrophy of the interventricular septum. The hypertrophy results in a dynamic subaortic obstruction during ventricular contraction. However, not all patients with the disorder experience outflow obstruction; in those who do not, symptoms of CHF can predominate.

Certain maneuvers can help in differentiating among murmurs (Table 3-16). The hemodynamic changes resulting in exertional syncope due to hypertrophic cardiomyopathy are similar to the changes that occur when going from a squatting to a standing position. During exercise, ventricular inotropy increases, followed by a decrease in ventricular volume immediately after exertion, when arterial resistance in the extremities is reduced and venous return is no longer augmented by the legs' muscular contraction. This combination of enhanced inotrophy and reduced preload maximizes the dynamic outflow obstruction.

Many young people have a so-called flow, or innocent, murmur. To avoid performing unnecessary diagnostic tests in such people, it is important to

Table 3-15. Systolic murmurs

Diagnosis	Auscultation	Other findings
Flow murmur	No other abnormalities; murmur > supine than when sitting	Individual less than 20 years old; high cardiac output (e.g., anemia, fever, and pregnancy)
Aortic stenosis	Ejection murmur at base with radiation to the carotids; A_2 soft ± ejection click, S_4 present, paradoxical splitting of S_2	Symptoms of angina, syncope, and CHF; delayed carotid upstroke; PMI sustained and LV lift; murmur usually does not change much with maneuvers; LAE and LVH on ECG; calcium in aortic valve on chest radiograph
Aortic "sclerosis" of the elderly	Radiation to carotids, early peaking ejection murmur at base	Elderly patient; absence of findings of aortic stenosis
Mitral regurgitation	Holosystolic murmur at apex with radiation to the axilla	Can be symptoms of slowly progressive CHF; LA enlargement and mitral valve calcification on chest radiograph
Mitral valve prolapse	Mid to late systolic murmur at apex; systolic click	Young women; positive family history; can be associated with connective tissue diseases (e.g., Marfan's and Ehlers-Danlos syndromes)
Atrial septal defect	Wide, fixed splitting of S_2; systolic murmur at base (due to increased pulmonic flow)	Palpable PA and RV lift, incomplete RBBB on ECG
Hypertrophic cardiomyopathy	Systolic ejection murmur at base; A_2 normal; S_4 present	LV lift; characteristic change in murmur with maneuvers (increases with Valsalva and going from squatting to standing); LVH on ECG

LAE = left atrial enlargement; LVH = left ventricular hypertrophy; LA = left atrial; PA = pulmonary artery; RBBB = right bundle-branch block.
LA = left atrium; RV = right ventricle; LV = left ventricle; ECG = electrocardiogram

know the characteristics of these murmurs. Flow murmurs are heard best when the person is supine, because the stroke volume is highest in that position. In addition, no stigmata of other causes for the murmur are present, such as fixed splitting of S_2, sustained PMI, or an increase in the murmur intensity in response to maneuvers that decrease ventricular volume. Other possible causes of a systolic murmur in a young person are mitral valve prolapse and an atrial septal defect (Table 3-16). Mitral valve prolapse is characterized by a midsystolic click or late systolic murmur, or both. Although endocarditis prophylaxis is indicated for all affected by mitral valve prolapse, the severe complications (need for valve replacement, ventricular arrhythmias, and sudden death) primarily occur among older men with the disorder.

Aortic stenosis can cause chest pain, syncope, CHF, and sudden death. Because many elderly people have systolic ejection murmurs, clinicians have tried to identify indicators of hemodynamically significant aortic stenosis. Unfortunately, the "classic" findings, (such as prolonged carotid upstroke, a late peaking murmur, single S_2, sustained PMI), are neither sensitive nor specific.

Table 3-16. Maneuvers and heart murmurs

		Effect on murmur			
Maneuver	Physiologic effect	IHSS	Aortic stenosis	Mitral regurgitation	Mitral valve prolapse
Valsalva straining	↓Venous return ↓Left ventricular volume	↑	±	↓	Click occurs earlier; murmur prolonged
Squatting	↑Venous return ↑Left ventricular volume	↓	±	↑	Click occurs later in systole; murmur shorter
Immediate standing from squatting	↓Venous return ↓Left ventricular volume	↑↑	±	↓	Click occurs earlier; murmur prolonged
Handgrip	↑Peripheral vascular resistance ↑Left ventricular volume	↓	↓or no change	↑	Click occurs later; murmur shorter

Although systolic murmurs can be a normal finding, diastolic murmurs are never normal. The two most frequent diastolic murmurs (aortic regurgitation and mitral stenosis) usually can be differentiated because they have unique characteristics (see Table 3-17). Murmurs from the right side of the heart are increased by inspiration.

Athletes can have "abnormal" cardiac examination findings that reflect the effects of exercise rather than a cardiac abnormality. Their heart rate often is slow, and the PMI can be displaced laterally and sustained. Both third and fourth sounds can be heard in approximately half of highly trained athletes. In addition, innocent murmurs can be heard in 40% of such people, because of their increased stroke volume.

Vignette Follow-ups

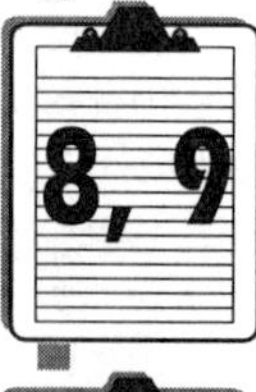

HB and DD each undergo electrocardiography and echocardiography. HB's echocardiogram shows mitral valve prolapse but no evidence of aortic root dilatation. Although DD shows increased voltage on his electrocardiogram, his echocardiogram is normal.

ET is admitted to the hospital and monitored by telemetry. Her electrocardiogram shows voltage and ST-T wave changes characteristic of LV hypertrophy and left atrial enlargement. She is found to have critical aortic stenosis and undergoes aortic valve replacement.

Table 3-17. Diastolic murmurs

Diagnosis	Auscultation	Other findings
Aortic regurgitation	High-pitched descrescendo murmur at base and left sternal border; A_2 can be decreased	Wide pulse pressure; displaced diffuse PMI and LV lift; signs of wide pulse pressure, such as visible capillary pulsations and "pistol shot" heard over femoral arteries
Mitral stenosis	Opening snap, middiastolic low-pitched rumble with presystolic accentuation at apex (with sinus rhythm)	Gradually increasing dyspnea on exertion; can acutely worsen with arrhythmia, infection, or pregnancy; RV lift, LA enlargement on ECG and chest radiograph

Vignette 11

Cardiac tamponade: a condition in which a pericardial effusion is causing hemodynamically significant restriction of cardiac filling.

WM is a 65-year-old woman who is seen emergently because of chest pain and shortness of breath. Her history is significant for squamous cell carcinoma of the larynx, diagnosed 1 month previously when hoarseness developed. A biopsy specimen of a laryngeal lesion showed squamous cell carcinoma. She has had no cardiac history, until 2 days before admission, when a nocturnal cough, orthopnea, and PND developed. She reports experiencing intermittent anterior chest discomfort that is 3/10 in severity. The pain is not positional and does not radiate. She also has noted progressive dysphagia for solids over the past 4 weeks and she has modified her diet to liquids only. She has a 100-pack year history of smoking and has rarely consumed alcohol.

Physical examination reveals an alert woman who is in mild distress and sitting upright. Her **blood pressure** is 110/85 mm Hg, and the **heart rate** is 125 beats/min. Her **respiratory rate** is 25 breaths/min, and her **temperature** is 36.8°C. A pulsus paradoxus is noted at 25 mm Hg. **HEENT** examination reveals bilateral, firm cervical adenopathy. **Chest:** scattered rhonchi; no rales or wheezes. **Cardiac:** jugular venous pressure at 12 cm of H_2O; carotids are 2+, with brisk but low-volume upstrokes; PMI cannot be palpated; auscultation reveals a tachycardia and distant heart sounds; a 2/6 ejective murmur is audible at the base; no rub is heard. **Abdomen:** soft without organomegaly or masses. **Extremities:** trace of pitting edema.

Vignette Objectives

1. What are the symptoms of pericarditis? How does pericardial pain differ from ischemic cardiac pain?
2. What are the physical examination findings indicative of cardiac tamponade?

Pericardial Effusions

The pain caused by pericardial inflammation is similar in location to that of angina. However, the pain usually is described as being sharp, rather than a sensation of pressure or squeezing. The pain is often continuous and affected by position, rather than by exertion. Sitting up and leaning forward can relieve the pain, and lying back increases the chest discomfort. Pericardial rubs can have one, two, or three components. They are heard best in a patient who has exhaled and is leaning forward.

Tamponade is a severe restriction of cardiac filling resulting from a pericardial effusion. Pericarditis is associated with cardiac tamponade if the pressure from the pericardial effusion limits RV filling. Accordingly, whether an effusion causes tamponade depends on both the effusion volume and pericardial distensibility. For example, a rapidly accumulating, small effusion and a nondistensible pericardial space (as might result from prior radiation) could result in tamponade. A history of an intrathoracic malignant tumor or chest trauma especially should alert examiners to the possibility of a pericardial effusion.

With tamponade, the neck veins show an elevated jugular venous pressure (JVP) and Kussmaul's sign (an increase in JVP with inspiration, rather than the usual inspiratory decrease). The PMI can be decreased or not palpable, but this finding is not specific, because the PMI is not palpable in approximately 15% of normal subjects. The pericardial fluid reduces transmission of the heart sounds, resulting in distant or muffled tones, and a pericardial friction rub can be present. A rub results from friction between the visceral and parietal pericardial surfaces, and it often is absent in the presence of a large effusion. The sensitivity of these findings is limited, however, and the finding of pulsus paradoxus is a key to the existence of pericardial tamponade. In addition to pulsus paradoxus, the restricted cardiac filling can result in reduced blood pressure.

Cardiac tamponade is a medical emergency, and distinguishing between CHF and cardiac tamponade is critical because the appropriate treatment for CHF would exacerbate tamponade. For patients with CHF, the immediate treatment is to reduce venous return and cardiac preload (usually with intravenous furosemide and nitrates). However, for patients with tamponade, cardiac output is critically dependent on adequate preload (filling pressure), and therefore any decrease in preload would cause a further decrement in cardiac filling and output.

Vignette Follow-up

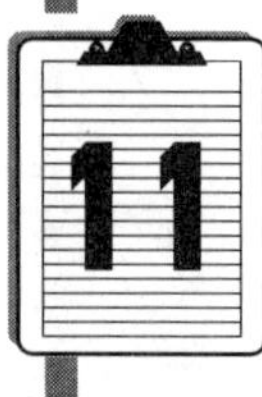

An echocardiogram shows WM to have a malignant pericardial effusion, and she undergoes a pericardiectomy.

Vignette 12

SW is a 28-year-old intravenous drug user who is seen in the emergency room with a fever and myalgias. She has been using intravenous drugs (both cocaine and heroin) intermittently for 12 years, and she supports her drug dependency by prostitution. Over the past 6 years she has had hepatitis B infection and four episodes of sexually transmitted diseases. She reports that she had an HIV antibody test 6 months ago and says that the result was negative.

Her physical examination is remarkable for a **temperature** of 102°F (38.8°C) orally; her **blood pressure** is 120/60 mm Hg, her **pulse** is 110 beats/min. and **respiratory rate** is 18 breaths/min. **Skin:** "tracks" but no Osler or Janeway lesions. **HEENT:** fundi are normal without Roth spots. **Chest:** normal breath sounds. **Cardiac:** no jugular venous distention, a dynamic PMI, normal S_1 and S_2, and a 2/6 systolic murmur at the base. **Abdomen:** no tenderness or organomegaly; **pelvic** examination findings are normal. **Neurologic** examination findings are normal.

Vignette Objectives

1. What potential sequelae of intravenous drug abuse can be detected by history and physical examination?
2. What physical examination findings are associated with bacterial endocarditis?
3. What physical examination findings indicate the presence of narcotic withdrawal?

Endocarditis

The symptoms and signs of endocarditis vary depending on the infecting organism, patient age, presence and extent of pre-existing cardiac disease, and the site of the infection. Over half of patients with endocarditis have cardiac conditions, such as valvular disease and congenital heart disease, that predispose to the development of infection. If endocarditis is suspected, it is important to obtain historical information about cardiac disease and reasons for a bacteremia (e.g., recent dental procedure or IV drug use). Endocarditis is associated with the general symptoms of a bacteremia, such as fever, myalgias, and arthralgias. The infection can cause valve dysfunction and extend to involve the cardiac conducting system. In addition, approximately half of patients with endocarditis have a complication that can involve any organ system, because of metastatic infection, emboli, and immune complexes. Problems that can result from endocarditis are listed in Table 3-18.

Table 3-18. Problems associated with endocarditis

System	Problems
General	Fever
Skin	Osler's nodes, Janeway lesions, petechiae, subungual splinter hemorrhages (today, endocarditis usually is caused more by virulent organisms, resulting in a shorter illness duration and a lower prevalence of peripheral manifestations)
Cardiac	Most patients with left-sided endocarditis have a murmur at or soon after hospital admission; can develop valve insufficiency, heart failure, pulmonary edema, conducting system involvement, myocardial abscess
Pulmonary	Septic pulmonary emboli with right-sided endocarditis
Renal	Septic emboli, immune complex glomerulonephritis, renal failure
Gastrointestinal	Splenomegaly, splenic infarction
Musculoskeletal	Myalgias and back pain can be present initially; septic arthritis and osteomyelitis
Neurologic	Roth spots on funduscopic examination; septic emboli can cause cerebral infarction and hemorrhage, mycotic aneurysms, meningoencephalitis, and brain abscess

Intravenous Drug Abuse

The complications of IV drug abuse can involve any organ system. Users often seek care when a fever develops, and bacterial endocarditis is a frequent diagnostic consideration. Occasionally the fever's cause is evident on the basis of the history and physical examination findings. However, no constellation of symptoms and signs has proved to be of use in separating those with and without endocarditis. In particular, the absence of a heart murmur does not exclude endocarditis. Among patients who present with endocarditis, 90% are febrile but only 55% to 85% have a heart murmur. In addition, a fever can cause an innocent flow murmur as the result of increased inotropy and the hyperdynamic state. Accordingly, febrile IV drug users usually are admitted to the hospital and treated empirically with antibiotics, while the results of blood cultures are awaited.

Intravenous drug users especially are predisposed to the development of right-sided endocarditis caused by *Staphylococcus aureus.* The septic pulmonary emboli that result from right-sided endocarditis can cause cough, hemoptysis, and pleuritic chest pain, and multiple infiltrates are seen on the chest radiographs obtained in such patients. HIV illness also is a frequent consideration in patients who use illicit IV drugs, and HIV positivity raises the possibility of an opportunistic infection in a febrile IV drug abuser. The mnemonic **LIKE 2 SHOOT** can be used to recall the many complications of IV drug use (Table 3-19).

Table 3-19. Consequences of IV drug abuse: LIKE 2 SHOOT

Lung: pulmonary edema can be a direct effect of intravenous heroin use; septic emboli result from right-sided endocarditis; pulmonary vascular disease results from talc injection; pneumonia from aspiration
IHIV
Kidney: glomerulonephritis resulting from endocarditis; heroin rarely causes nephrotic syndrome
Endocarditis; myocardial infarction and arrhythmias with cocaine; rule out endocarditis for any febrile patient, with at least **2** (and preferably 3) sets of blood cultures
Skeletal: localized cutaneous abscess, osteomyelitis, rhabdomyolysis, septic or immune complex arthritis
Hepar (liver): hepatitis
Other organ involvement
Overdose
in**T**egument: injection site scarring; cellulitis, abscess; thrombophlebitis; need for tetanus prophylaxis

Opiate Withdrawal

A person with a history of opiate abuse can require treatment of withdrawal. The symptoms and signs of differing severities of withdrawal are presented in Table 3-20. The occurrence of more severe symptoms of withdrawal indicates that greater methadone doses are needed to alleviate the symptoms.

Table 3-20. Stages of opiate withdrawal and treatment

Grade 1: Lacrimation, rhinorrhea, diaphoresis, yawning, and insomnia
Grade 2: Myalgia, arthralgia, abdominal pain, mydriasis, piloerection, and muscle twitching
Grade 3: Anorexia, nausea, restlessness, fever, tachycardia, hypertension, and tachypnea
Grade 4: Vomiting, diarrhea, findings of dehydration, and hypotension

Vignette Follow-up

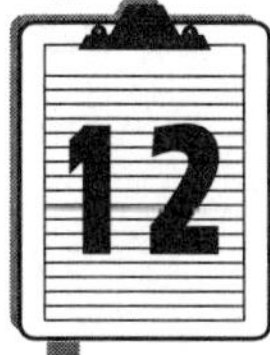

SW has blood cultures performed that are positive for *S. aureus*. She is treated successfully for endocarditis with intravenous antibiotics.

Objectives Review

1. What are the symptoms of orthostatic hypotension?
2. What is the sequence of pulse and blood pressure changes that occur with increasing intravascular volume depletion?
3. How do normal blood pressure values vary with age?
4. What evidence of long-standing hypertension can be detected during a physical examination?
5. What findings from the history and physical examination help determine the appropriate management for hypertension?
6. What aspects of the history are important in predicting the cause of a patient's chest pain?
7. What questions would you ask to assess cardiac risk factors?
8. Chest pain due to angina or cardiac ischemia can be classified as new onset, stable, unstable, or as a myocardial infarction. What questions can help in characterizing these types of anginal pains?
9. List the findings characteristic of peripheral arterial occlusive disease and define the ankle brachial index.
10. How would a patient's history and physical examination findings distinguish among the causes of syncope?
11. What are the symptoms of CHF?
12. What questions would you ask to clarify the cause of new-onset CHF and define the cause of an exacerbation of chronic CHF?
13. What are the physical examination findings associated with CHF?
14. What features are used to decide whether a murmur is originating from the aortic or mitral valve?
15. What are the characteristics that distinguish among an innocent flow murmur and the murmurs of aortic stenosis, asymmetrical septal hypertrophy, and an atrial septal defect?
16. What features of the history and physical examination indicate that a systolic ejection murmur represents hemodynamically significant aortic stenosis?
17. What are the symptoms of pericarditis? How does pericardial pain differ from ischemic cardiac pain?
18. What are the physical examination findings indicative of cardiac tamponade?
19. What potential sequelae of intravenous drug abuse can be detected by history and physical examination?
20. What physical examination findings are associated with bacterial endocarditis?
21. What physical examination findings indicate the presence of narcotic withdrawal?

Suggested Reading

Belmin J, Visintin J-M, Salvatore R, et al. Osler's maneuver: absence of usefulness for the detection of pseudohypertension in the elderly population. *Am J Med* 1995;98:42–9.
Osler's maneuver is not uncommon among the elderly; these authors found it was not predictive of individuals with pseudohypertension.

Birdwell BG, Hebers JE, Kroenke K. The patient's presentation style alters the physician's diagnostic approach. *Arch Intern Med* 1993;153:1991–5.
Patients' style in relating their history influences how the information is interpreted. Physicians tended to discount information from "histrionic" patients and rated the probability of coronary disease as less than that for a more "business-like" historian giving the same information.

Cook DJ, Simel DL. Does this patient have abnormal central venous pressure. *JAMA* 1996;275:630–4.
The authors review bedside assessment of the jugular venous pressure and the measurement's precision and accuracy.

Devereau RB, Kramer-Fox R, Kligfield P. Mitral valve prolapse: causes, clinical manifestations, and management. *Ann Intern Med* 1989;111:305–7.
The authors summarize findings from 800 patients and from the literature pertaining to the findings associated with mitral valve prolapse.

Ewy GA. The abdominojugular test: technique and hemodynamic correlates. *Ann Intern Med* 1988;109:456–7.
This study clarified the significance of this finding and its relationship to an elevated pulmonary artery wedge pressure; it also can occur with a right ventricular infarct.

George KP, Wolfe LA, Gurggraf GW. The 'athletic heart syndrome.' *Sports Med* 1991; 11:300–31.
Extensive review of the physical and laboratory findings in athletes. The authors also present information concerning the mechanisms for the cardiac changes resulting from athletic training.

Guberman BA, Fowler NO, Engel PJ, et al. Cardiac tamponade in medical patients. *Circulation* 1981;64:633–40.
Description of 56 patients with cardiac tamponade. Three quarters had pulsus paradoxus and only 29% had a rub.

Hurst JW. The examination of the heart: the importance of initial screening. *Dis Mon* 1990;36:245–4.
This monograph contains an extensive review of the "low-technology" cardiac evaluation, consisting of the history, physical examination, electrocardiogram, and chest radiograph.

Kapoor WN. Evaluation and management of the patient with syncope. *JAMA* 1992;268: 2553–60.
Review article that points out approximately half of patients have no diagnosis established. When an etiology is defined, the 85 percent are established with the history and physical examination.

Lembo NJ, Dell'Italia LJ, Crawford MH, O'Rourke RA. Bedside diagnosis of systolic murmurs. *N Engl J Med* 1988;318:1572–8.
Describes characteristics of different systolic murmurs revealed by different bedside maneuvers.

Mansur AJ, Ginberg M, Lemos da Luz P, Bellotti G. The complications of infective endocarditis: a reappraisal in the 1980s. *Arch Intern Med* 1992;152:2428–32.

O'Connor PG, Samet JH, Stein MD. Management of hospitalized intravenous drug users: role of the internist. *Am J Med* 1994;96:551–8.
Review of previous articles on the medical problems among this group of patients, including behavioral problems and the problems associated with drug withdrawal.

Reisberg B. Infective endocarditis in the narcotic addict. *Prog Cardiovasc Dis* 1979;22: 193–04.

This review article contains information about the presentation and complications of and the prognosis for endocarditis and relates these features to the site of infection and organism.

Smith ND, Raizada V, Abrams J. Auscultation of the normally functioning prosthetic valve. *Ann Intern Med* 1981;95:594–8.

The authors describe the findings for ball, disk, porcine, and bileaflet valves.

Sox HC Jr, Hickam DH, Marton KI, et al. Using the patient's history to estimate the probability of coronary disease: a comparison of primary care and referral practices. *Am J Med* 1990;89:7–14.

The authors relate different aspects of assessment to the presence of coronary disease and identify features that are indicative of coronary artery disease.

4 Pulmonary Problems

Objectives

List history and physical examination findings for the following problems:

- Acute bacterial pneumonia
- Asthma
- Bronchiectasis
- Chronic bronchitis
- Chronic cough
- Chronic obstructive pulmonary disease
- Cystic fibrosis
- Deep venous thrombosis
- Emphysema
- Hemoptysis
- Lung cancer
- Pleural effusion
- Pleuritic chest pain
- Pulmonary embolus
- Shortness of breath or dyspnea on exertion
- Sleep apnea
- Tuberculosis

Pertinent Points

History

Any lung problems?
Current or former smoker?
- Packs per day × years
- Interest in quitting
- Prior attempts at quitting
- Problems resulting from smoking, such as cough or exertional dyspnea

Any history of asthma?
- Onset, duration, progression
- What medications were/are used
- Treatment with oral corticosteroids
- Self-monitoring of flow rates
- Recent upper respiratory tract infection (URI), change in medications, or exposure to specific allergen
- History of allergic rhinitis, eczema, or urticaria
- Aspirin sensitivity
- History of sinus infections or gastroesophageal reflux

Ever have pneumonia?
- Circumstances
- Treatment

For patients who may have pneumonia:
- Onset and progression of symptoms
- Character and color of sputum
- Fever, rigor, night sweats, chest pain
- Prior pneumococcal vaccine
- History of loss of consciousness
- Alcohol intake, drug use
- Antecedent symptoms of viral URI or influenza
- Systemic complaints (malaise, myalgia)
- Prior infection or exposure to tuberculosis (TB), prior TB skin tests
- HIV risk factors

For patients with hemoptysis:
- Onset
- Quantity of blood
- Associated symptoms (purulent sputum, URI, pleuritic chest pain)
- Smoker
- Asbestos exposure
- Leg pain or swelling
- History of deep venous thrombosis (DVT)
- Heart murmurs or other cardiac problems
- History of tuberculosis (TB) infections or exposure, prior TB skin tests
- Hematuria

For patients with chronic obstructive pulmonary disease (COPD):
- Onset, progression
- Limitations due to dyspnea, exercise tolerance
- Smoking, passive smoke exposure
- Sputum production (amount, when)
- Medications, requirement for antibiotics
- Hospitalizations and emergency room visits
- Family history of pulmonary disease
- Exposure to pulmonary irritants or toxins, occupation

For patients with suspected pulmonary emboli:
- Onset of dyspnea
- Cough, chest pain, hemoptysis
- Leg pain or swelling
- History of DVT
- Reason for venous stasis (such as bed rest, casting, prolonged sitting)
- Reasons for being in hypercoagulable state (e.g., malignancy, family history of thrombosis, postpartum)

Physical Examination

Vital Signs
- Blood pressure, pulsus paradoxus, heart rate and regularity, respiratory rate

Inspection
- Ability to talk without dyspnea
- Nutritional state
- Use of accessory muscles to breathe
- Central cyanosis

HEENT
- Inspection of nasal mucosa (edema, septal ulceration, polyps)
- Cervical and supraclavicular nodes

Chest
- Inspection for configuration and symmetry of chest expansion
- Percussion
- Auscultation

Cardiac
- Jugular venous pressure (JVP)
- Precordial palpation for pulmonary artery impulse, right ventricular (RV) lift, location of point of maximal impulse (PMI)
- Auscultation for heart sounds, murmurs, and extra sounds

Extremities
- Cyanosis
- Clubbing
- Thigh and calf circumference (asymmetry, >2 cm difference)
- Venous cord
- Homans' sign (calf pain with dorsiflexion of foot)
- Edema

Vignette 1

Bronchial breath sounds: respiratory sounds normally heard when auscultating over the trachea and main bronchi; both inspiration and expiration are audible and similar in duration; if heard over the lung periphery, these indicate the presence of consolidation.

Bronchophony: finding of pulmonary consolidation; spoken words normally are muffled when auscultating the lung periphery; words are amplified in the presence of consolidation.

Crackles: see rales.

Egophony: finding of pulmonary consolidation; the patient says "eeeee," as in bee but if auscultating over an area of consolidation, one hears "aaah" as in say.

Rales: high-pitched, discontinuous, crackling sounds, heard during auscultation; they are abnormal sounds that indicate the presence of either fluid in small airways or pulmonary fibrosis.

Rhonchi: low-pitched, gurgling sounds, suggestive of the presence of fluid in the larger airways; can clear or change quality after a cough.

Stridor: long, whooping musical sound caused by upper airway obstruction.

Vesicular breath sounds: sounds normally heard during auscultation of the lung periphery (away from the main bronchi); the inspiratory phase is heard well and lasts longer than the quiet expiratory phase.

Whispered pectoriloquy: whispered words are conducted better through solids than through air; therefore whispered words sound louder if one is listening over pulmonary consolidation.

EB is a 48-year-old man admitted to the hospital for treatment of a "cough" and "shaking chills." The patient was drinking alcohol heavily before admission and still was intoxicated when seen in the emergency room. He relates that for 2 days he has had a cough productive of green sputum. He has not taken his temperature, but says he has felt warm. On the day of admission, he describes having had a shaking chill, during which his teeth rattled. He also has felt more short of breath, and his sputum has become blood streaked. Because he was feeling progressively worse, he called the paramedics and was brought to the emergency room. He has no history of loss of consciousness or seizures. He has smoked one-and-a-half packs of cigarettes a day for over 30 years.

Regarding his alcohol use, the patient relates that he began drinking heavily in his 20s. After his divorce at age 32, he began drinking even more heavily and started moving around the country. Currently he is not employed full time but works intermittently doing odd jobs. He reports having no medical problems stemming from his alcoholism. He has been through detoxification programs twice, but neither has resulted in a prolonged period of abstinence. His family history is remarkable for a father and uncle whom he describes as "alcoholics."

Physical examination reveals a thin, diaphoretic man, lying on a gurney, wearing nasal prongs, and smelling of alcohol. His vital signs include an oral **temperature** of 38.5°C, **blood pressure** of 96/72 mm Hg, **heart rate** of 110 beats/min; and **respiratory rate** of 22 breaths/min. Orthostatic changes are not recorded. **HEENT:** head is free of trauma; extraocular movements are full, without nystagmus; tympanic membranes are clear; poor dentition and periodontal disease are found upon examination of his oropharynx. His neck is supple without adenopathy, and the trachea is midline. **Chest:** normal anteroposterior (AP) diameter; normal expansion on the left, but decreased excursion is noted for the right side of his chest. There is dullness to percussion in the right base. Breath sounds are bronchial over the dullness, with rales and "e" to "a" changes (egophony). **Cardiac:** no JVD; PMI is in normal position and of normal size; S_1 is normal; S_2 is physiologically split. There are no murmurs, gallops, or rubs. **Abdomen:** bowel sounds are present, and his abdomen is nontender. The liver span is 11 cm to percussion, palpable one finger breath below the right costal margin and mildly tender. There is no splenomegaly or mass. Stool is occult-blood negative. **Genitourinary** examination reveals a circumcised male; testes are reduced in size but of normal consistency. **Extremities:** no cyanosis, clubbing, or edema. **Neurologic** exam reveals he is alert and oriented to person, place, and time. His speech is slurred, and he does not cooperate with other aspects of the mental status examination. Reflexes are 2+ and symmetrical. Sensory examination is not performed. Chest radiograph shows a right lower lobe infiltrate.

Vignette Objectives

1. Outline the components of the pulmonary examination.
2. How do history and physical examination findings help predict the pathogen causing a pneumonia?
3. What conditions could result in this patient's hypotension, and what findings pertain to each diagnosis?
4. Describe the pulmonary examination findings that help differentiate a right lower lobe pneumonia and a right pleural effusion.

Pulmonary Examination

Components of the pulmonary examination are listed in Table 4-1. Despite what skeptics say, the pulmonary examination is a useful skill. Certain components are more useful than others. The interobserver reliability has been found to be greatest for dichotomous findings (i.e., for items recorded as present or

Table 4-1. Pulmonary examination

Component	Finding and its implications
INSPECTION	
Chest configuration	Anteroposterior diameter increased in chronic obstructive pulmonary disease; severe kyphosis associated with restrictive lung disease
Chest expansion	Normal increase in circumference is 4 to 6 cm; reduced in emphysema (due to hyperinflation) and rib immobility (e.g., ankylosing spondylitis)
Accessory respiratory muscles	Using these muscles indicates moderate to severe respiratory disease
PERCUSSION	Normal percussion note is resonant; dullness indicates a pulmonary infiltrate or pleural effusion; a hyperresonant sound (similar to percussion of gastric air bubble) results from hyperinflation or a pneumothorax
PALPATION	
Tactile fremitus	Vibrations that can be felt when the patient says "ninety-nine"; consolidation increases the vibration's transmission
AUSCULTATION	
Normal respiration sounds	Normal lung sounds are bronchial, bronchovesicular, and vesicular; vesicular sounds (long inspiration, quiet expiration) are heard over the lung periphery; bronchial sounds are found over the trachea (both inspiration and expiration are heard to a similar degree)
Whispered pectoriloquy	Whispered "sixty-six" is amplified over pulmonary consolidation
Egophony	Spoken sound "e" as in "bee," is heard as a long "a" as in say, when listening over consolidation

absent). Graded findings (e.g., coarseness of rales and loudness of breath sounds) are least reliable. Developing physical examination skills and "calibrating" findings with a range of normal and abnormal findings increases an examiner's reliability.

Pneumonia

A diagnosis of pneumonia is indicated by the presence of: (1) fever, (2) purulent sputum, (3) leukocytosis, and (4) a chest radiograph demonstrating a pulmonary infiltrate. Patients with pneumonia should be assessed for factors that predispose to pneumonia and findings indicating potential infecting organisms. Risks for pneumonia are (1) altered immunocompetence (e.g., myeloma, malnutrition, corticosteroid treatment, alcoholism, and HIV disease); (2) changes in the lung anatomy (e.g., a denuded respiratory epithelium resulting from influenza and partial obstruction of a bronchus); and (3) increased exposure to pathogens, as occurs with chronic aspiration.

More than 85% of patients with pneumonia have a cough, two thirds have chest pain, and hemoptysis occurs in approximately 15%. Symptoms and signs of pneumonia sometimes are classified as either typical (bacterial pneumonias) or atypical (caused by organisms such as *Mycoplasma pneumoniae, Legionella, Chlamydia,* or *Moraxella*). In general, atypical pneumonias are associated with a nonproductive cough, fewer signs of pulmonary consolidation, patchy infiltrates on chest radiograph, and a greater likelihood of abnormalities in other organ systems (e.g., headache, diarrhea, bullous myringitis, abnormal hepatic function, and hyponatremia). The different clinical features of pneumonia are listed in Table 4-2. Not included in the table, however, are the additional diagnoses that must be considered in immunosuppressed patients, such as those with HIV disease.

The decision to hospitalize a person for the treatment of pneumonia is determined on the basis of (1) the host's ability to fight infection and the "fragility" or general state of his or her health; (2) the severity of the pneumonia, as shown by symptoms, signs, and laboratory results; and (3) the ability to monitor a patient's status. Other host considerations that would favor hospitalization include age over 65 and the presence of other acute or chronic problems (e.g., diabetic ketoacidosis, congestive heart failure exacerbation, or azotemia).

Elderly people are less able to fight infection, and gram-negative and *Staphylococcus aureus* infections are more prevalent in this group of individuals. Findings indicating a severe illness are a heart rate of more than 120 beats/min, hypotension, a respiratory rate of more than 30 breaths/min, altered mental status, and historical evidence for infection with an organism not sensitive to antibiotics usually prescribed for a community-acquired infection. Several laboratory findings can also indicate the presence of a severe infection (e.g., hypoxemia, hyponatremia, neutropenia, and azotemia).

The finding of percussion dullness at a lung base can indicate the presence of either pneumonia or a pleural effusion. The ability to use the pulmonary examination to distinguish these might prompt a request to have a lateral decubitus film done in addition to the initial radiograph, if an effusion is expected. The different lung examination findings noted in the settings of consolidation and a pleural effusion are given in Table 4-3. Although percussion dullness is noted for both, the two conditions differ in terms of other aspects of the examination.

The chest radiograph findings in a patient who has had pneumonia often lag behind the clinical signs of resolution and can take up to 8 weeks to resolve. Documenting resolution of the infiltrate on chest radiograph reduces the likelihood that the pneumonia was associated with obstructing lung neoplasm.

Fever and Hypotension

The patient in Vignette 1 has hypotension, which necessitates immediate management. The findings associated with hypotension due to cardiac dysfunction, hypovolemia, and sepsis are listed in Table 3-1. This patient's history and physical examination findings do not indicate a cardiac disorder, making cardiogenic shock less likely. His history does indicate the possibility of sepsis, hypovolemia, or both. Orthostatic vital signs would be important in determining his intravascular volume. Although septic shock is associated with vasodilation,

Table 4-2. Clinical findings in pneumonia

Etiologic agent	Cough and sputum production	Other features
Pneumococcus (*Streptococcus pneumoniae*)	Productive cough in 75%; sputum purulent, rusty, blood streaked; pleuritic chest pain can occur	Often single shaking chill at its onset; most common community-acquired pneumonia; often a preceding upper respiratory tract infection; lobar consolidation; Gram's staining of sputum about 60% sensitive
Mycoplasma pneumoniae (similar symptoms with other atypical pneumonias*)	Persistent, nonproductive cough; pleurisy rare; sputum scant	Gradual onset; *Mycoplasma* infections occur among young, healthy people; prominent myalgias and headaches; *Mycoplasma*-associated bullous myringitis; *Legionella* species associated with myalgia, headaches, diarrhea, and abnormal hepatic function; *Moraxella* among elderly, smokers, and patients with COPD
Aspiration pneumonia	Cough usually productive; sputum purulent and can be foul smelling	Poor dentition (edentulous people are rarely affected); reason for aspiration (such as alcohol or drug abuse), loss of consciousness, and impaired swallowing; usual sites are apical segments lower lobes (right > left)
Influenza A	Dry cough; sputum is scant or bloody	Rigors are unusual; headache; myalgias; marked dyspnea; occurs during "flu season"; can be followed by *Staphylococcus* or *Haemophilus influenzae* infection
Haemophilus influenzae	Productive cough; wheezing common in children; sputum purulent and "apple green"	Most common in alcoholics or patients with chronic lung disease
Escherichia coli	Prominent cough; sputum is thick and purulent	Usually associated with preexisting chronic debilitating illness and a reason for colonization with gram-negative pathogens (such as nursing home residence or recent hospitalization)
Klebsiella pneumoniae	Productive cough; severe pleuritic pain; sputum purulent, thick, can be bloody	More common in patients with alcoholism and diabetes; reasons for colonization similar to those for *E. coli*
Staphylococcus aureus	Productive cough; sputum purulent and blood streaked; occasionally gross hemoptysis	Increased risk after viral influenza; patients often debilitated

**Legionella* species, *Moraxella catarrhalis, Chlamydia pneumoniae.*

Table 4-3. Differentiating between pulmonary consolidation and a pleural effusion

Pulmonary exam	Pleural effusion	Consolidation
Percussion	Dull	Dull
Palpation	Tactile fremitus decreased	Tactile fremitus increased
Auscultation	Absent breath sounds*	Rales; bronchial breath sounds over consolidation; egophony and whispered pectoriloquy

*Compression of lung tissue by an effusion can result in a narrow band of pulmonary consolidation above a pleural effusion.

Vignette Follow-up

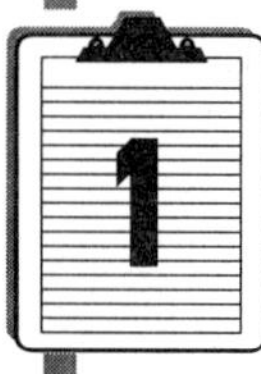

EB's sputum shows gram-positive, lancet-shaped diplococci. Pneumococcal pneumonia seems likely. However, in similar situations, culture confirmation of this organism is obtained in only half to two thirds of patients. Because Mr. B is at risk for infection with other pathogens, he is treated initially with broad-spectrum antibiotics, then switched to penicillin when blood cultures grow. *S. pneumonia.* He becomes afebrile after 2 days and is discharged after 3 days of therapy. He does not return for follow-up.

Vignette 2

AW is a 25-year-old woman, who comes to clinic complaining of fever, night sweats, fatigue, anorexia, and dysuria. Her past history is notable for polysubstance abuse (alcohol and occasional intravenous heroin). However, for the past 3 weeks, she has been in a rehabilitation program, and she reports no drug use during that time. She denies exposure to TB and had a 7-mm TB skin test result 7 months ago.

AW is found to have a bacterial urinary tract infection, which resolves with antibiotic treatment. Purified protein derivative (PPD) testing, done as part of her initial evaluation, yields 19-mm of induration, but her chest radiograph findings are normal. Because of her recent skin test conversion, she is begun on prophylactic isoniazid (INH). When seen 5 weeks later, she again reports fever and night sweats. A repeat chest radiograph shows new hilar and right peritracheal adenopathy. Three sputum smears are negative for acid-fast bacilli (AFB).

Vignette Objectives

1. What historical findings identify people who should undergo skin testing for TB?
2. What are the clinical features of different "types" of TB (i.e., primary, reactivation, miliary)?

volume replacement only partially reverses the hypotension, and blood pressure will not return to presepsis levels until the underlying infection is treated.

Tuberculosis

TB has become more prevalent over the past 10 years, and drug-resistant organisms now are a significant problem. A Mantoux TB skin test, using PPD tuberculin, is appropriate for people with the characteristics listed in Table 4-4. Criteria for a "positive" test result in a patient with no risks for tuberculosis (i.e., the conditions listed in Table 4-4) is induration measuring more than 15 mm in diameter. An induration exceeding 10 mm is considered positive when a patient has risk factors for TB infection. An induration of only 5 mm is considered positive in patients who are HIV positive, people recently exposed to active TB, and those with healed TB, as confirmed by findings on chest radiography. An increase of more than 10 mm of induration is needed for sequential test results to be interpreted as showing conversion of a TB skin test from negative to positive. Recent conversion is associated with a 5% risk of active TB developing during the next 2 years.

Individuals with a positive skin test should obtain sputum smears and a chest radiograph to identify those requiring treatment for active TB. Three to six sputum smears are only about 60% sensitive in revealing AFB. While culture results are awaited, the clinical history and chest radiograph findings are used as the basis for deciding whether to begin adults on treatment for active TB.

Primary TB usually involves the lower lobes. Most primary infections are contained by the body's defenses and can result in the calcified Ghon lesion seen on chest radiographs. Overall, the life-time risk of a contained primary in-

Table 4-4. Skin testing for tuberculosis (who should be tested)

Condition	Comments
Symptoms or signs of TB	Any of presentations outlined in Table 4-5
Recent contact with people suspected or known to have TB	County health officials (and hospital epidemiologist) identify and skin test contacts
Medical, demographic, and occupational conditions that predispose to TB	(1) Alcohol and IV drug use; (2) foreign born; (3) homeless; (4) health care workers; (5) previous gastrectomy, corticosteroid or other immunosuppressive therapy, myeloproliferative disorder, chronic renal failure, and silicosis
HIV positivity	HIV-positive people require prophylactic therapy if skin test positive; as HIV progresses, anergy and false-negative skin tests are more common; PPD testing should be a component of initial evaluation
Nursing-home dwellers	Rate of reactivation is more than ten times that of noninstitutionalized elderly people; TB can reactivate in the elderly without the usual symptoms of active infection

fection reactivating is approximately 10%. The symptoms of reactivation TB are nonspecific. The manifestations of different stages of TB are listed in Table 4-5.

Dyspnea

Dyspnea is the subjective experience of difficulty in breathing, and patients can describe it as a smothering sensation, chest tightness, and an inability to

Vignette Follow-up

Unfortunately, Ms. W resumes substance abuse and is lost to follow-up. After 8 weeks, one of the sputum cultures is found to be growing *Mycobacterium tuberculosis* and she is reported to the county health department as a case of active tuberculosis. She is located approximately 1 month later. At that time, her chest radiograph shows upper lobe infiltrates and hilar adenopathy. One of three sputum smears is positive for AFB, and at 3 weeks, two specimens are growing *Mycobacterium tuberculosis.* Ms. W refuses HIV testing. She is begun on four-drug therapy with INH, rifampin, ethambutol, and pyrazinamide, and is to be followed closely by the county's TB clinic.

Table 4-5. Classification of active tuberculosis

Type of infection	Manifestations
Primary infection	More than 90% of patients are asymptomatic; can heal with calcified peripheral granuloma and hilar node; occasionally localized infiltrate and symptoms of pneumonia; subpleural infection can rupture into the pleural space and cause an exudative effusion
Pulmonary reactivation (most common in apical-posterior section of upper lobes)	Progressive weight loss, cough, fever, and sputum production; in U.S., reactivation most common in those >60 years old and those with HIV disease
Extrapulmonary reactivation (organisms are disseminated with the primary infection and can reactivate in areas of high oxygen tension, such as the renal cortex, vertebra, meninges, peritoneum, GI tract, renal cortex, and GU tract)	Accounts for approximately 15% of active cases of TB; if patient HIV positive, then twice as likely to have extrapulmonary site; CXR normal in half; symptoms vary with location; can be indolent infection with local tissue destruction and minimal fever and weight loss
Miliary tuberculosis	Can manifest as FUO; CXR abnormal in 90%, with diffuse, small nodules (syndrome's name comes from these millet seed–sized nodules); infection is widespread, and sites can be lung, liver, meninges, and lymphatic system; bone marrow involvement can result in leukemoid reaction or pancytopenia

CXR = chest x-ray study; FUO = fever of unknown origin.

Vignette 3

Dyspnea: subjective awareness of difficulty breathing.

PT is a 64-year-old woman who recently was discharged from a local hospital after treatment for a "blood clot to my lungs." Because her symptoms have not resolved, she comes to clinic seeking a second opinion concerning the diagnoses rendered during her recent hospitalization. Before her hospitalization, Ms. T had been in her usual state of health, but during the week before admission, progressive shortness of breath, cough, and dark yellow sputum had developed. About 2 days before admission, her sputum became "bloody" and she went to the hospital emergency room for evaluation. At that time, her arterial blood gases were as follows: PaO_2, 68 mm Hg; $PaCO_2$, 48 mm Hg; and pH, 7.41; her hematocrit was 51%. A chest radiograph showed increased bronchovesicular markings in the bases. A lung scan showed matched defects, and the findings were interpreted as indicating a low to moderate probability of pulmonary embolus. She was treated with low-flow oxygen, broad-spectrum antibiotics, and heparin. After 5 days, she was discharged off antibiotics and put on warfarin therapy.

Ms. T has been out of the hospital for 14 days and currently complains of increased sputum production and dyspnea on exertion. Her history is significant for smoking two packs of cigarettes a day for 33 years. She has had an intermittent cough and sputum production for the past 5 years, especially during the winter months. She gradually has reduced her level of physical activity because of exertional dyspnea.

Physical examination reveals a slender woman looking older than her stated years. Vital signs: **blood pressure** is 110/62 mm Hg; **heart rate** is 92 beats/min; and **respiratory rate** is 24 breaths/min. **HEENT:** supple neck, with a midline trachea; she has no adenopathy or thyromegaly. Her mouth and throat are clear, without postnasal discharge. **Chest:** percussion note is hyperresonant; bibasilar rhonchi and occasional wheezes are present. **Cardiac:** JVP is elevated slightly at 11 cm H_2O; S_1 is normal, S_2 has a loud pulmonic component, and an S_4 is present; no S_3 or murmur is heard. **Abdomen:** nontender, with no organomegaly or masses. **Extremities:** 1+ dependent edema of lower extremities; pulses are present and symmetrical; no clubbing; no calf or thigh tenderness; and no palpable venous cords; leg circumferences are symmetrical.

Spirometry reveals a forced expiratory volume at 1 second (FEV_1) of 42% of predicted and a forced vital capacity (FVC) of 74% of predicted. A chest radiograph shows increased lower lobe markings. PaO_2 is 74 mm Hg, $PaCO_2$ is 42 mm Hg, and pH is 7.41. These results were similar to valves during her hospitalization.

Vignette Objectives

1. Dyspnea is a nonspecific symptom. List the cardiac and pulmonary causes of dyspnea and patient findings relevant to each diagnosis.
2. List findings in patients with COPD due to emphysema and chronic bronchitis.

catch their breath. Acute dyspnea is due to problems that develop over a few hours to a few days, such as pneumonia, bronchospasm, pulmonary emboli, a spontaneous pneumothorax, or the sudden onset of severe congestive heart failure (CHF).

Chronic dyspnea develops more slowly, and the causes can be divided into three major categories: pulmonary, cardiac, and other (e.g., severe anxiety or hyperventilation) (Table 4-6). Examples of conditions causing gradually progressive dyspnea are COPD, interstitial lung disease, and chronic CHF. Often more than one problem coexists.

The accuracy of the history in establishing the cause of dyspnea has been estimated to be 70%. Certain historical features are useful for distinguishing between cardiac and pulmonary dyspnea. Those with CHF are more likely to describe a "smothering" or "suffocating" sensation. Those with pulmonary disease frequently complain of chest "tightness" or "feeling wheezy" and that it is more work to breath. The different findings in those with pulmonary and cardiac dyspnea are given in Table 4-6.

Table 4-6. Causes of dyspnea

	Cardiac disease	Pulmonary disease		
	Congestive heart failure	Pneumonia	Pulmonary Emboli	Asthma
History	Positive fluid balance; reason for new onset or exacerbation of CHF (such as new medication reducing contractility, recent chest pain/ischemia, nonadherence to medication regimen); may describe dyspnea as smothering or suffocating	Predisposing condition (such as aspiration, immunocompromised state or preceding viral URI); sputum, fever, rigor	Risks for thrombosis (such as postoperative state or malignancy); leg swelling; pleuritic pain, cough	Cough precipitated by exercise in cold weather; exposure to allergen or URI; may report wheezing and that it is more work to breathe
Exam	Weight increase; elevated JVP; S_3; rales; peripheral edema	Fever; dullness to percussion; rales and signs of consolidation	Other than tachycardia, findings can be normal; leg swelling	Pulsus paradoxus; wheezing, prolonged expiratory phase
ECG	New ischemia or arrhythmia	No change	Classic pattern is an S wave in lead I and a Q wave in lead III	No change
Chest radiograph	Cardiomegaly and pulmonary vascular congestion; can have pleural effusions	Infiltrate with air bronchogram; can have effusion	Can be normal; wedge-shaped infiltrate with pulmonary infarction	Normal or hyperinflation

Chronic Obstructive Pulmonary Disease

Chronic Bronchitis and Emphysema

COPD is a nonspecific term and can refer to chronic bronchitis, emphysema, asthma (also termed *reactive airway disease*), and bronchiectasis. All these diseases result in limitations in air flow, an increased work of breathing, and reduced gas exchange.

COPD usually develops as the result of smoking cigarettes. Among susceptible people, smoking doubles the usual 30 mm per year decrement in FEV_1, and the severity of the COPD is proportional to the number of pack years (years smoked × packs per day). Although the incidence of COPD is highest in men, it is becoming more prevalent among women as more women smoke. COPD is uncommon among those less than age 40. A younger individual with COPD should be assessed for alpha-1-antitrypsin deficiency, which predisposes smokers to lung damage and results in early-onset COPD. This deficiency accounts for approximately two percent of patients with emphysema.

The classic clinical presentations of COPD include the "pink puffer," characteristic of emphysema, and the "blue bloater," characteristic of chronic bronchitis (Table 4-7). In reality, patients usually have a mix of different types of COPD.

Emphysema is a pathologic condition characterized by the formation of enlarged air spaces distal to the terminal bronchi and destruction of the alveolar septa. This destruction is reflected in loss of the lung's elastic recoil ability and prolonged expiration. Emphysematous pink puffers are so called because of their ability to maintain adequate resting oxygenation, without significant carbon dioxide retention. Patients are tachypneic, often use accessory respiratory muscles, and expire against pursed lips, to keep their airways from collapsing. Their hyperinflated lungs are associated with depressed diaphragms and reduced chest expansion. These patients can have a barrel chest resulting from an increased AP diameter. However, the utility of this finding is not clear, and the apparent increase in the AP diameter may only reflect the slender body habitus of patients with emphysema.

Table 4-7. Differentiating chronic bronchitis and emphysema

	Emphysema ("Pink Puffer")	Chronic bronchitis ("Blue Bloater")
Patient appearance	Thin, using accessory muscles to breathe through pursed lips	Obese, central cyanosis, plethora
History	Shortness of breath on exertion	Predominant cough, sputum production, frequent tracheobronchitis
Physical examination	Increased resonance; decreased breath sounds	Rhonchi ± wheezing; elevated neck veins and peripheral edema due to chronic hypoxia causing right ventricular failure

Blue bloaters have chronic bronchitis, defined by a clinical history of 3 months of daily sputum production occurring in 2 successive years. The excessive tracheobronchial mucus causes airway obstruction and predisposes to the development of infection. Patients are "blue" as the result of their hypoxemia, which results in secondary polycythemia and central cyanosis. Those with chronic bronchitis often have an elevated $PaCO_2$. Expiration also is prolonged in these patients, but this is due to airway obstruction rather than to loss of lung elastic recoil.

The dyspnea provoked by different levels of exertion helps quantitate the reduction in ventilatory capacity. As the FEV_1 decreases from 70% to 30% of normal, dyspnea occurs in response to progressively shorter exertional distances, and a patient who experiences dyspnea at rest usually has an FEV_1 of less than 30% of predicted. *Central cyanosis* refers to blueness of the lips and mucous membranes, and its finding indicates severe COPD and hypoxemia, with an oxygen saturation of less than 75%. The detection of cyanosis depends on the hemoglobin content, skin perfusion, and lighting; it is not a sensitive indicator of severe pulmonary disease.

Bronchiectasis

Bronchiectasis is the irreversible dilatation of the bronchial wall. Cystic fibrosis (CF) is the most common condition leading to bronchiectasis, and it is the ongoing infections associated with the disease that result in progressive lung destruction. Findings manifested by adults with CF are listed in Table 4-8. Occasionally, bronchiectasis can result from other causes, such as a healed pneumonia or prior TB.

Table 4-8. Manifestations of cystic fibrosis

Findings	Comment
Cough and chronic daily sputum production	Bronchiectasis is present in 95% and is a major cause of morbidity and mortality; a quarter of patients also have a component of reactive airway disease
Minor and massive hemoptysis	Minor bleeding is common (60% of patients); massive hemoptysis is less frequent (7%)
Pneumothorax	Can cause acute worsening of respiratory status; overall incidence, 16%
Sinusitis and nasal polyps	Most patients have chronic sinusitis, with polyps in approximately half
Clubbing	Universal finding; associated with bronchiectasis of any cause
Steatorrhea	Pancreatic insufficiency present in 95% of adult patients
Failure to thrive	Height and weight usually lower limits of normal; however, 7% are overweight, and an occasional patient can be tall

Vignette Follow-up

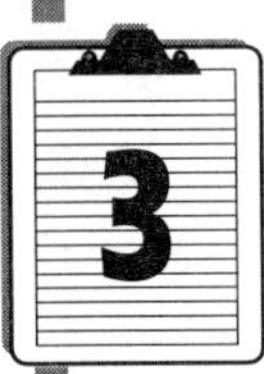

Chronic bronchitis is diagnosed in PT. Although patients with COPD can have pulmonary emboli, a review of her prior hospitalization findings reveals that pulmonary embolus is an unlikely diagnosis. Warfarin therapy is therefore discontinued. The patient participates in smoking cessation classes, and she successfully stops smoking. She begins using inhaled bronchodilator therapy on an as-needed basis. Five years later, she is more active and attends exercise classes three times a week. She continues to have a morning productive cough.

Vignette 4

Status asthmaticus: severe, prolonged asthmatic episode, refractory to the usual therapy.

Wheezing: high-pitched, musical, continuous sounds that indicate partial airway obstruction.

TS is a 50-year-old man who complains of increasing shortness of breath. He had been well until about 8 years ago when "bronchopneumonia," characterized by fever and respiratory distress, developed. At that time he was hospitalized for approximately a week and recalls that, over the subsequent month, shortness of breath, wheezing, and cough developed. He saw his physician and was told that he had "asthma." He then quit smoking, having smoked three packs a day for 30 years. Since then, he has experienced recurrent "asthma attacks," usually precipitated by respiratory tract infections.

He has no history of eczema or childhood asthma. Most recently, TS has been feeling well, using his bronchodilator medications, and doing farm work without dyspnea. About 3 days before his appointment, he developed a "runny nose," mild sore throat, and a nonproductive cough. He then noted increasing shortness of breath and began using his inhaler four to six times a day. The night before being seen, he was unable to sleep lying down because of shortness of breath. In addition to respiratory complaints, Mr. S has a 3-year history of an "acid stomach." Occasionally, he is awakened by heartburn and a sour taste in his mouth.

Physical examination reveals a well-nourished man in moderate respiratory distress and using his accessory muscles to breathe. Vital signs: his **heart rate** is 92 beats/min, and his **blood pressure** is 128/80 mm Hg, with 15 mm of pulsus paradoxus. His **respiratory rate** is 32 breaths/min, and his oral **temperature** is 98.4°F (36.8°C). **Skin:** actinic keratoses are noted over his face. **HEENT:** nasal passages are clear without polyps. His neck shows no adenopathy or thyromegaly. **Chest:** clear to percussion, diffuse expiratory wheezes, no rales. **Cardiac:** no JVD; his PMI is not palpable, and heart tones are distant. S_1 and S_2 are normal, and no additional sounds are present. **Abdomen:** nontender; no organomegaly or masses. **Rectal:** prostate is 1+ enlarged, stool is occult-blood negative. **Extremities:** no cyanosis, clubbing, or edema.

Vignette Objectives

1. List the causes of wheezing and the history and physical examination findings that help when distinguishing among those causes.
2. List the causes of an exacerbation of reactive airway disease and the history and physical examination findings relating to each.
3. Which historical and physical examination findings indicate the severity of respiratory distress?
4. What is the relationship between esophageal reflux and reactive airway disease?

Asthma or Reactive Airway Disease

Asthma is a defined as a reversible airway obstruction. Dyspnea, cough, and wheezing are the common symptoms. For most patients, acute asthmatic episodes, lasting hours to days, are separated by periods of remission, during which symptoms are reduced or absent.

An asthma exacerbation or episode is an acute worsening of symptoms. Respiratory secretions become thick and difficult to expectorate, and the air flow obstruction leads to high-pitched inspiratory and expiratory wheezes and hyperinflation. The history and physical examination often identify a triggering event leading to an exacerbation. The major triggers are infection, exposure to respiratory irritants or allergens, noncompliance with medication regimen, exposure to medications that can exacerbate symptoms (e.g., beta-blockers and aspirin), CHF, spontaneous pneumothorax, and pulmonary emboli. Rare considerations are an aspirated foreign body and an endobronchial tumor.

Historical features suggesting an allergic component include prior allergic rhinitis, seasonal symptoms (pollens and outdoor molds), wheezing with pet contact (dander), and exacerbation caused by certain exposures (such as making beds [mites], cleaning a stable [molds], and spending time in a damp basement [molds]). Identifying patients with allergen sensitivity allows environmental controls to be implemented to reduce and prevent exposures.

Measurement of lung volumes and peak expiratory flow are a means to monitor the illness. Patients often record their peak expiratory flow rate (PEFR) as part of management. Those with moderate asthma (FEV_1 and PEFR 60% to 80% of predicted) who suffer attacks more than twice a week are candidates for inhaled steroids, along with bronchodilators. More severe asthma can be an indication for long-term oral corticosteroid therapy.

In general, the tempo of an exacerbation's onset is proportional to the rapidity of its resolution. That is, an acute attack coming on abruptly often can be reversed quickly. Slowly worsening symptoms are associated with inspissated mucous plugs, as well as bronchospasm. These subacute exacerbations take longer to resolve.

Severe disease is suggested when an individual reports a history of prior intubation for asthma, more than three emergency room visits a year for asthma, and hospitalization in the last month. Other indices of severity are inability to talk in complete sentences because of the dyspnea, a heart rate of more than 120 beats/min, and a respiratory rate of more than 30 breaths/min. During an exacerbation, patients generate greater negative intrapleural pressures to overcome air flow obstruction, which can result in a pulsus paradoxus. Usually, the finding of a pulsus paradoxus indicates a decrement in the FEV_1 of more than 50%. Status asthmaticus is a severe, prolonged asthmatic episode that is unresponsive to standard therapy.

Patients experiencing an asthma exacerbation typically are found to have diffuse wheezing, that can be expiratory only or expiratory and inspiratory. The distribution and characteristics of the wheezing indicate the severity of the airway obstruction. Expiratory wheezes indicate less severe disease; expiratory and inspiratory wheezes indicate more severe disease. However, wheezes should be interpreted in the context of other findings, in that a decrease in the intensity of wheezes could mean either an improved air flow or just the opposite, with the reduced air movement and reduced wheezing resulting from more severe obstruction and patient fatigue.

Most patients with asthma experience bronchospasm with exercise, but some only have symptoms after exertion. This latter disorder (exercise-induced asthma) can result in cough, shortness of breath, or wheezing that begins during or within minutes after exercise. The accelerated loss of heat and moisture from the airways during exercise is thought to precipitate the bronchospasm. This explains why symptoms frequently are provoked by exposure to cold, dry air (such as running in the cold), whereas exercise in warm moist air (as in a swimming pool) can be tolerated without problems.

The patient in Vignette 4 probably has gastroesophageal reflux disease (GERD). GERD can cause acid to enter the tracheobronchial tree while the patient is supine, causing bronchospasm. Unfortunately, medications that relax airway smooth muscle (i.e., those used to treat bronchospasm) also relax the gastroesophageal sphincter, and this only worsens GERD.

Airway obstruction caused by a tracheal or laryngeal tumor can result in a clinical presentation simulating asthma, but a comparison of the maximum inspiratory and expiratory flow rates can differentiate between the two conditions. In asthma, air flow is obstructed primarily during expiration, whereas in upper airway obstruction, both inspiratory and expiratory flow rates are reduced and the stridor is loudest in the region of the obstruction.

Vignette Follow-up

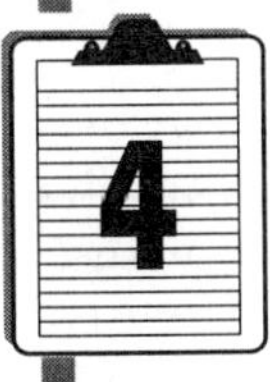

TS is treated for acute bronchitis. He receives a brief course of oral corticosteroids, and as they are tapered, inhaled steroid treatment is initiated, in addition to his bronchodilator treatment. His GERD is managed with elevation of the head of his bed, avoiding eating for 2 hours before retiring, and antacid use. He continues to be followed for asthma.

Vignette 5

Pleural friction rub: coarse rubbing sound heard on chest auscultation, usually due to an inflammatory process causing friction between the visceral and parietal pleurae.

Pleuritic pain: discomfort resulting from pleural inflammation; it usually is described as a sharp pain, made worse with respiratory movements.

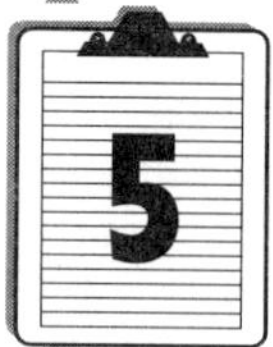

AM is a 24-year-old woman who has experienced the sudden onset of right-sided pleuritic chest pain 9 days postpartum. She describes the chest pain as being sharp and worse with inspiration. She also complains of shortness of breath and a nonproductive cough. She does not report fever or other pulmonary symptoms.

Nine days before she gave birth to a healthy 8 lb, 2 oz. girl in an uncomplicated vaginal delivery, and they spent less than 48 hours in the hospital. Ms. M was discharged feeling well and has been home for a week. Her only prior hospitalization was for the birth of her first child 3 years ago.

Physical examination reveals a healthy-appearing woman. Her **blood pressure** is 120/70 mm Hg, her **heart rate** is 100 beats/min, and her **respiratory rate** is 20 breaths/min. Her oral **temperature** is 37.5°C. **HEENT:** normal findings. **Chest:** clear to percussion and auscultation; no rub; no chest wall tenderness. **Cardiac:** no JVD; normal S_1, physiologically split S_2, and no murmurs, gallops, or rubs. **Abdomen:** soft without organomegaly or mass; bimanual examination reveals a nontender postpartum uterus. **Extremities:** no cyanosis or edema. Tenderness is present over the proximal right femoral area, and the circumference of the right thigh measures 39 cm and the left, 35 cm. There is no asymmetry at the calf. Homans' sign is negative, and no venous cords are palpable. Arterial blood gases measured, while breathing room air, are as follows: pH, 7.5; $PaCO_2$, 30 mm Hg; PaO_2, 90 mm Hg.

Vignette Objectives

1. List the causes of pleuritic chest pain and how the history and physical examination findings relate to each diagnosis.
2. List the classic findings in patients with a DVT. How sensitive and specific are physical examination findings in detecting a DVT?

Pleuritic Chest Pain

Pleuritic chest pain ("pleurisy") is caused by irritation of the visceral or parietal pleura. The inflammation prevents the normal, smooth movement of the pleural surfaces, resulting in a grating sound on chest auscultation (pleural rub) and pleuritic pain. Pleuritic pain often is described as sharp and increased by respiratory movements. Causes of pleuritic pain are listed in Table 4-9.

Table 4-9. Causes of pleuritic pain

Condition	Findings
Viral pleuritis	Fever and symptoms of a URI; patients usually less than 40 years old; no conditions predisposing to thromboembolic disease
Acute pneumonia	Fever, cough, purulent sputum; signs of pulmonary consolidation; infiltrate ± effusion on chest radiogram; TB can manifest as a unilateral effusion
Pulmonary embolus	Risk factors for thromboembolic disease; signs of DVT; occasionally fever and hemoptysis
Immune-mediated pleuritis	SLE can be associated with serositis Dressler's syndrome is an immune-mediated pleuropericarditis that can develop 2 to 4 weeks after a myocardial infarction or cardiac surgery
Spontaneous pneumothorax	Acute-onset dyspnea and pain; can be idiopathic among young men, due to trauma, or associated with COPD
Chest wall trauma	History of rib or intercostal muscle trauma; usually associated with chest wall tenderness; can be point tenderness and ecchymosis
Neuropathic pain	Pain in radicular distribution; can have cutaneous hypersensitivity; causes include herpes zoster, radiculopathy of compression fractures, and diabetic neuropathy

SLE = systemic lupus erythematosus.

Chest wall disorders can cause a similar pain; however, those problems are associated with local chest wall tenderness.

The physical findings typical of a pleural effusion are given in Table 4-3. As with ascites, pleural fluid characteristics are used to identify a transudate (usually due to CHF, cirrhosis, or nephrotic syndrome) and exudates (related to infection, malignancies, trauma, pancreatitis, and immune-mediated serositis). When a patient presents with pneumonia and pleural effusion, a thoracentesis is needed to obtain pleural fluid to be used to differentiate an infected exudative empyema from a sterile transudate or "sympathetic" effusion.

Pulmonary Embolus

Identifying risks for a pulmonary embolus can help determine its likelihood. Risks for thromboembolic disease are (1) venous stasis (such as that caused by immobility, casting, bed rest, and CHF), (2) a hypercoagulable state (e.g., an inherited disorder [such as deficiency of protein S or C and antithrombin III], recent surgery, long-bone fracture, malignancy, postpartum state, and presence of lupus anticoagulant or anticardiolipin antibody); and (3) venous damage (as can occur in patients with hip or pelvic fractures or those who have undergone pelvic surgery).

Pulmonary emboli are a frequent diagnostic consideration (see Figure 4-1, p. 108), and they have been associated with many symptoms and signs. However, none of these findings are sensitive for or specific to the diagnosis. Depending

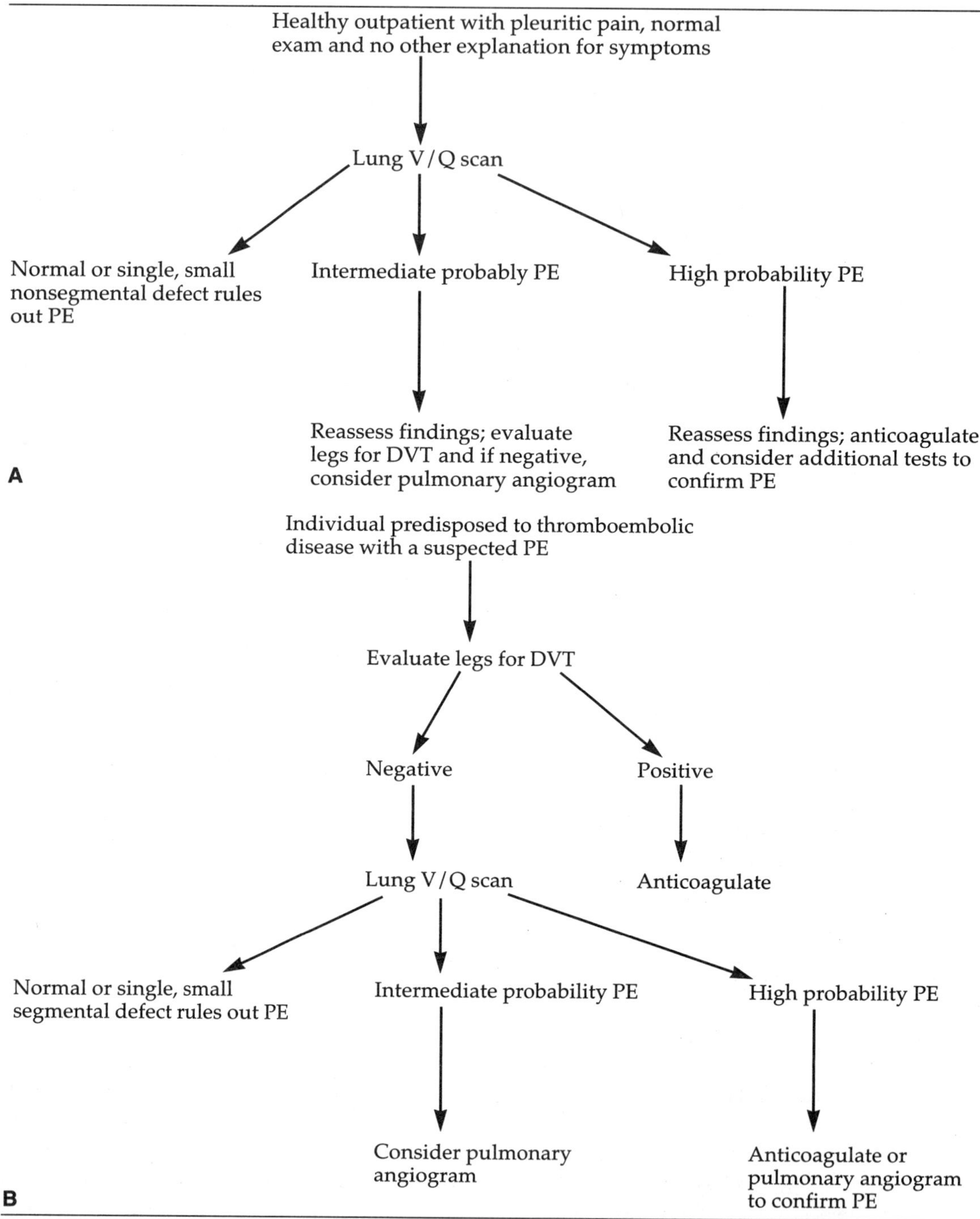

Figure 4-1. Algorithms for evaluating patients with a suspected pulmonary embolus (*PE*) address two categories of patients: A. Outpatients with pleuritic pain, in whom the differential diagnosis primarily is between pulmonary emboli and viral pleuritis. B. Patients at risk for thromboembolic disease, who often also have underlying cardiac or pulmonary disease. (*V/Q* = ventilation-perfusion, *DVT* = deep venous thrombosis.)

on the extent of the emboli and the patient's underlying pulmonary status, dyspnea can vary from mild to severe. Other potential symptoms are cough, pleuritic chest pain, and hemoptysis (the last occurs with pulmonary infarction). Physical examination findings can include tachypnea, tachycardia, fever, and a pleural rub. Algorithms (Fig. 4-1) have been suggested that can be used to sequentially assess patients in whom the diagnosis is suspected.

A lung ventilation-perfusion scan is sensitive in detecting pulmonary emboli and is an important test to exclude the disorder. Among healthy adults less than 40 years old, pleuritic chest pain usually is not due to a pulmonary embolus if (1) the chest radiograph is normal, (2) the patient has no conditions that predispose to thromboembolism, and (3) the lower extremity exam reveals no signs of a DVT.

Deep Venous Thrombosis

The physical examination for DVT is neither sensitive nor specific. Approximately half of patients with a proven DVT have normal physical examination findings and a third with findings suggestive of a DVT have problems other than venous thrombosis. Findings suggestive of a DVT include leg pain, calf tenderness, a palpable "cord" (due to the thrombosed vein), edema (detected by measuring leg circumferences at the calf and thigh), fever, and, uncommonly, Homans' sign (calf pain elicited by passive ankle dorsiflexion). A thigh or more proximal thrombosis is of greatest concern, because it leads to pulmonary emboli. DVTs confined to the calf usually do not result in pulmonary emboli, unless the clot propagates above the knee.

A swollen extremity that is not due to a DVT is referred to as *pseudothrombophlebitis*. Conditions causing these findings include a ruptured popliteal cyst (often, but not always, associated with an inflammatory arthritis of the knee), torn calf muscles (plantaris or gastrocnemius), unilateral lymphatic obstruction, or incompetent venous valves.

Vignette Follow-up

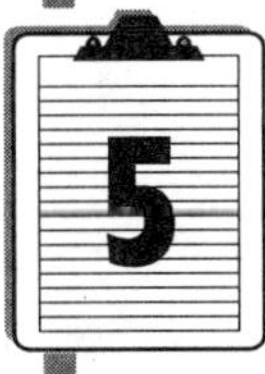

AM is found to have a DVT, as documented by venous Doppler studies, and a presumed pulmonary embolus. She is anticoagulated for 3 months and does well.

Vignette 6

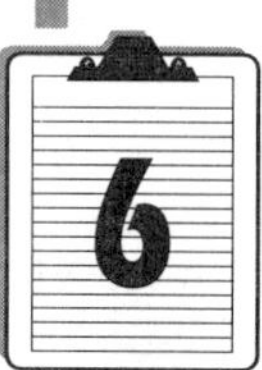

RG is a 31-year-old woman who has been pregnant for 37-weeks. For 24-hours, she has experienced headache, nausea, vomiting, and fever. She has also noted low back and abdominal pain and thought that she might be in labor. She is thought to have a viral syndrome and is admitted for hydration and observation. Ms. G's general health is good, and she has no medical problems. However, four previous pregnancies have ended in spontaneous abortions, and this pregnancy has been complicated by cervical incompetence, requiring cervical cerclage at 16 weeks. She smokes one pack of cigarettes each day, but she does not drink alcohol or use drugs.

On admission, her **blood pressure** is 80/40 mm Hg, her **heart rate** is 110 beats/min, and her **temperature** is 38.2°C. When seen initially, her **chest** is clear to auscultation, and the **cardiac** examination reveals a normal S_1 and S_2, with a 2/6 systolic ejection murmur heard at the base. Her **extremity** exam reveals 1+ edema below the knees, and **reflexes** are 2+, without clonus. The **fetal heart rate** is in the 160s.

Two days later, her symptoms have abated, but generalized edema and facial puffiness develop. Although her blood pressure is only 110/80 mm Hg, the edema raises concern about preeclampsia and labor is induced. During the pitressin infusion, 4+ reflexes develop and intravenous magnesium therapy is instituted. Labor fails to progress, and she undergoes a cesarean section with epidural anesthesia, with delivery of a healthy infant.

Forty-eight hours postoperatively, she complains of shortness of breath and a dry cough. At that time, her **cardiac** examination reveals a tachycardia but additional sounds are obscured by respiratory noises. Her neck veins cannot be seen. **Pulmonary** examination reveals the presence of diffuse rhonchi and wheezing. Generalized edema is present. Her blood gases measured when breathing room air are as follows: PaO_2, 63 mm Hg; $PaCO_2$, 35 mm Hg; and pH, 7.43. A portable chest radiograph shows diffuse pulmonary infiltrates. Her cardiac diameter appears appropriate for an AP view.

Vignette Objectives

1. List conditions that can result in the adult respiratory distress syndrome (ARDS). For each, describe historical events that might precede the development of ARDS.
2. How useful are the physical examination findings in differentiating cardiac from noncardiac pulmonary edema?

Adult Respiratory Distress Syndrome

ARDS is characterized by hypoxemia (PaO_2, <50 mm Hg with an inspired oxygen concentration of ≥60%) and the chest radiograph finding of diffuse pulmonary infiltrates, not attributable to heart failure (pulmonary artery wedge pressure, ≤18 mm Hg). The potential causes are listed in Table 4-10. Most of these conditions cause lung damage and lead to the entrance of fluid into the alveoli. Because the left ventricular end-diastolic pressure is not elevated, as it would be in pulmonary edema stemming from heart disease, the condition sometimes is referred to as *noncardiac pulmonary edema.*

The clinical features of cardiac and noncardiac pulmonary edema are listed in Table 4-11. Excluding heart failure as a cause for findings can be difficult, and bedside examination findings often fail to correctly distinguish the two types of pulmonary edema. Experienced ICU physicians have been found to only agree half of the time as to whether heart failure is present. Physical examination indicators of heart failure are not sensitive, and it may be necessary to perform an invasive hemodynamic assessment to distinguish cardiac from

Table 4-10. Causes of ARDS

Condition	Findings
Septic shock	Fever, hypotension; site for origin of infection (e.g., pneumonia, pyelonephritis, cholangitis)
Pneumonia	Viral pneumonia and occasionally an atypical pneumonia cause diffuse lung involvement and ARDS; *Pneumocystis carinii* pneumonia can cause ARDS in immunosuppressed patients
Pancreatitis	Usually severe episode of pancreatitis, as evidenced by other laboratory findings (e.g., leukocytosis, falling hematocrit, rising BUN, and hypocalcemia)
Smoke inhalation	Smoke and toxic gas (such as chlorine gas) inhalation; onset can be delayed up to 48 hours; especially consider if burns to scalp, face, or nostrils
Aspiration of gastric contents	Condition predisposing to aspiration; bacterial infection can follow chemical pneumonitis
Narcotic overdose	Idiopathic reaction to intravenous narcotics and rarely cocaine; onset up to 24 hours after drug injection
Near drowning	Pulmonary edema develops in 75%, in addition to hypoxic acidemia, bronchospasm, and hypothermia

Table 4-11. Clinical features of the pulmonary edema syndromes

	Noncardiac pulmonary edema (lung damage and leaky capillaries)	Hydrostatic pulmonary edema (left ventricular failure and an elevated pulmonary artery wedge pressure)
Clinical setting	Sepsis, trauma, multiple-organ failure (see Table 4-10)	Acute onset of CHF or an exacerbation of chronic CHF
Chest radiograph	Diffuse infiltrates, peripheral prominence, no Kerley's B lines, clear lung bases	Patchy infiltrates, perihilar prominence, Kerley's B lines, obscured lung bases, cardiomegaly
Pulmonary capillary wedge pressure	Not elevated	Elevated

noncardiac pulmonary edema. Cardiomegaly on a chest radiograph usually indicates the presence of cardiogenic pulmonary edema, but the finding is not sensitive and can be absent in acute-onset heart failure.

Vignette Follow-up

Initial diagnostic considerations in Ms. G include both cardiac and noncardiac causes of the pulmonary edema. The primary cardiac concern is a peripartum cardiomyopathy. Potential noncardiac causes are aspiration during anesthesia, sepsis, and preeclampsia. Pulmonary emboli are a rare cause of ARDS, but because of her postpartum hypercoagulable state and bed rest, those also are considerations.

The patient receives an intravenous dose of furosemide, and she is moved to the intensive care unit. Although diuresis may not be an appropriate therapy for noncardiac pulmonary edema and risks reducing her blood pressure, this patient's underlying diagnosis is not clear, and her vital signs are being monitored closely. Any decline in the blood pressure would be detected immediately. On balance, the benefits of diuresis seemed to outweigh the risks, and those caring for her are prepared to administer fluids if her blood pressure drops. Ultimately, an echocardiogram demonstrates normal cardiac function. Her ARDS resolves over 48 hours and is attributed to preeclampsia.

Vignette 7

DP, a 56-year-old woman, is a retired nurse. She recently has moved to be near her children and has made a clinic appointment to establish care and for a "check-up." She currently is feeling well and has no complaints.

Her past medical history is significant for hypertension, with reportedly good control on lisinopril treatment (10 mg per day). She has smoked one-and-a-half packs of cigarettes per day, beginning at age 17. She does not drink alcohol. She has been divorced for 12 years. Currently, she is not physically active, although she reports that "the grandchildren keep me running around."

Physical examination reveals a healthy-appearing woman whose **height** is 65 inches (1.6 m), and **weight** is 172 pounds (77 kg). Her vital signs include a **blood pressure** of 140/80 mm Hg and a **heart rate** of 76 beats/min. **HEENT:** mild arteriolar narrowing; oropharynx notable for a small amount of leukoplakia on the right buccal mucosa. Her neck is without adenopathy. **Chest:** percussion is resonant and clear to auscultation. **Cardiac:** normal S_1 and S_2; an S_4 is heard at the apex. **Breasts:** no masses or tenderness. **Abdomen:** soft without organomegaly, masses, or bruits. **Pelvis:** atrophic vaginal mucosa, normal bimanual examination findings. Stool is occult-blood negative. **Extremities:** no edema or clubbing; peripheral pulses are all present and symmetrical.

Vignette Objectives

1. List questions that are used to help people quit smoking.
2. List the symptoms and signs of lung cancer.

Smokers

Tobacco use is assessed by asking patients about their smoking and smokeless-tobacco use. Nicotine-stained fingers and the smell of stale cigarette smoke can identify smokers. In addition, heavy smokers can have a characteristic smoker's facies, which demonstrate many fine wrinkles. A deep cough and "husky" voice also support a history of smoking cigarettes.

Surveys have shown that fewer than 44% of smokers report being advised by their physicians to stop smoking. Evidence from randomized studies have shown that as little as 3 minutes of interaction can influence patients to attempt to stop smoking. They should be reassured that prior failed attempts to stop are not a reason for becoming discouraged; in fact, repeated efforts to quit increase the likelihood of ultimate success. The sequence of questions outlined in Table 4-12 are used to identify smokers and help them stop smoking.

Helping a person stop smoking is the most cost-effective health promotion activity. Ninety percent of people who stop smoking experience an unpleasant nicotine withdrawal syndrome. Withdrawal is most severe for those who

Table 4-12. Helping people stop smoking

1. **ASK** about smoking at every opportunity.
- "Do you smoke?"
- "How much?"
- "How soon after waking do you have your first cigarette?"
- "Are you interested in quitting?"
- "Have you ever tried to stop before?" If so, "What happened?"

2. **ADVISE** all smokers to stop.
- State your advice clearly and personalize the benefits of quitting; for example. "As your physician, I must advise you to stop smoking. I know that stopping would reduce your risk for a heart attack."

3. **ASSIST** patients in stopping.
- Set a quit date. Help the patient pick a date within the next 4 weeks, acknowledging that no time is ideal.
- Provide self-help materials (e.g., call 1-800-4-CANCER for National Cancer Institute's *Quit for Good* materials).
- Consider prescribing nicotine patches or gum, especially for highly addicted patients (those who smoke more than one pack per day or those who smoke their first cigarette within 30 minutes of waking).

4. **ARRANGE** follow-up visits.

Table 4-13. Condition associated with asbestos exposure

Condition	Findings
Mesothelioma	80% are associated with asbestos exposure, with a latency of approximately 35 years; risk not further increased by smoking; symptoms are chest pain, dyspnea, weight loss, and cough; illness usually rapidly progressive, with death in 6 months
Lung cancer	Risk increases with smoking; asbestos exposure in nonsmokers may not increase risk
Asbestosis	Pulmonary fibrosis associated with dyspnea, cough, basilar rales; when severe, can cause cyanosis and clubbing
Benign pleural disorders (effusions, calcified plaques, and pleural fibrosis)	Often asymptomatic; can have pleural pain and dyspnea

smoke more than 26 cigarettes per day or who smoke within 30 minutes of awakening, are more dependent on nicotine and can have even more severe withdrawal symptoms.

Asbestos-related Pulmonary Disease

Asbestos exposure can cause a spectrum of respiratory disorders (Table 4-13). Benign conditions include pulmonary fibrosis and pleural disorders. The development of malignant mesothelioma is associated with asbestos exposure, and smokers with asbestos exposure greatly increase their risk of lung cancer.

Cough

Cough can be a symptom of inflammation or of irritation of the airways. Usually a cough of recent onset is due to a respiratory tract infection. Causes of chronic cough (often defined as a cough persisting for more than 3 weeks) are listed in Table 4-14, according to the mnemonic **BAD MASS,** which is what one hopes is not found on the chest radiograph.

Lung Cancer

Patients with lung cancer manifest symptoms and signs late in their illness. To date, routine testing to detect early lung cancers has not been successful. Neither chest radiographs nor sputum cytologies are useful screening tests for lung cancer in asymptomatic smokers. The risk for lung cancer is greater among smokers, and it is even higher in those also exposed to asbestos.

Lung cancer can have various clinical consequences, depending on both the local and paraneoplastic effects. Symptoms suggestive of primary lung cancer include weight loss, cough, and blood-streaked sputum, but these frequently are late manifestations. Tumors at the lung's apex, referred to as *Pancoast's tumors,* can invade the brachial plexus and cervical sympathetic ganglion, caus-

Table 4-14. Conditions causing chronic cough: BAD MASS

Condition	Findings
Bronchitis	Daily sputum production for 3 months for 2 consecutive years; usually smoker; rhonchi
Asthma and ACE inhibitors	History of childhood allergies or asthma; exacerbated by exercise, especially in the cold; can be wheezes with forced expiration, but finding of clear lungs does not exclude diagnosis; ACE inhibitors can cause cough, possibly due to their effect of the kinin (bradykinin) system
Dysfunction of the left ventricle (CHF)	History of cardiac problems; exertional dyspnea; abnormal cardiac examination findings
Malignancy	Smoker; asbestos exposure; weight loss; hemoptysis; clubbing
Aspiration (nocturnal) aspiration due to gastroesophageal reflux)	Symptoms of reflux esophagitis; chronic sore throat or dental problems (loss of enamel) due to nocturnal reflux
Sinusitis and chronic postnasal drip	Symptoms begin after URI; unilateral nasal discharge; worse in morning after awakening
Smoking cigarettes or other respiratory irritants	Smoker; occupational or recreational exposure to respiratory irritants

ACE = angiotensin-converting enzyme.

ing arm pain or numbness and Horner's syndrome (unilateral miosis, ptosis, and anhidrosis), respectively. Tumors can cause a postobstructive pneumonia, and their direct extension to the pericardium or mediastinum can lead to cardiac tamponade and superior vena cava obstruction. Metastatic disease involving the central nervous system or bones also can be the first evidence of a primary lung tumor.

Lung cancer can be associated with several paraneoplastic conditions, including a hypercoagulable state and thromboembolic events, the syndrome of inappropriate antidiuretic hormones, hypercalcemia, ectopic ACTH with rapid development of symptoms and signs of hypercortisolism, and hypertrophic osteodystrophy (approximately 20% of patients with lung cancer have clubbing, hypertrophic osteodystrophy's most common manifestation). Paraneoplastic disorders are discussed further in Chapter 6.

Vignette Follow-up

DP has tried to quit smoking cigarettes twice, each time with only short-term success. She is congratulated for her attempts and what she has learned. She is being encouraged in her continued efforts to stop smoking. She is referred to an ENT consultant for biopsy of her oral lesion.

Vignette 8

Hemoptysis: coughing up or expectorating blood.

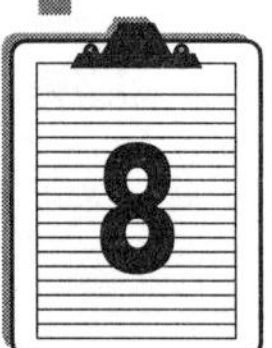

CF is a 57-year-old woman admitted to the hospital because of hemoptysis. She was in her usual state of health until 2 days before hospitalization. At that time, she recalls a feeling of warmth (she did not take her temperature) and the onset of a nonproductive cough. Several hours later, she had two coughing episodes, both associated with hemoptysis. She initially coughed up about "two tablespoons" of blood, and about 2 hours later, it occurred again. She is unsure how much she expectorated, but it seemed to "fill her mouth." After the second episode, she went to the emergency room and was admitted.

The patient has no prior history of chronic cough or hemoptysis. She has a 40 pack-year history of smoking and quit 2 years ago. She had pulmonary TB as a young teenager but is uncertain about events relating to that illness. She remembers being told that she had TB, spent several months in a hospital sanitorium, and later was given medication for about a year.

Physical examination reveals an anxious woman receiving oxygen by nasal prongs. Vital signs: **blood pressure** is 130/80 mm Hg, and her **heart rate** is 80 beats/min. No orthostatic changes are present. Her oral **temperature** is 99.2°F (37.3°C), and her **respiratory rate** is 20 breaths/min. **Skin:** normal without ecchymosis or telangiectasias. **HEENT:** clear oropharynx; no thyromegaly or adenopathy. Her trachea is midline and movable. **Chest:** decreased respiratory excursion of the right hemithorax. The percussion note is dull in the right midlung field, and rales are present in that area. An expiratory wheeze is audible over the right midlung field. **Cardiac:** no JVD; the PMI is nondisplaced and nonsustained; normal S_1 and S_2; a 1/6 systolic ejection murmur is heard at the left upper sternal border. **Breast** exam: normal without dimpling, nipple retraction, mass, or discharge. **Abdomen:** soft without organomegaly or masses. Her liver percusses to a span of 8 cm. Stool is occult-blood negative. **Extremities:** no cyanosis or edema. There is a slight sponginess of her fingernail beds but no definite clubbing. **Neurologic** examination findings are normal. A chest radiograph shows a right middle lobe infiltrate, with volume loss in that area.

Vignette Objectives

1. List the distinguishing features of hemoptysis and hematemesis.
2. What questions can help determine the severity of hemoptysis, and what volume denotes massive hemoptysis?
3. List the potential causes of hemoptysis and the history and physical examination findings that relate to these diagnoses.

Hemoptysis

The complaint of **hemoptysis,** or "coughing up blood," must be differentiated from hematemesis and, occasionally, epistaxis. Hemoptysis usually does not

Table 4-15. Distinctive characteristics of hemoptysis and hematemesis

Hemoptysis	Hematemesis
Associated with coughing	Associated with nausea, vomiting, and other GI symptoms
Blood mixed with sputum	Blood mixed with food or gastric contents
Blood often bright red	Blood usually dark ("coffee grounds")
History of pulmonary disease	History of gastrointestinal disease
Patient describes "blood from lungs"	Patient describes "blood from stomach"

result in blood in the nasopharynx, which distinguishes it from nasal bleeding. The features of hemoptysis and hematemesis are presented in Table 4-15.

The volume of the hemoptysis is important in determining both the prognosis and the management strategy. Massive hemoptysis is defined as more than approximately 500 ml of bleeding in 24 hours. Although it accounts for less than 5% of all cases of hemoptysis, it is a life-threatening condition with a mortality of 7% to 32%. Although the hemodynamic consequences of losing 500 ml of blood are not severe, that volume in the airways can cause asphyxiation. Management can necessitate ICU admission and urgent bronchoscopy.

The various causes of hemoptysis and the associated findings are listed in Table 4-16, organized according to the mnemonic **I BET I'M BUFF.** The extent to which to pursue an evaluation in a patient with hemoptysis and normal chest radiograph findings is controversial. For those individuals, an age over 40 and more than 40 pack-years of smoking are indications for bronchoscopy.

TB can cause hemoptysis as the result of the following mechanisms: (1) active pulmonary TB, (2) bronchiectasis resulting from healed TB and rupture of a small bronchial artery aneurysm, (3) aspergillosis in pulmonary cavity, and (4) "scar carcinoma" in an area of healed disease.

Vignette Follow-up

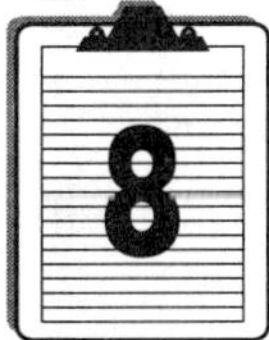

CF dies of massive hemoptysis, despite aggressive efforts at diagnosis and management, including urgent bronchoscopy, intubation, angiography, and an attempted embolization. Postmortem examination reveals the cause of her bleeding is squamous cell carcinoma, with vessel invasion.

Table 4-16. Causes of hemoptysis: I BET I'M BUFF

Condition	Findings
Idiopathic	Several rare causes are possible; approximately 10% of cases are "idiopathic," with no established diagnosis, despite a thorough evaluation
Bronchitis (acute or chronic)	Cough, purulent sputum; hemoptysis in those with chronic bronchitis usually occurs during an acute exacerbation
Embolism	Risks for thromboembolic disease; pleuritic chest pain; dyspnea; only 10% of patients with a pulmonary embolus experience hemoptysis
Tuberculosis	Exposure history; chronic cough, fever, weight loss; hemoptysis can result from cavitating active disease or old, healed disease
Immune-mediated pulmonary-renal syndromes	Wegener's granulomatosis: vasculitis affecting middle-aged people, glomerulonephritis and necrotizing granulomas of the upper and lower airways (including pulmonary infiltrates, cavitation, and hemoptysis); Goodpasture's syndrome: illness of young men due to antibodies against basement membrane antigens; antibodies produce alveolitis and lung hemorrhage; hemoptysis often first manifestation, rapidly progressive glomerulonephritis
Malignancy	Risks for lung cancer (e.g., smoking and asbestos exposure); cough; weight loss; more than 90% of patients with hemoptysis and lung cancer have a lesion on chest radiograph
Bronchiectasis	Chronic sputum production; recurrent pulmonary infections; cystic fibrosis is most common cause of bronchiectasis; clubbing can be caused by bronchiectasis (in addition to pulmonary malignant tumors and cyanotic congenital heart disease)
Usual pulmonary infection (pneumonias)	Fever, cough, sputum production; rales and signs of pulmonary consolidation; see Table 4-2 for characteristics pneumonia
Failure (cardiogenic pulmonary edema)	History of heart disease; reason for acute onset or exacerbation of CHF; "silent" mitral stenosis can first manifest as hemoptysis; sputum of person with pulmonary edema is "pink, frothy"; cyanotic congenital heart disease can cause polycythemia and hemoptysis; chronic pulmonary hypertension can lead to rupture of small vessels and hemoptysis
Fungus ball (mycetoma)	Pulmonary cavity in which a fungus ball grows

Vignette 9

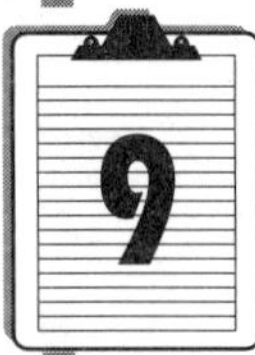

DC is a 55-year-old man who is admitted with the chief complaint of several months of "increasing fatigue" and bilateral "leg swelling." He first noted increasing dyspnea 7 years ago but did not seek medical care. Approximately 3 years ago he was admitted to another hospital for evaluation of a hematocrit of 62%. At that time, he was noted to have an FEV_1 of 1.60 liters, an FVC of 1.95 liters, and the following arterial blood gas values measured while breathing room air: pH, 7.42; $PaCO_2$, 56 mm Hg, PaO_2, 40 mm Hg. He was thought to have COPD, with secondary hypoxemia, hypercapnia, cor pulmonale, and erythrocytosis. He was treated with inhaled beta-agonists, diuretics, and supplemental oxygen.

He initially noted some improvement but continued to experience chronic daytime somnolence. Mr. C also reports experiencing agitated sleep, snoring, morning headaches, and progressive weight gain. He has been obese "all his life" but has gained 20 pounds (9 kg) in the past 3 weeks. He has a 120 pack year history of smoking and still smokes two packs daily. He drinks one "stiff drink" each evening. The remainder of his history is noncontributory.

Physical examination reveals a cyanotic morbidly obese man. Vital signs: **blood pressure** of 104/74 mm Hg, **heart rate** of 100 beats/min, **respirations** are shallow and the rate is 30 breaths/min; his oral **temperature** is 37.0°C. His **height** is 70 inches (1.75 m) and his **weight** is 306 pounds (138 kg). **Cardiac:** JVP is estimated to be 12 cm H_2O; normal S_1, S_2 demonstrates an increased P_2 component, and an S_4 is present. **Chest:** decreased breath sounds and bibasilar crackles. **Extremities:** 2+ symmetrical lower extremity edema to the thighs. **Neurologic** examination reveals that the patient is somnolent and dozes when not engaged in conversation; otherwise his mental status is normal. Motor, sensory, and cerebellar findings are normal. No asterixis is present. The initial chest radiograph is interpreted to show biventricular enlargement and possible pulmonary hypertension; the peripheral lung fields are clear.

Vignette Objectives

1. List the symptoms and signs of obstructive sleep apnea.
2. What is meant by morbid obesity?
3. What conditions are associated with obesity?

Obstructive Sleep Apnea

When erythrocytosis is found in association with hypoxia, obstructive sleep apnea is one of the diagnoses to consider. (The evaluation of patients with polycythemia and erythrocytosis is presented in Chapter 6.) Obstructive sleep apnea is characterized by the cessation of inspiratory air flow, despite persistent diaphragmatic effort. Findings predictive of sleep apnea include snoring, daytime somnolence, and a bed partner's description of apneic spells (additional findings are listed in Table 4-17). Exacerbating factors, especially alcohol consumption and the use of central nervous system depressants, can increase the number of obstructive events and prolong their duration. However, none of these history or exam findings, either singly or in combination, are sensitive or specific for obstructive sleep apnea. Sleep studies are needed to establish the diagnosis.

Approximately two thirds of patients with sleep apnea are obese, and a substantial weight loss can reverse the disorder. However, the pathogenic link between obesity and sleep apnea is not clear. In its most full-blown state, as illustrated by this patient, the disorder is called *pickwickian syndrome* (obesity, daytime somnolence erythrocytosis, and right ventricular failure due to pulmonary hypertension resulting from chronic hypoxia). The name comes from a character named Joe in the novel by Charles Dickens entitled *Posthumous Papers of the Pickwick Club*, and Sir William Osler, in 1918, was the first to use the term to describe this clinical picture.

Table 4-17. Features of obstructive sleep apnea

Finding	Comments
Restless sleep, loud snoring	Information from bed partner best identifies these symptoms and characterizes nocturnal apneic episodes
Daytime somnolence, intellectual and personality changes	Chronic deprivation of rapid eye movement sleep can cause mental status changes
Morning headache	Carbon dioxide retention causes dilation of cerebral vessels, leading to morning headaches
Elevated JVP, edema, and erythrocytosis	Chronic hypoxia leads to secondary erythrocytosis, pulmonary hypertension, and findings of right ventricular failure

Obesity

Obesity is defined as being 20% above a desirable body weight and usually amounts to 30 to 40 pounds (13.5 to 18 kg) above the desirable weight. Desirable levels are determined from actuarial insurance data and listed in standard height-and-weight charts. *Morbid obesity* is a term reserved for the small fraction of people who are more than 100 pounds (45 kg) overweight, or twice their desirable body weight. Morbidity and mortality are greatly increased in morbidly obese people.

An increased body weight is associated with several medical problems (Table 4-18), and these associated conditions have been identified on the basis of population data. For any individual person, however, the precise risk associated with obesity is difficult to define. Achieving and maintaining a weight loss is difficult, but even a relatively small weight loss (e.g., a 15-pound [6.75 kg] loss in a person who would need to lose 60 pounds [27 kg] to achieve a desirable weight) can alleviate conditions associated with obesity.

Table 4-18. Conditions associated with obesity

Condition	Comments
Type II diabetes mellitus	Prevalence increased approximately threefold
Hypertension	Risk highest among young people; prevalence increased approximately threefold
Osteoarthritis	Altered body mechanics and increased joint stress can accelerate degenerative joint disease
Hyperlipidemia	Twice the likelihood of a total cholesterol of >259 mg/dl
Cholelithiasis	Pathogenesis may relate to repeated attempts at weight loss
Malignancy	Men's risk of prostate cancer increased; women at increased risk for breast, endometrial, and gallbladder cancer

Vignette Follow-up

Three years before, DC was noted to have an elevated hematocrit reading, severe hypoxemia, and CO_2 retention, all findings compatible with COPD. However, the FEV_1/FVC ratio was not reduced, which is not consistent with COPD. The reduced lung volumes indicate ventilatory restriction, probably as a consequence of his massive obesity and limited chest wall movement. Sleep studies documented Mr. C's obstructive sleep apnea. He then loses 60 pounds [27 kg] on a medically supervised modified fast. He is able to stop smoking and discontinue his alcohol intake. His room air PaO_2 increases to 62 mm Hq, and the symptoms and signs of cor pulmonale are no longer present.

Objectives Review

1. Outline components of the pulmonary examination.
2. How do history and physical examination findings help predict the pathogen causing a pneumonia?
3. Describe the pulmonary examination findings that help differentiate a right lower lobe pneumonia and a right pleural effusion.
4. What historical findings identify people who should undergo skin testing for TB?
5. What are the clinical features of different "types" of TB (i.e., primary, reactivation, miliary)?
6. Dyspnea is a nonspecific symptom. List the cardiac and pulmonary causes of dyspnea and patient findings relevant to each diagnosis.
7. List findings in patients with COPD due to emphysema and chronic bronchitis.
8. List the causes of wheezing and the history and physical examination findings that help distinguish among the causes.
9. List the causes of an exacerbation of reactive airway disease and the history and physical examination findings relating to each.
10. Which historical and physical examination findings indicate the severity of respiratory distress?
11. What is the relationship between esophageal reflux and reactive airway disease?
12. List the causes of pleuritic chest pain and how the history and physical examination findings relate to each diagnosis.
13. List the classic findings in patients with a DVT. How sensitive and specific are the physical examination findings in detecting a DVT?
14. List conditions that can result in the adult respiratory distress syndrome (ARDS). For each, describe historical events that might precede the development of ARDS.
15. How useful are the physical examination findings in differentiating cardiac from noncardiac pulmonary edema?

16. List questions that are used to help people quit smoking.
17. List the symptoms and signs of lung cancer.
18. List the distinguishing features of hemoptysis and hematemesis.
19. What questions can help determine the severity of hemoptysis, and what volume denotes massive hemoptysis?
20. List the potential causes of hemoptysis and the history and physical examination findings that relate to these diagnoses.
21. List the symptoms and signs of obstructive sleep apnea.
22. What is meant by morbid obesity?
23. What conditions are associated with obesity?

Suggested Reading

Badgett RG, Tanaka DJ, Hunt DK, et al. Can moderate chronic obstructive pulmonary disease be diagnosed by historical and physical findings alone? *Am J Med* 1993;94: 188–96.

COPD is unlikely if patient has no history of smoking, normal breath sounds, and peak flow exceeding 200 L/min; diminished breath sounds are the only physical finding that has utility in addition to the patient's history for detecting patients with COPD.

Blumberg S, Kantrowiz FG. The pseudothrombophlebitis syndrome: a reappraisal. *Semin Arthritis Rheum* 1981;10:278–81.

Symptoms and signs of a DVT can be due to a ruptured popliteal cyst; it can occur as an isolated finding in patients without an underlying rheumatologic disorder.

Cromartie RS III, Parker EF, May JE, Metcalf JS, Bartles DM. Carcinoma of the lung: a clinical review. *Ann Thorac Surg* 1980;30:30–5.

di Sant'Agnese PA, Davis PB. Cystic fibrosis in adults: 75 cases and a review of 232 cases in the literature. *Am J Med* 1979;66:121–30.

Overall, minor hemoptysis occurs in 60%, massive hemoptysis in 7%, pneumothorax in 16%, sinusitis in 100%, and nasal polyps in 48%; the authors point out that older patients can look well, and a high index of suspicion can be needed to diagnose cystic fibrosis among adults.

Edelson JD, Rebuck AS. The clinical assessment of severe asthma. *Arch Intern Med* 1985;145:321–23.

Gennis P, Gallagher J, Falvo C, Baker S, Than W. Clinical criteria for the detection of pneumonia in adults: guidelines for ordering chest roentgenograms in the emergency department. *J Emerg Med* 1989;7:263–8.

Patients with pneumonia usually have at least one abnormal vital sign, that is temperature, >37.8°C [100°F]; heart rate, >100 beats/min, or respirations, >20 breaths/min; approximately 20% with pneumonia have normal chest examination findings.

Hoffstein V, Szalai JP. Predictive value of clinical features in diagnosing obstructive sleep apnea. *Sleep* 1993;16:118–22.

Report on 594 patients referred to a sleep clinic; although clinical criteria could explain over half the variability between affected and nonaffected subjects, sleep studies were needed to establish the diagnosis.

Hull RD, Raskob GE, Carter CJ, et al. Pulmonary embolism in outpatients with pleuritic chest pain. *Arch Intern Med* 1988;148:838–44.

One fifth of patients seen in the emergency room with pleuritic chest pain were found to have a pulmonary embolism; sensitivity and specificity of clinical findings are limited in establishing the diagnosis; and a ventilation/perfusion scan and impedance plethysmography often are needed.

Hyde L, Hyde CI. Clinical manifestations of lung cancer. *Chest* 1974;65:299–306.
Discusses four groups of symptoms: (1) direct tumor effects (cough, hemoptysis, and obstruction), (2) extension and metastasis, (3) systemic symptoms (fever and weight loss), and (4) remote effects (hormonal, paraneoplastic, and thrombotic).

Katz RS, Zizic TM, Stevens MB. The pseudothrombophlebitis syndrome. *Medicine* 1977; 56:151–64.

Kollef MH, Schuster DP. The acute respiratory distress syndrome. *N Engl J Med* 1995; 332:27–34.
Brief review of the causes; most of the review is devoted to a discussion of medical management and ventilator use.

Kral JG. Morbid obesity and related health risks. *Ann Intern Med* 1985;103(6 pt 2):1043–7.
This article is from a supplement about obesity; morbid obesity is associated with increased mortality and unique morbidities, such as sudden unexplained death, ventilatory disorders, and severe functional limitations.

Martin L, Khalil H. How much reduced hemoglobin is necessary to generate central cyanosis? *Chest* 1990;97:182–5.
Brief summary of information on this topic.

McFadden ER Jr, Gilbert IA. Asthma. *N Engl J Med* 1992;327:1928–36.
Review of pathophysiology, natural history, and management of asthma.

Mossman BT, Gee BG. Asbestos-related diseases. *N Engl J Med* 1989;320:1721–9.
Review of mesothelioma, lung cancer, pulmonary fibrosis, and four types of pleural disease.

Mulrow CD, Dolmatch BL, Delong ER, et al. Observer variability in the pulmonary examination. *J Gen Intern Med* 1986;1:364–7.
Study findings document the limited interobserver reliability when physical exam findings are compared; findings assessed as present/absent were more reliable than graded findings.

Mulrow CD, Lucey CR, Farnett LE. Discriminating causes of dyspnea through clinical examination. *J Gen Intern Med* 1993;8:383–92.
Clinical examination findings (history of pulmonary disease, description of breathlessness, and signs of left ventricular failure) are useful in differentiating pulmonary from cardiac dyspnea, with an accuracy of approximately 70%.

Nachman RL, Silverstein R. Hypercoagulable states. *Ann Intern Med* 1993;119:819–27.

National Asthma Educational Program: *Expert Panel Report. Executive summary: guidelines for the diagnosis and management of asthma* (Publication No. 91-3042A). Washington: U.S. Department of Health and Human Services, 1991.
Extensive review, including guidelines for medical management, patient education, environmental control, and treatment of special situations, such as asthma and pregnancy, older patients, aspirin sensitivity, and gastroesophageal reflux.

Pomilla PV, Brown RB. Outpatient treatment of community-acquired pneumonia in adults. *Arch Intern Med* 1994;154:1793–1800.
Review of the past 30 years' worth of articles on this topic; discusses the limitations of patient findings in predicting the cause and the indications for obtaining radiograms and hospitalizing patients; approaches to therapy are presented.

Pratter MR, Bartter T, Akers S, DuBois J. An algorithmic approach to chronic cough. *Ann Intern Med* 1993;119:977–83.

Study of nonsmokers referred to pulmonary clinic; postnasal drip was the most common cause of chronic cough, and initial antihistamine-decongestant therapy resolved the problem in most patients.

Schneider IC, Anderson AE Jr. Correlation of clinical signs with ventilatory function in obstructive lung disease. *Ann Intern Med* 1965;62:477–85.
Even 30 years ago, clinicians' abilities to detect emphysema showed variations and limitations.

The pickwickian syndrome. Medical Staff Conference, University of California, San Francisco. *West J Med* 1977;127:24–31.

Van Itallie TB. Health implications of overweight and obesity in the United States. *Ann Intern Med* 1985;103(6 pt 2):983–8.
The author presents the health risks and illnesses associated with obesity; he also describes how race and socioeconomic status relate to body weight and points out that being overweight as a young adult is more dangerous than becoming obese as an older adult.

5 Urinary and Renal Problems

Objectives

List history and physical examination findings for the following problems:

- Benign prostatic hypertrophy
- Bladder incontinence
- Bladder outlet obstruction
- Cystitis
- Decreased urine output (oliguria / anuria)
- End-stage renal disease / uremia
- Essential hypertension
- Flank pain
- Hypercalcemia
- Hyponatremia
- Incontinence
- Nephrolithiasis
- Pain on urination (dysuria)
- Prostate cancer
- Pyelonephritis
- Red urine
- Vaginitis
- Urethritis

Pertinent Points

History

History of kidney or bladder problems?
Infections of kidney or bladder?
- Frequency of infection
- Symptoms (pain, burning, urgency)
- Fever, flank pain
- Treatment
- Women:
  - Sexually active
  - Use of diaphragm, cervical cap
  - Void after intercourse
  - Postmenopausal
  - Incontinence
  - History of vaginal infections or discharge
  - (Pelvic infections are covered in Chapter 9)
- Men:
  - Prior kidney and bladder evaluation
  - Sexual activity, condom use
  - Symptoms of bladder outlet obstruction
  - Infections of prostate or urethra
  - Force of stream, nocturia, dribbling
  - For patients with urethral discharge, associated symptoms (fever, arthralgias, skin lesions), sexual activity, prior sexually transmitted diseases (STDs)

History of red or cola-colored urine?
- Renal colic or dysuria
- Urinary tract infections
- Sickle cell trait
- Trauma, muscle injury or pain
- Exposure to carcinogens
- Symptoms of prostatic hypertrophy

For patients with renal stones:
- Family history
- Symptoms of gout
- Hypercalcemia
- Intake of fluids, calcium, vitamin D, antacids

Trouble leaking or losing urine?
- Volume of urine
- Loss during straining or coughing
- Symptoms of bladder outlet obstruction
- History of neurologic disease
- Parity
- Estrogen status

History of frequent urination:
- Volume of urine per void
- Thirst and fluid intake
- Nocturia
- Medications (diuretics, lithium)
- History of diabetes
- History of renal problems

For patients with low urine output:
- Serial weights
- Thirst
- Prior renal problems
- History of conditions with low renal perfusion (congestive heart failure [CHF], cirrhosis, nephrotic syndrome)
- Exposure to nephrotoxins (drugs, contrast agents, myoglobin)
- Symptoms of bladder outlet obstruction (difficulty voiding, bladder spasms)

For patients with chronic renal disease:
- Anorexia, nausea, vomiting
- Pruritus
- Dyspnea on exertion
- Easy bruising, bleeding
- Muscle cramps, weakness, dysesthesia
- Prior evaluation of renal function (urinalysis, serum chemistries)
- History of hypertension, diabetes, nephritis, or analgesic use

Physical Examination

Inspection
- Skin turgor
- Assessment for pigmentation, ecchymosis, purpura

Weight

Vital signs
- Blood pressure, heart rate; orthostatic change (intravascular volume status)

Respiratory rate

Temperature

Fundi (findings characteristic of hypertension and diabetes)
Nasopharynx Nasal mucosa ulceration (Wegener's syndrome), hydration of mucous membranes
Chest
- Percuss lung fields
- Ausculate breath sound
- Unusual conditions can involve kidney and lung (Wegener's syndrome, Goodpasture's syndrome)

Cardiac
- Jugular venous pressure (JVP)
- Point of maximal impulse (PMI) location, size
- S_1, S_2, S_4, S_3, murmur and rub

Abdomen
- Aortic, renal artery bruits
- Suprapubic tenderness
- Palpable kidneys
- Palpable bladder distention
- Percuss costovertebral angle
- Occult-blood in stool

Genitourinary (male)
- Inguinal nodes
- Palpate testes and intrascrotal structures
- Inspect glans, ureteral meatus (discharge, lesions)
- Digital prostatic examination
- Perineal sensation, cremasteric reflex
- Palpate inguinal nodes

Pelvic (female)
- Inspect perineum, perineal sensation
- Inspect vagina and cervix and character of discharge, if present
- Bimanually palpate uterus and adnexa
- Effect of Valsalva's maneuver on cystocele and continence
- Palpate inguinal nodes

Extremities
- Edema (anasarca versus dependent)
- Pulses
- Palpate for arteriovenous fistula thrill (hemodialysis access)
- Tophi (gout)
- Tenosynovitis, arthritis, skin lesions, rash

Mental status (especially if uremia, hypertensive encephalopathy, or metabolic disorder suspected)
Neurologic
Cranial nerves: VIII (deafness associated with hereditary renal disease)
Motor/sensation: Peripheral neuropathy associated with uremia
- Asterixis

Suspicion of nephritic or nephrotic syndromes, electrolyte disorders, or uremia can prompt a focused evaluation of other organ systems

Vignette 1

Adherence or **compliance:** concordance between what is advised and what a patient does.

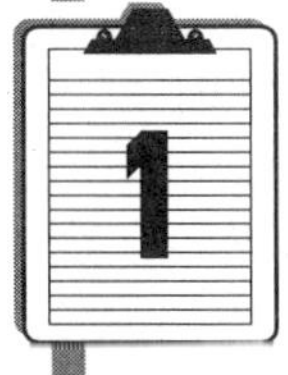

AW is a 42-year-old man who was first told he had hypertension 3 weeks ago, when his blood pressure was taken at a shopping mall health fair. This is his third office visit, and at each visit his blood pressure has been elevated at a level of 155/100 mm Hg. He takes no medications or drugs, and he has no findings indicating a secondary cause of elevated blood pressure, such as an abdominal mass (polycystic renal disease); weight loss, episodic headaches, and orthostasis (pheochromocytoma); abdominal bruit (renovascular disease); truncal obesity, stria, and easy bruising (hypercortisolism), or goiter, tremor, and lid lag (hyperthyroidism). He exercises regularly and is not overweight. Today you plan to start him on antihypertensive therapy and your task is to explain the medication side effects to him and to assess his ability to adhere to treatment. Mr. W has heard that blood pressure medications can make a person feel lethargic, reduce exercise capacity, and affect sexual function. He is concerned and asks, "Will I have to take this medicine for the rest of my life?"

Vignette Objective

1. What communication strategies are useful when talking with patients about a treatment plan? What strategies improve patients' adherence to treatment plans?

Talking with Patients about Medications

Patients' adherence to medication regimens depends on many factors, and the rate varies between 20% and 80%. Elevated blood pressure provides an example of a situation in which patient education and a good physician-patient relationship are needed for therapy to be effective. In part this is because hypertension, especially in its early stages, is asymptomatic, whereas its treatment can cause problematic side effects. This in turn helps explain why most "refractory" hypertension is due to patients not taking their medications.

Communication skills that improve adherence are listed in Table 5-1. The best way to assess medication compliance is to ask the patient about it. Some patients are reluctant to admit difficulties with taking medication. Phrasing questions in such a way as to give patients "permission" to admit noncompli-

Table 5-1. Communicating with patients about medications

- Evaluate the patient's understanding and beliefs concerning high blood pressure and management.

  Avoid asking, "How much do you know about hypertension?," which might be perceived as disrespectful; instead say, "Let's be sure that we are working together. Tell me what you understand about hypertension." The patient's interpretations and personal beliefs can affect adherence and therapeutic decisions.

- Be concrete and specific, and state important information concisely.

  Studies have shown that, immediately after the visit, patients remember only 50% of the information physicians provide. Even less information is retained several weeks later. Keeping the message simple and supplementing it with patient education material improves patient understanding.

- Ask the patient to repeat a plan, and identify the patient's concerns. Reach a mutually agreed upon approach to management.

  This assesses patient understanding, acknowledges the difficulty in following directions, and allows concerns and potential problems to be addressed. The technique increases patient satisfaction, accurate recall of information, and the sense of partnership between patient and physician.

ance is useful. For instance, you might say, "Some people have trouble taking this sort of medication. How did it go for you?"

Objective measures also can be used to assess medication use. One strategy is to ask patients to bring their pill bottles with them to their appointment. A check of the bottles' contents can give the physician an idea of whether the appropriate number of pills have been taken. For some drugs, measuring serum medication levels and direct observation of a drug's physiologic response (e.g., heart rate reduction in response to a beta-blocker) also are means to assess adherence.

Assessing adherence is an essential component of follow-up care, and each visit is a chance to identify side effects, address patient concerns, and reinforce the need for adherence. Changing to another agent and simplifying medication scheduling (qd versus tid) can enhance adherence and treatment efficacy. Finally, patients should be informed of the effects of sudden discontinuation of a medication, in that a "rebound" elevation in blood pressure or accelerated worsening of angina can occur if certain antihypertensive and antianginal medications are discontinued abruptly.

Vignette Follow-up

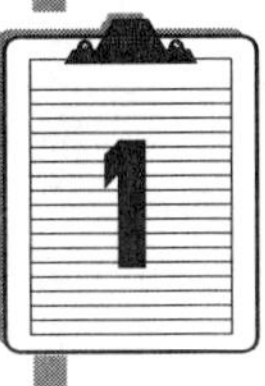

After discussion, Mr. W is begun on lisinopril (10 mg qd). At three successive monthly follow-up visits his average blood pressure is 122/80 mm Hg. His renal function and serum potassium are normal and do not change after therapy. He denies dizziness, cough, rash, or angioedema. AW probably will need ongoing pharmacologic treatment for hypertension, because he has already been practicing first-line nonmedication therapies (weight loss, exercise, avoidance of alcohol, and low sodium intake).

Vignette 2

Azotemia: elevation of nitrogenous waste products, reflected by an elevation in blood urea nitrogen and serum creatinine levels.

End-stage renal disease: chronic decline in renal function, such that renal replacement therapy (dialysis or transplantation) is necessary.

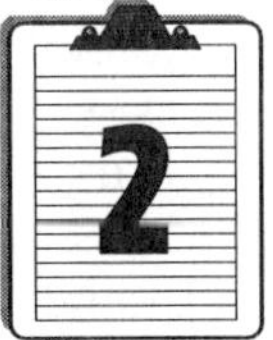

CU, a 47-year-old male research chemist, has a history of chronic renal disease. At age 18, he had a "strep throat" that was followed by the appearance of "cola-colored" urine. At age 21, he had an episode of gross hematuria and was told that he had "red cell casts." Urinalysis performed over the next 20 years intermittently revealed red blood cells on microscopic examination. His blood pressure during this period is reported to have been normal.

CU relates that he began to have headaches 2 years ago, which prompted him to see a physician, who told him that his blood pressure was "very high" and started him on treatment with two antihypertensive medications (a beta-blocker and diuretic). During the following year, Mr. U felt well and his blood pressure remained normal on medication. In the past 3 months, however, he has noticed episodic lower extremity swelling and has taken an extra diuretic pill when this has occurred. Over the prior month, he has experienced progressive fatigue and intermittent nausea and vomiting. He takes no other prescribed or over-the-counter medications.

Today he is found to be a thin, pale man who appears chronically ill. Vital signs: **blood pressure** is 165/95 mm Hg, **heart rate** is 80 beats/min without orthostatic changes, and **respiratory rate** is 18 breaths/min. His **breath** has a particular odor. **Skin:** normal, other than pallor. **HEENT:** funduscopic exam shows moderate narrowing of retinal arteries, without hemorrhages, exudates, or papilledema. **Chest:** rales are present at the right base. **Cardiac:** full neck veins with jugular venous pressure of at least 14 cm H_2O; no Kussmaul's sign. His PMI is in the anterior axillary line and sustained. A loud to-and-fro, scratchy sound is heard over the precordium, obscuring S_1 and S_2. **Abdomen:** liver span is 12 cm to percussion, with an edge palpated one finger breadth below the right costal margin. The spleen is not palpable. **Genitourinary:** normal male genitalia. **Rectal:** stool is occult-blood negative. The prostate is slightly enlarged, without nodules. **Extremities:** no edema; peripheral pulses are present and symmetrical. **Neurologic:** normal mental status, symmetrical 2+ reflexes, and no asterixis.

Vignette Objectives

1. What history and physical examination findings are associated with end-stage renal disease?
2. Uremic pericarditis is a complication of end-stage renal disease, and tamponade is a life threatening complication of pericarditis. Does this patient have findings indicative of cardiac tamponade?

End-Stage Renal Disease

The most common causes of chronic renal failure are diabetes, hypertension, and chronic glomerulonephritis. Most patients with progressive renal dysfunction are identified prior to developing end-stage renal disease (ESRD), because the manifestations of the illness (e.g., an elevated blood pressure or abnormal urinalysis) bring the renal dysfunction to light. If it is diagnosed before the "end stage" is reached, blood pressure control, a reduction in dietary protein consumption, and avoidance of nephrotoxins may slow disease progression. However, renal dysfunction can manifest few symptoms until late in its course (when function is less than 25% of normal), and these patients come to medical attention when there is little chance to retard or reverse their advanced renal disease.

When azotemia is detected initially, a patient's elevated creatinine level could be due either to potentially reversible acute problems or to chronic renal abnormalities. Long-standing renal dysfunction is indicated by chronic complaints of fatigue, anorexia, or pruritus and a history of renal disease or hypertension. Laboratory results indicating the presence of chronic renal disease include anemia or the finding of small kidneys on renal ultrasound studies.

The uremia of ESRD affects all organ systems, and Table 5-2 outlines these findings. An important preventable cause is analgesic nephropathy. Long-term use of NSAIDs, aspirin-phenacetin preparations, or acetaminophen can lead to irreversible renal damage.

Vignette Follow-up

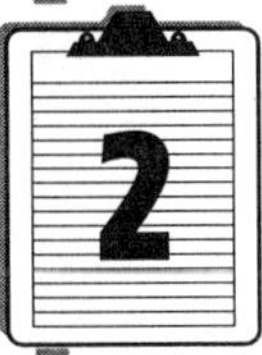

CU is admitted to the hospital and is found to have congestive heart failure and a pericardial effusion that is not hemodynamically significant. The absence of pulsus paradoxus and Kussmaul's sign indicates that tamponade is not present, and this is substantiated by an echocardiogram obtained the following day. Because of the presumed uremic pericarditis, he begins urgent hemodialysis. His history of gross hematuria during viral infections suggests his problem may have been IgA nephropathy (Buerger's disease). Although the patient's renal dysfunction is irreversible, identifying its cause allows estimation of the results of a subsequent renal transplant and can suggest the need to screen family members for the disorder.

Table 5-2. Potential effects of uremia

Problem	History	Physical examination
General	Weight gain, weakness, fatigue	Uremic breath odor
Cardiovascular	Hypertension, chest pain, angina, edema and other symptoms of CHF	*Hypertension:* sustained PMI, S_4 *CHF:* rales, elevated JVP, displaced PMI, S_3, edema *Pericarditis:* pericardial rub, rarely tamponade with low blood pressure, muffled cardiac sounds, elevated JVP with Kussmaul's sign
Pulmonary	Dyspnea on exertion (due to anemia, CHF)	Rales resulting from CHF
Gastrointestinal	Anorexia, nausea, vomiting, abnormal taste (dysgeusia)	Occult-blood positive stool
Urinary tract	Reduced urine output, nocturia	—
Skin	Pruritus, easy bruising	Increased pigmentation, bruising
Central nervous system	Difficulty concentrating, restless legs, muscle twitching	Abnormal mental status, myoclonic jerks, asterixis
Hematologic	Fatigue, bruising, or bleeding	Pallor (anemia), bruises, gingival bleeding

Vignette 3

Oliguria: urine output of less than 400 ml in 24 hours or less than 20 ml per hour.
Anuria: urine output of less than 50 ml in 24 hours.

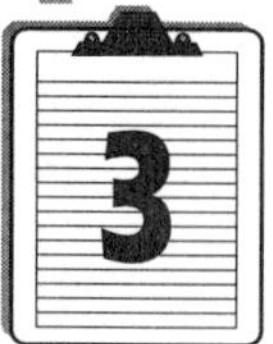

It is 11:00 P.M., and you are on call. The nurse pages you to see Mr. P because he has not voided during the past two 8 hour shifts. Mr. P is an 88-year-old man, hospitalized 3 days ago with cellulitis of his left foot. He is being treated with intravenous nafcillin. He also has chronic congestive heart failure, due to coronary artery disease, for which he takes furosemide, enalapril, and digoxin. Initial physical assessment reveals a frail man who is lying comfortably in bed. His height is 5 feet, 5 inches (1.6 m) and weight is 115 pounds (52 kg). His **blood pressure** is 136/88 mm Hg, **heart rate** is 88 beats/min, and oral **temperature** is 37.3°C.

Vignette Objective

1. What aspects of a patient's evaluation are most important for establishing the cause of oliguria or a low urine output?

Oliguria

An algorithm can be useful in organizing the assessment of people with oliguria (Fig. 5-1), though it can also oversimplify a situation. Each patient requires some individualization. There are three categories of renal dysfunction: prerenal, postrenal, and intrinsic. Prerenal dysfunction is due to hypovolemia or conditions causing low renal perfusion. Postrenal dysfunction is due to collecting system obstruction. Intrinsic renal dysfunction can involve four renal structures: vasculature, glomeruli, tubules, and interstitium.

The assessment seeks findings consistent with one of the three categories of abnormalities and its specific cause. In addition, the evaluation focuses on problems that are immediately reversible or life-threatening, such as bladder outlet obstruction, hypovolemia, the use of offending drugs, and hyperkalemia. Laboratory data of immediate importance are the urinalysis findings, serum chemistry values, and spot urine electrolyte and creatinine levels.

Vignette Follow-up

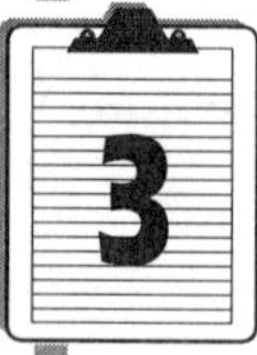

Mr. P is found to have a distended bladder and a large prostate on digital examination. A urinary catheter is inserted, and 1200 ml of urine is drained from his bladder. His blood pressure remains stable after catheter insertion and bladder drainage, and there is no postobstructive diuresis. Subsequent urologic consultants recommend that Mr. P undergo a transurethral resection of the prostate for the treatment of his bladder outlet obstruction.

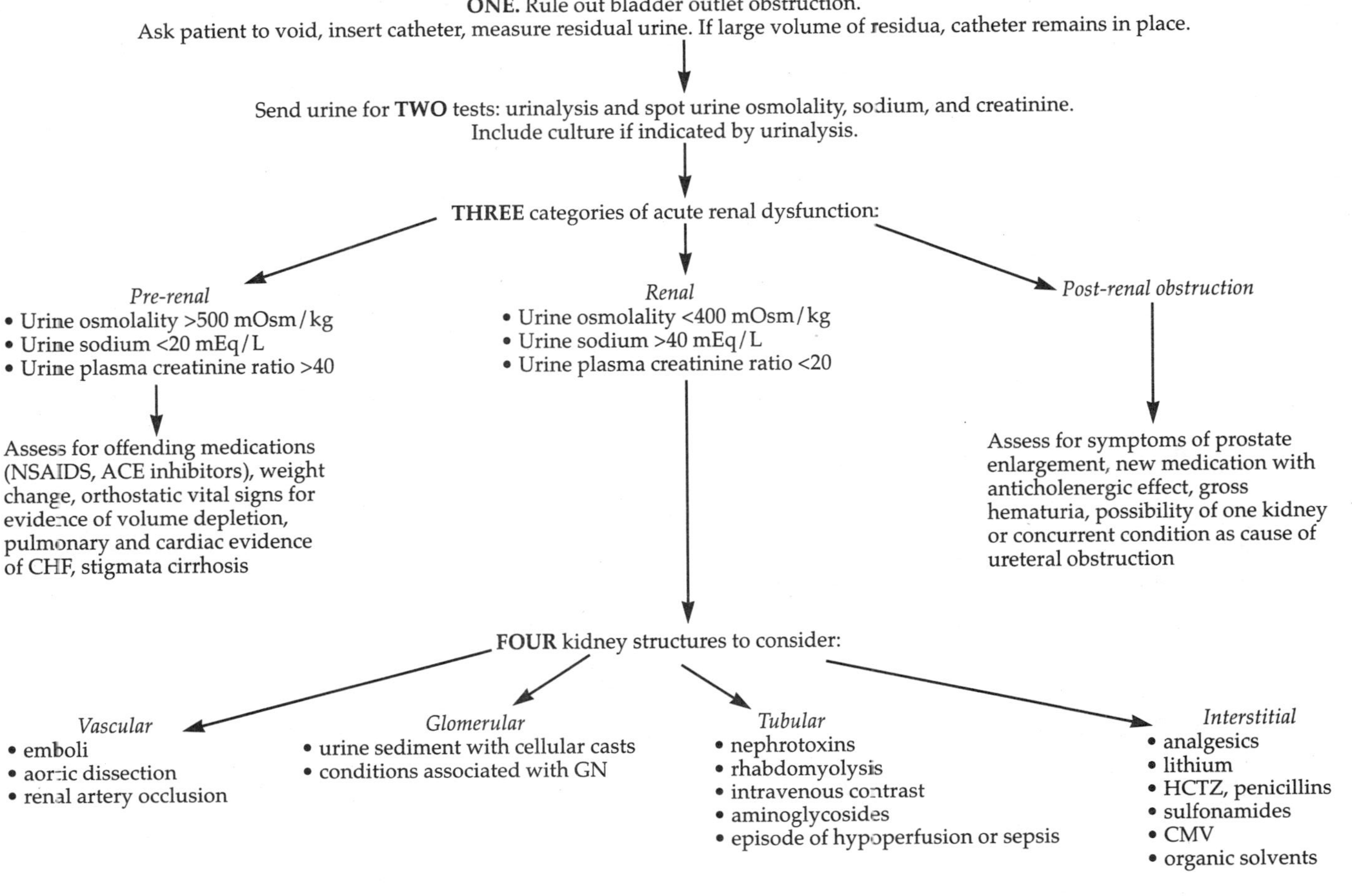

Figure 5-1. The evaluation of declining renal function or inability to void follows a one (rule out bladder outlet obstruction), two (obtain urine for urinalysis and chemistries), three (prerenal, postrenal, and renal categories), and four (four renal structures) sequence. *CHF* = congestive heart failure; *HCTZ* = hydrochlorothiazide; *CMV* = cytomegalovirus.

Vignette 4

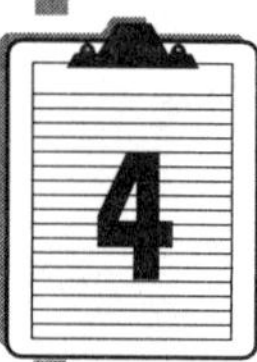

TO is a 42-year-old man admitted with "complicated pneumonia." His current problems began 6 months ago, when progressive bilateral lower extremity edema developed and he was found to have nephrotic syndrome. Before the current problem, Mr. O had been well. He was taking no medications or drugs and had no family history of renal disease. No other systemic problems were identified, and he began a trial of every-other-day, high-dose corticosteroid therapy. So far, however, he has not noted any clinical improvement and continues to have edema and an 8 gm of proteinuria/24 hr.

Two weeks ago, Mr. O complained of pleuritic pain and cough. His local physician was concerned about a pneumonia (especially in light of his corticosteroid treatment) and began erythromycin treatment. However, the symptoms persisted and a chest radiograph showed a wedge-shaped infiltrate. He was referred to the University Hospital.

Physical examination reveals a cushingoid man who is tachypneic but in no distress. His **blood pressure** is 156/90 mm Hg, **heart rate** is 86 beats/ min, **respiratory rate** is 24 breaths/min, and oral **temperature** is 37.4°C. **HEENT:** moon facies; clear oropharynx and tympanic membranes; no cervical adenopathy. **Chest:** splinting of left chest, clear to percussion; rales in left base but no rub or signs of consolidation. **Cardiac:** no JVD; PMI not palpable; S_1 and S_2 are normal; no gallop, murmur or rub. **Abdomen:** liver, 9-cm percussion span in midclavicular line, nontender; no masses or splenomegaly. **Extremities:** 1+ edema bilaterally; symmetrical circumferences at the thigh and calf; pulses are present and symmetrical.

Vignette Objectives

1. How do the findings differ in patients with lower extremity edema due to congestive heart failure, cirrhosis, nephrotic syndrome, and venous obstruction?
2. What are the most frequent causes of nephrotic syndrome and how does the assessment differ for each?

Nephrotic Syndrome

Lower-extremity edema can be due to several causes: congestive heart failure, nephrotic syndrome, cirrhosis, venous or lymphatic obstruction, or venous insufficiency. The findings in patients with these various problems are listed in Table 5-3.

Nephrotic syndrome is defined by proteinuria of >2.5 gm/24 hr, hypoalbuminemia, and edema. The most common causes of nephrotic syndrome are diabetic nephropathy, membranous glomerulonephritis, lipoid or minimal-change nephropathy, and focal glomerulosclerosis. However, many other problems can also cause the disorder (Tables 5-4 and 5-5).

Table 5-3. Assessments of patients with bilateral lower extremity edema

Etiology	History	Physical examination
Congestive heart failure (CHF)	Dyspnea on exertion, orthopnea, history of cardiac problems or severe COPD (if isolated right ventricular failure)	Elevated JVP, displaced PMI, S_3; rales and dullness at bases
Nephrotic syndrome	Diabetes, certain medications, intravenous drug abuse	No JVD; examination findings can be normal except for lower extremity edema; can have diffuse edema (anasarca)
Cirrhosis (portal hypertension)	History of liver disease, chronic alcohol use; prior episode of jaundice; exposure to hepatotoxins	Palmar erythema, spider angiomas, ecchymosis, ascites, splenomegaly
Venous or lymphatic obstruction	Weight loss or fever with malignant tumor	Adenopathy; distention of abdominal veins with flow toward head (opposite to that of portal hypertension)
Venous insufficiency	History of varicose veins; lower extremity pain; edema resolves overnight and increases when upright	Varicosities, increased skin pigmentation (stasis dermatitis); no evidence of other problems

Table 5-4. Common causes of nephrotic syndrome

Etiology	Comments
Diabetic nephropathy	Usually coincident diabetic retinopathy; nonnephrotic range of proteinuria and hypertension usually precede nephrotic syndrome
Membranous glomerulonephritis	Rare in children; half of cases in nephrotic adults; usually not hypertensive; can have associated malignant tumor; can respond to corticosteroid and other immunosuppressive treatment
Focal glomerulosclerosis	Clinically similar to minimal change nephropathy, but histologically different; most cases slowly progressive; recurs in half of renal transplant patients
Minimal-change nephropathy	80% of cases in children; 15% in nephrotic adults; hypertension infrequent; 90% of cases resolve with corticosteroid therapy

Other than proteinuria, the urinalysis findings in patients with the nephrotic syndrome often are normal. This distinguishes these "nephrotic" findings from nephritic disorders. In the latter, proteinuria is accompanied by hematuria and the finding of cellular casts, and usually patients are hypertensive. The common causes of proteinuria, hematuria, and cellular casts are listed in Table 5-6.

Patients with nephrotic syndrome are at increased risk for infection and atherosclerotic disease as the result of their elevated serum lipid levels. They also lose antithrombin III (as well as other proteins) through the glomeruli, resulting in a reduction in its concentration in the renal vein. This mechanism partially explains the frequent association of renal vein thrombosis with nephrotic syndrome. These thrombi can extend into the inferior vena cava and result in pulmonary emboli. However, whether to anticoagulate all patients with nephrotic syndrome and how to screen for thromboembolic events are controversial issues.

Table 5-5. Additional causes of proteinuria

TRANSIENT PROTEINURIA
- Exercise
- Orthostatic (only present when upright)
- Fever

PERSISTENT PROTEINURIA
- Renal glomerular: membranous, focal glomerulonephritis; membranoproliferative glomerulonephritis; postinfectious glomerulonephritis
- Diabetes
- Medications: gold, penicillamine, ACE inhibitors, heroin, analgesics, antibiotics
- Malignant tumor: colon, lung, breast, lymphoma
- Amyloidosis
- Hereditary: sickle cell, Alport's syndrome, hereditary amyloidosis
- Systemic immunologic disease: systemic lupus erythematosus, Goodpasture's syndrome, rheumatoid arthritis

Table 5-6. Acute glomerulonephritis causing nephritic urinalysis findings

Condition	Comments
Acute poststreptococcal glomerulonephritis	Immunologic evidence of prior streptococcal infection; most patients hypertensive; most cases resolve spontaneously
Membranoproliferative glomerulonephritis	Young adults; usually slowly progressive
Systemic lupus erythematosus	Syndrome criteria presented in Chapter 10
Rapidly progressive glomerulonephritis	Diagnosis associated with many conditions: immune complex (bacterial endocarditis, visceral abscess); systemic lupus erythematosus; vasculitis; Henoch-Schönlein purpura
IgA nephropathy	Microscopic hematuria, some with gross hematuria during viral infections; males > females; can be slowly progressive; most common cause chronic glomerulonephritis; recurs in half of transplant patients
Henoch-Schönlein purpura	Rash
Vasculitis	Polyarteritis nodosa; Wegener's granulomatosis

Vignette Follow-up

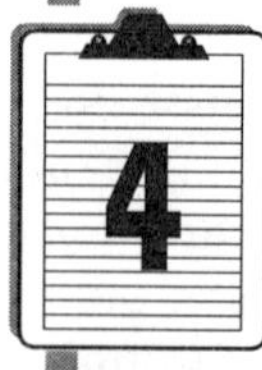

Mr. O is found to have a pulmonary embolus and renal vein thrombosis. He is anticoagulated and continues to be followed for nephrotic syndrome.

Vignette 5

BR is a 57-year-old dentist who recently was hospitalized for the treatment of depression and was given amitriptyline. He has a history of hypertension, for which he takes hydrochlorothiazide. He comes to clinic because his wife has noticed that, since coming home 7 days ago, he has been confused and lethargic.

Physical examination reveals a confused, lethargic middle-aged man. His **blood pressure while sitting** is 124/80 mm Hg, and **pulse** is 80 beats/min (seated). His **standing blood pressure** is 100/56 mm Hg, with a **heart rate** of 105 beats/min. He is oriented to person but does not know the place or date. He knows the names of the president, his wife, and children but cannot perform the serial 7 test. The remainder of the physical examination findings are normal. Laboratory data obtained just before the visit include a serum sodium level of 116 mEq/L and a creatinine level of 1.5 mg/dl.

Vignette Objective

1. Describe how patient assessment allows determining the cause of hyponatremia.

Hyponatremia

Hyponatremia is defined as a serum sodium level of less than 134 mEq/L. However, a patient's symptoms are related to the degree and rate of sodium reduction, and not necessarily the absolute serum sodium concentration. Symptoms usually do not occur until values are less than 125 mEq/L; whereas, levels below 120 mEq/L can result in seizures. A low serum sodium level is appropriate in the setting of an elevated blood glucose or serum triglyceride level (pseudohyponatremia).

The cause of true hyponatremia is established by assessing the intravascular volume, which identifies whether a patient is euvolemic, hypovolemic, or edematous (hypervolemic) (Table 5-7). In hypovolemic patients, the intravascular volume is preserved at the expense of serum osmolarity. A decreased effective renal perfusion (despite hypervolemia and an increased total body sodium level) is associated with congestive heart failure, cirrhosis, and the nephrotic syndrome. Certain drugs (such as NSAIDs and ACE inhibitors) can exacerbate these conditions and also result in hyponatremia. However, the treatment is the opposite of that for hypovolemia (i.e., water restriction rather than the replacement of volume deficits).

Most hyponatremic, euvolemic patients have the syndrome of inappropriate antidiuretic hormone (SIADH). However, before making that diagnosis, hypothyroidism and adrenal insufficiency should be excluded. Hypothyroidism

Table 5-7. Assessment of patients with hyponatremia

Condition[a]	History	Physical examination
Euvolemia (syndrome of inappropriate antidiuretic hormone [SIADH])*	History of lung disorders CNS, disease, or use of certain drugs (e.g., chlorpropamide, narcotics, barbiturates, vincristine, haloperidol, phenothizines, tricyclic antidepressants)	No orthostatic change in blood pressure or heart rate; no findings of CHF, cirrhosis, or nephrotic syndrome
Hypovolemia	History of vomiting, diarrhea; thirsty; light-headedness when upright	Significant orthostatic blood pressure and heart rate changes; reduced skin turgor; dry mucous membranes
Edematous (hypervolemia)	Symptoms of CHF, liver disease, or nephrotic syndrome; weight gain; lower extremity swelling	*CHF:* elevated JVP, displaced PMI, S_3; rales; edema *Cirrhosis:* palmar erythema, spider angiomas, ascites, dilated abdominal veins, splenomegaly, ascites, edema *Nephrotic syndrome:* lower-extremity or generalized edema; proteinuria on urinalysis

[a] When considering SIADH, hypothyroidism and adrenal insufficiency must be excluded.

results in a reduced ability to excrete a water load, and adrenal hormones are needed for appropriate sodium and volume regulation.

Vignette Follow-up

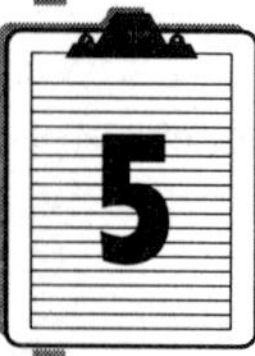

Dr. R has several reasons for his hyponatremia. Although he shows orthostatic changes in his initial vital signs, this could be a side effect of the amitriptyline. He has no history of cardiac, hepatic, or renal problems, and none are suggested by his examination findings. He is taking hydrochlorothiazide, which can result in hyponatremia, but it is elderly women who are most prone to the hyponatremia associated with use of this drug, and it would be unusual for this side effect to develop after several years of treatment. In addition, use of the tricyclic antidepressant amitriptyline can cause SIADH. BR is admitted to the hospital, treated with free water restriction, and the diuretic and tricyclic antidepressant are discontinued. His serum sodium level increases over a 3-day period.

Vignette 6

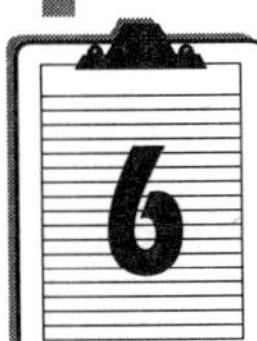

GH is a 68-year-old Asian man whose previous primary care physician has retired. The patient has long-standing, difficult-to-control hypertension. Currently he takes a diuretic (50 mg of hydrochlorothiazide per day), along with the alpha-beta blocker labetalol. He also takes two to four calcium carbonate tablets daily for the relief of heartburn.

His medical history is significant for prostate cancer, treated with radiation therapy 2 years ago. His prostate-specific antigen (PSA) levels are measured every 6 months and have been within the normal range. He has no bone pain, arthralgias, or arthritis. He relates that, over the past few months, he has been more constipated than usual, but otherwise feels well. He is a retired electrical engineer and remains physically active by taking 3-mile walks daily and working in his garden.

Vignette Objectives

1. List the manifestations of hypercalcemia that are independent of its cause.
2. How do the history and physical examination findings relate to the different causes of hypercalcemia?

Hypercalcemia

Primary hyperparathyroidism is the most common cause of hypercalcemia among outpatients. Malignancy predominates as the cause of severe hypercalcemia necessitating hospitalization and can cause hypercalcemia by means of several mechanisms: direct involvement of bone and elaboration of parathyroid-like hormones, osteoclast-activating factors, and other substances affecting bone homeostasis.

Potential causes of hypercalcemia are listed in Table 5-8. Marked hypercalcemia usually is associated with hypovolemia (as a consequence of anorexia, decreased fluid intake, and increased sodium and water excretion), which accentuates the disorder. Volume replacement is an important component of management, independent of hypercalcemia's cause.

Vignette Follow-up

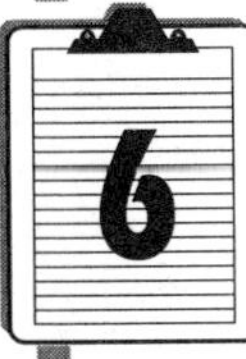

GH has several potential causes for his hypercalcemia: hydrochlorothiazide use, excess calcium intake, prior malignancy, and a new diagnosis of either hyperparathyroidism or another condition causing hypercalcemia. Subsequent evaluation determines that GH has primary hyperparathyroidism.

Table 5-8. Causes of hypercalcemia*

Etiology	History	Physical examination
Primary hyperparathyroidism	Often asymptomatic; "bones, stones, abdominal groans, and psychological moans," relate to findings of osteoporosis, nephrolithiasis, peptic ulcer disease, and vague complaints, respectively	Hypertension, band keratopathy, hyporeflexia
Malignant tumor: spread to bone (usually breast, lung, myeloma, lymphoma, or prostate); hormone-mediated (squamous cell of lung, head and neck, transitional cell of bladder or ovarian)	Bone pain, history of malignant tumor	Bone pain in response to palpation; pathologic fractures; evidence of metastatic disease almost always present
Drugs	Hydrochlorothiazide; lithium; calcium and bicarbonate ("milk alkali" syndrome); vitamin D intoxication	—
Immobilization	Occurs among children; rarely those with Paget's disease or hyperthyroidism	—

*Granulomatous disease also can cause hypercalcemia (e.g., sarcoidosis, tuberculosis)

Vignette 7

Incontinence: involuntary loss of urine.

KW is a 50-year-old woman who comes to clinic for her annual Pap smear. Although she is in good general health, review of systems discloses a history of urinary urgency and "losing urine" when she coughs or sneezes. She continues to have regular menses and believes her bleeding has become heavier. She is gravida 1, para 1. She was widowed last year and is not sexually active.

Abnormalities revealed by the physical examination are limited to the **pelvic** examination. Her external genitalia, vagina, and cervix appear normal. A cystocele is demonstrable with a Valsalva's maneuver. Her uterus is enlarged, firm, movable, and nontender. Adnexa cannot be appreciated because of uterine enlargement.

Vignette Objective

1. How can you obtain information about continence? What additional information would help establish the problem's cause?

Incontinence

Incontinence is a prevalent disorder that occurs most frequently among older people, women, and those whose functional status is reduced. Among adults living in senior citizen communities, 15% to 40% experience incontinence; over half of the institutionalized elderly have the disorder.

Questions concerning continence usually are introduced during the genitourinary review of systems and can include such questions as: "Do you have any trouble with urination?" To clarify what urination means, however, one may need to ask instead: "Do you ever lose urine or wet yourself?" or "Are there times when you lose your urine before you reach the bathroom?"

In general, there are four types of incontinence, but history and physical examination findings are not specific enough to accurately differentiate among these (Table 5-9) and conditions often coexist. Identifying the cause of incontinence can be assisted by the patient keeping a diary of fluid intake, medication use, voiding, and incontinence. Catheterizing the patient, after he or she voluntarily empties the bladder, and assessing the postvoid residual is appropriate for most patients. Both bladder outlet obstruction and a large flaccid bladder result in a high (>100 ml) postvoid volume; in either case, referral to a urologist is needed.

In addition to suggesting a cause, patient assessment can identify intercurrent problems that can exacerbate incontinence. The mnemonic DDIAPERS is useful to remember these factors (Table 5-10).

Table 5-9. Evaluation of patients with incontinence

Type of incontinence	History	Physical examination
"URGENCY INCONTINENCE" Detrusor instability due to bladder irritation resulting from infection or inflammation, or an uninhibited bladder due to loss of central nervous system control	Inability to make it to the toilet; small volume of urine; urgency, nocturia, frequency; incomplete emptying; history of stroke or other central nervous system disorder; complete spinal cord lesions at T-7	Other neurologic abnormalities, such as dementia or residua from prior CVAs
"STRESS INCONTINENCE": Due to sphincter dysfunction	Loss of small amounts of urine when straining, laughing, or coughing; inability to stop the urinary stream while voiding; associated with multiparity, obesity, menopause, and aging	Cystocele may be present
"BOO AND OVERFLOW INCONTINENCE": Incontinence due to bladder outlet obstruction (BOO)	Frequency, nocturia, hesitancy initiating stream, decreased stream force, bladder fullness; worsened by use of drugs with anticholinergic effects	Elderly man (BPH) with large prostate; distended bladder (suprapubic mass); postvoid residual volume of ≥300 ml
"FLACCID OVERFLOW INCONTINENCE": Large flaccid bladder due to a neuropathy	Diabetes, multiple sclerosis; loss of bladder sensation; results in urinary tract infections due to "stagnant" urine; worsened by use of drugs with anticholinergic side effects	Distended bladder; increased postvoid residua; other neurologic abnormalities

Table 5-10. Factors exacerbating incontinence: DDIAPERS

Drugs: diuretics, sedatives, and medications with anticholinergic effects
Delirium
Infection
Atrophic vaginitis due to estrogen deficiency
Psychological disorders, especially depression
Endocrine: hyperglycemia causing an osmotic diuresis
Restricted mobility, so that it becomes more difficult to get to a toilet
Stool impaction can cause acute bladder outlet obstruction

Vignette Follow-up

KW undergoes an abdominal hysterectomy for removal of a large uterine fibroid and surgical correction of her stress incontinence. She is doing well 6 months after surgery.

Vignette 8

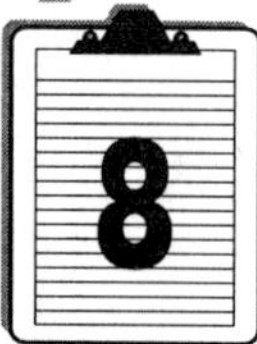

LG is a healthy 31-year-old man who urinates what he thought was blood. The episode occurred after jogging his typical 2 to 3 miles, which he does three to four times a week. When he returned home, LG voided red urine, but his next void was clear. He denies running on a new surface, wearing new shoes, or changing any of his routine. He has no excessive muscle soreness, flank pain, or other urinary complaints. He has no history of trauma and no use of medications. The patient does not smoke and has not been exposed to toxic chemicals. His family history is notable for a father with kidney stones.

Approximately a week after the first episode, the symptom occurs a second time and he comes to clinic for evaluation. Mr. G's **vital signs** and **general physical examination** findings are normal. Findings from urinalysis (performed 3 days after the second episode) are normal except for 5 to 10 red blood cells/high-power field.

Vignette Objective

1. How do the history and physical examination findings relate to possible causes of "red urine"?

Hematuria

Hematuria is a common problem with many potential causes. It is initially categorized as either gross (blood visible on inspection) or microscopic (red blood cells seen only with dipstick and microscopic evaluation). The relative frequency of the different diagnoses varies for the two types of hematuria and also with the patient's age and sex. The patient's history and physical examination provide information to guide management. However, not all red, dark, or smokey urine is due to the presence of red blood cells. Myoglobin (resulting from muscle breakdown) and certain drugs (e.g., rifampin, quinine, and levadopa) can also cause this finding. Causes of "red urine" are listed in Table 5-11, and the categories of disorders causing hematuria can be remembered by the mnemonic R(enal stone) HITT (Table 5-12). The possible diagnoses in patients with either gross or microscopic hematuria are presented in Table 5-13.

Nephrolithiasis causing gross hematuria usually is associated with severe flank pain or renal colic. Rarely it can cause asymptomatic hematuria. If the renal function is normal and urinalysis findings are not suggestive of an acute in-

Table 5-11. Categories of disorders causing red urine

Disorder	Cause
Pigmenturia without hematuria (positive dipstick, without RBCs)	Beets, certain drugs, myoglobin from muscle breakdown; hemoglobinuria
Hematologic	Coagulopathies, sickle cell trait
Kidney, prostate, and collecting system	Acute and chronic glomerulonephritis; Buerger's (IgA) nephropathy; polycystic kidneys; genitourinary stones; infection; arteriovenous malformation; neoplasms: bladder (60%), renal (40%); benign prostatic hypertrophy; direct renal trauma; bladder trauma; and factitious

Table 5-12. Disorders causing hematuria: RHITT

Category	Comments
Renal stones: nephrolithiasis	Usually associated with severe renal colic and dysuria; history of nephrolithiasis
Hemoglobinopathy: sickle trait and rarely coagulopathies	Family history; sickle cell trait usually asymptomatic
Infection (cystitis, prostatitis or pyelonephritis)	Frequency, dysuria, fever, flank pain
Transitional cell tumor or renal cell (hypernephroma)	Risk for transitional cell tumor increases with tobacco use, analgesic abuse, cyclophosphamide, exposure to certain dyes, and pelvic irradiation; bladder tumors often asymptomatic; renal cell carcinoma can be associated with bruit or palpable mass
Trauma	History of trauma, flank ecchymosis
Other (benign prostatic hypertrophy [BPH], polycystic kidney disease)	Symptoms of BPH (decreased stream, nocturia); family history (polycystic kidney disease)

Table 5-13. Possible diagnoses in patients with hematuria

Condition	Comments
GROSS HEMATURIA	
Infection (most common)	Acute onset of dysuria, frequency; pyuria with hematuria
Benign prostatic hypertrophy	Elderly men; prostatic enlargement found on digital rectal examination
Urologic malignant tumor	Risk increases with age and exposure to carcinogens (tobacco, analgesic abuse, cyclophosphamide, dyes)
Nephrolithiasis	Usually symptomatic with flank pain, renal colic
Other	Sickle cell trait, trauma, polycystic kidney disease, malignant tumor
MICROSCOPIC HEMATURIA	
Urologic malignancy	More common if male and >50 years old
Nephrolithiasis	Rarely asymptomatic; most cases associated with acute renal colic
Benign prostatic hypertrophy	Elderly men; prostatic enlargement found on digital rectal examination
Glomerulonephritis	Hypertension; urinalysis shows proteinuria and cellular casts
Polycystic kidney disease	Autosomal dominant inheritance, flank mass
No diagnosis established	Persistent hematuria makes this less likely

fection or glomerulonephritis, it is important to evaluate all patients for malignancy, which requires an intravenous pyelogram and cystoscopy.

Exercise alone has been associated with hematuria, but its mechanism is not known. It is thought to result from bladder trauma, caused as the empty bladder strikes the prostate gland. The disorder is more common among men, and the exercise resulting in hematuria usually is intense or prolonged.

Vignette Follow-up

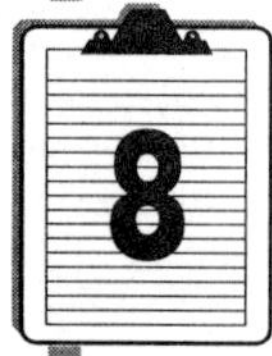

LG had cystoscopic resection of a low-grade, transitional cell cancer of the bladder and has not had recurrence by surveillance cystoscopy over the past six years.

Vignette 9

Renal colic: severe pain located in the flank or costovertebral angle (not in the lumbar area or low back).

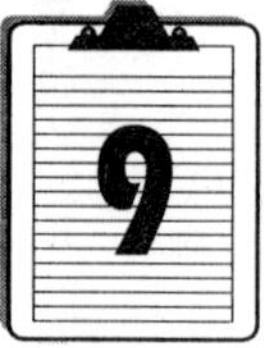

PZ is a 43-year-old man who was vacationing with his family, when right-sided "back pain," associated with nausea and vomiting, developed. He had no chills, fever, dysuria, trauma, or history of renal stones. The pain caused him to writhe, and he did not feel comfortable in any position. He describes the pain as constant, but its intensity fluctuates from "tolerable" to severe. The pain radiates from his right flank to the right lower quadrant. He called his brother-in-law to take him to the emergency room.

Physical examination reveals an uncomfortable man who is frequently changing positions on the gurney. His **blood pressure** is 136/86 mm Hg, and his **heart rate** is 88 beats/min. His **temperature** is 37.0°C. The only abnormal physical finding is **right flank tenderness** in response to fist percussion.

Vignette Objectives

1. What are the symptoms of a kidney stone and renal colic?
2. How do the findings of renal colic differ from the findings of an "acute abdomen"?

Renal Colic

Symptomatic nephrolithiasis is characterized by the sudden onset of severe flank pain. The pain is constant but can vary in intensity. It can radiate to the labia or testes. The peritoneal irritation of acute abdominal conditions is increased with movement, and patients prefer to lie still. Unlike patients with an intraabdominal process, patients with renal colic (with retroperitoneal pain) often writhe in an attempt to find a comfortable position. Although patients with renal colic can show mild tenderness in response to abdominal palpation, peritoneal signs are absent and the greatest tenderness is produced by percussing the costovertebral angle.

The history assists in defining the cause of nephrolithiasis. Most stones consist of calcium oxalate. A high intake of calcium-containing foods or antacids should be sought in patients suspected of having stones. A family or personal history of renal stones, gout, or recent urinary tract infection with urea-splitting organisms *(Proteus mirabilis)* can lead to the formation of uric acid or struvite (magnesium-ammonia-phosphate) stones. If fluid intake is low, especially during hot weather or with prolonged physical activity, the urinary concentration of stone-producing substances can increase.

Vignette Follow-up

Mr. Z is given parenteral analgesics, and an intravenous pyelogram reveals a distal ureteral stone. Mr. Z also is treated with intravenous fluids (to increase urinary flow) and passes a calcium oxalate stone as an outpatient 1 day later.

Vignettes 10, 11, and 12

Pyelonephritis: infection of the kidney.
Cystitis: infection of the bladder epithelium.
Urethritis: inflammation of the urethra, usually due to infection.
Vaginitis: infection of the vaginal epithelium.
Prostatitis: infection of the prostate gland.

BW is a 57-year-old woman who is complaining of progressive burning pain with urination of 1 week's duration. She also is experiencing urinary frequency, such that she is getting up several times at night to void. She has felt "warm" but has not taken her temperature.

Her history is notable for rheumatic fever as a child. She has undergone mitral valve commissurotomies 15 and 5 years ago. Her cardiac rhythm is chronic atrial fibrillation, and she has been receiving anticoagulants since her initial mitral valve surgery. In addition, her blood glucose level has been slightly elevated (ranging from 110 to 155 mg/dl) for the past year. She is not on any drug therapy for hyperglycemia and has been trying to walk daily and decrease her caloric intake.

Physical examination reveals a moderately overweight woman. Vital signs: **temperature** is 38.9°C orally, **supine blood pressure** is 150/80 mm Hg, and **heart rate** is 108 beats/min; **seated values** are 130/70 mm Hg and 120 beats/min (irregularly irregular). **HEENT:** mild retinal artery narrowing; oropharynx is clear, with dry mucous membranes. **Chest:** rales at both bases. **Cardiac:** venous pressure is estimated to be 11 cm of H_2O. A 3/6 systolic murmur is heard at the left lower sternal border, radiating to the apex. No opening snap, diastolic murmur, or S_3 can be appreciated. **Abdomen:** active bowel sounds and no organomegaly or masses. Examination of her **back** reveals bilateral costovertebral tenderness. **Extremities:** 1+ lower extremity pretibial edema.

AT is a 62-year-old woman who calls to make an appointment because she thinks she has a "bladder infection." However, upon talking with Ms. T over the phone, it is found that her symptoms are primarily a foul-smelling vaginal discharge. She is g5, p4014 (full term pregnancies, premature births, abortions, [spontaneous and therapeutic], living children) and her menses stopped 6 years ago. She is sexually active with one partner, her husband. Intercourse is uncomfortable, however, and she notes persistent irritation at her introitus. She has not had similar symptoms previously, although she has had "yeast" infections associated with antibiotic use and had a couple of episodes of cystitis in her 20s. Her husband has no genitourinary tract symptoms.

AT is in good general health and takes no medications. She has never taken estrogen replacement therapy. Her physical examination abnormalities are confined to the **pelvic** examination. Inspection of the vaginal and cervical mucosa reveals that the mucosa is friable. Bimanual palpation reveals no cervical motion tenderness, a small antiflexed uterus, and nonpalpable ovaries.

SR is a healthy 27-year-old man complaining of a penile discharge and painful urination. The symptoms began abruptly yesterday, and these are his only

complaints. He specifically reports no fever, arthralgia, rash, and prior similar episodes. During the last four months, he had unprotected sexual contact with four women; as far as known, his partners have not had recent genitourinary infections. SR has not had a symptomatic sexually transmitted disease (STD). However, two years ago, based on blood tests done at a free clinic, he was treated for syphilis with a "penicillin shot." His test for HIV, at that time, was negative.

Physical examination reveals a man who appears to be healthy. His **blood pressure** is 135/78 mm Hg, **heart rate** is 82 beats/minute, and oral **temperature** is 37.0°C. **HEENT:** oropharynx is clear, no adenopathy. **Chest:** clear to auscultation. **Cardiac:** no jugular venous distention; PMI was within the midclavicular line; S_1 and S_2 were normal, without murmur or gallop. **Abdomen:** no tenderness, liver percussion span of 8 cm and not palpable; no mass. **Genitalia:** uncircumcised, without penile or scrotal skin lesions; no testicular or epididymal mass; purulent discharge expressed from the urethra; no inguinal adenopathy. **Rectal:** prostate mildly tender, without nodules and not fluctuant. **Extremities:** no evidence tenosynovitis or arthritis. **Skin:** no isolated skin lesions or rash.

Vignette Objectives

1. How do the history and physical examination findings help differentiate among potential diagnoses in a patient with dysuria?
2. How do the list of diagnoses differ for women and men with dysuria?
3. How do the history and physical examination findings help differentiate among the causes of vaginitis?
4. What are common causes of a urethral discharge and which aspects of the history and physical examination can help identify the cause?

Urinary Tract Infections

In both women and men, urinary tract infections can occur in the urethra, bladder (cystitis), or kidney (pyelonephritis). The different anatomic locations of genitourinary tract infections and their characteristics are presented in Table 5-14. In addition, prostatitis can develop in men, and vaginitis can cause dysuria and frequency of urination in women.

Cystitis usually causes dysuria, frequency, urgency of urination, and lower abdominal (suprapubic) discomfort. Although it is common in women (at least 20% of women experience cystitis), it is uncommon among men. This difference is likely due to the fact that men have a longer urethra, which increases the distance bacteria have to ascend to reach the bladder. Risk factors for women with cystitis include sexual activity and diaphragm and cervical cap use.

Not all dysuria is due to cystitis. The most common cause of dysuria among women is vaginitis. The symptoms of vaginitis and cystitis overlap, and a pelvic examination and urinalysis often are needed to differentiate between the

Table 5-14. Differentiating the location of urinary tract infections

Condition	History	Physical examination
Pyelonephritis	Dysuria; flank or costovertebral pain; high fever; nausea, vomiting	Costovertebral angle tenderness; temperature >101°F (38.3°C)
Cystitis (up to a third of cases can involve upper tract without any additional symptoms)	Dysuria, frequency; lower abdominal (suprapubic) pain; low-grade fever	Lower abdominal tenderness
Urethritis	Sexually active; dysuria (abrupt onset), usually within a few days of exposure (if gonococcus) or 1–2 weeks after exposure (if nongonococcal); urethral discharge copious (with gonococcus) versus scant with nongonococcal infections	Inguinal adenopathy; swelling and tenderness of scrotum (secondary epididymitis / orchitis)
Acute prostatitis	Age >35; dysuria, urethral discharge, frequency, and urgency; fever, chills; bladder outlet obstruction symptoms (frequency, dribbling, hesitancy)	Tender, boggy prostate; palpable bladder (if bladder outlet obstruction)

two. Vaginitis is usually due to candidiasis, *Trichomonas* infection, vaginosis associated with *Gardnerella vaginalis* infection, or nonspecific (i.e., no cause is identified). The characteristic features of the first three are listed in Table 5-15, and the last is a diagnosis of exclusion. However, the specificity of symptoms has been found to be limited, and microscopic examination of the discharge usually is needed to establish the diagnosis.

Estrogen deficiency results in thinning of the vaginal epithelium and decreased vaginal secretions. Estrogen therapy (discussed further in Chapter 9) may be needed to promote healing and cause the symptoms of vaginosis to resolve. Other less frequent causes of vaginal irritation include contact dermatitis caused by spermacides, douches, or deodorant sprays.

The symptoms of urethritis (Table 5-16) and cystitis are similar. Suprapubic discomfort may be a more prominent symptom among women with cystitis. In men, a urethral discharge can distinguish urethritis from cystitis. Acute prostatitis often is associated with severe perineal pain, a penile discharge, and an exquisitely tender, boggy prostate gland. Chronic prostatitis, however, usually is not accompanied by fever or the same marked prostate tenderness.

A man with a urinary tract infection proximal to the urethra requires a urologic evaluation to investigate for anatomic abnormalities leading to the infection. A suspected prostatic foci of infection can influence both the choice of antibiotic and the duration of therapy.

Table 5-15. Causes of vaginitis

Etiology	History	Physical examination	Comments
Candidiasis	Pruritus involving vagina and vulva; recent antibiotic use; glycosuria; HIV disease	Erythema, edema; vulvar involvement with satellite lesions	Thick, white discharge; pH <4.5
Trichomonal infection	Dysuria, frequency; multiple sexual partners; prior sexually transmitted infections	Petechiae of the cervix	Copious purulent discharge
Vaginosis (mixed infection with anaerobes and *Gardnerella vaginalis*)	Fishy smell, especially after intercourse	—	Thin, foul-smelling discharge; pH >4.5; amine odor (fishy smell) produced when potassium hydroxide added preparing the microscopic examination

Table 5-16. Causes of urethritis

Etiology	History	Physical examination
N. gonorrhoea	Abrupt onset of symptoms about 1 week after exposure; complaint of purulent discharge	Expressible purulent urethral discharge
Non-gonococcal urethritis (NGU) (*Chlamydia trichomatous* is the etiology for approximately 50%, and no etiology is defined for 20%)	Symptoms begin 10 to 14 days after contact; scant, clear or mucoid discharge; symptoms can be urethral itching rather than dysuria	Minimal expressible urethral discharge
Reiter's syndrome (also called reactive arthritis; this syndrome much less common than other two disorders)	Usually illness of young men; onset may be 1 to 3 weeks following venereal or enteric infection; approximately 50% of patients have urethritis as initial symptom; other manifestations can cause eye, rheumatologic, and skin complaints	Classic triad is urethritis, ocular findings (conjunctivitis or anterior uveitis), and arthritis (unilateral sacroilitis, synovitis of 1 to 6 large joints, and inflammation at insertion tendons on bone); mucocutaneous findings also can be present

Pyelonephritis is an upper genitourinary tract or kidney infection, but the symptoms and signs do not always distinguish an upper from a lower urinary tract infection. Lower urinary tract infections involve the urinary epithelium, and upper urinary tract infections affect the kidney parenchyma, resulting in systemic symptoms. Findings suggestive of upper urinary tract infection are high fever, costovertebral pain, and costovertebral-angle percussion tenderness. Pyelonephritis can be associated with bacteremia, and its manifestations can include septic shock.

Vignette Follow-ups

BW is admitted to the hospital, where parenteral antibiotic therapy is begun after blood and urine specimens are obtained for culture. Concern about a bacteremia seeding her mitral valve has prompted the acquisition of three sets of blood cultures before the start of the parenteral antibiotics. Urine culture grows more than 100,000 colonies of *Escherichia coli,* and blood cultures are sterile. After 2 days of intravenous antibiotics, Ms. W is switched to oral antibiotics and discharged. She completes a course of oral antibiotics. Besides the danger of endocarditis, Ms. R's diabetes puts her at increased risk for the complications of pyelonephritis, such as a perinephric abscess, papillary necrosis, and emphysematous pyelonephritis. Her symptoms resolve quickly, but persistent fever or flank pain would have prompted immediate radiographic visualization of her genitourinary system.

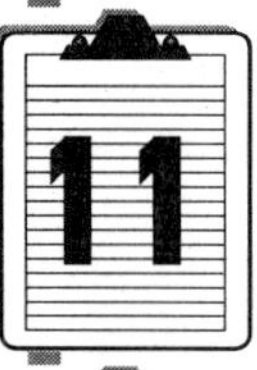

AT is thought to have vaginosis and atrophic vaginitis. She receives metronidazole and oral estrogens. Initially she prefers only short-term estrogen replacement in an effort to resolve her infection, but because she notes a reduction in the number of her rare hot flashes and a more restful sleep, she elects to continue with long-term combined estrogen and progesterone therapy.

As is the case for most cases of symptomatic gonococcal urethritis, intracellular gram negative diplococci were seen on microscopic examination of the discharge. Cultures for GC and an antigen test for *Chlamydia* were obtained. Because of the frequent coexistence of *N. Gonorrhoea* and *C. Trichomatous* infection, SR received an injection of ceftriaxone and oral doxycycline. He declined an HIV test and was counseled about notifying contacts and safe-sex behaviors.

Vignette 13

MR is a 39-year-old man with severe pain in the left side of his scrotum. He has pain with urination and a low-grade "fever" (he has felt hot but has not measured his temperature). He has no history of genitourinary trauma, no exposure to sexually transmitted disease and no symptoms of urinary outflow obstruction. Abnormal physical examination findings are limited to the **testes,** where an exquisitely tender, nodular mass is palpable at the posterosuperior aspect of the left testicle, extending down toward the lower pole. The mass cannot be transilluminated.

Vignette Objective

1. What are causes of acute scrotal pain and how can the history and physical examination findings differentiate among the conditions causing acute scrotal pain?

Acute Testicular Pain

Pain in the testes is a common complaint and can be due to infections (epididymitis and orchitis), trauma, malignancies, ischemia resulting from testicular torsion, and an incarcerated scrotal hernia. In addition, testicular pain can be referred pain from a renal or intraabdominal process. A feature that helps differentiate torsion from epididymitis is the effect of position on the pain. Pain is exacerbated when a patient with testicular torsion is in the supine position, whereas discomfort is reduced in a patient with epididymitis (Prehn's sign). Identifying torsion is critical because the ischemia results in irreversible damage within 24 hours of onset.

The causes of epididymitis vary with age. Sexually active, younger men with epididymitis often have sexually transmitted disease, whereas affected older patients (with progressive prostate enlargement) typically have a prostatic infection. The disorder can be distinguished from torsion on the basis of its more gradual onset, the fever associated with the infection, epididymal tenderness, and pyuria.

Usually, testicular malignancies and epididymal masses (spermatocele, tumor, and chronic syphilis or tuberculosis) are nontender. However, testicular tumors can cause pain, and the fact that a patient has testicular pain does not exclude a malignancy.

Vignette Follow-up

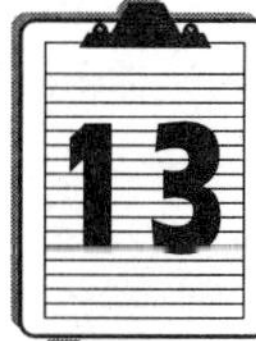

MR is thought to have epididymitis. He is treated with supine rest, elevation of the scrotum, oral antibiotics, and ibuprofen. He feels much better within 36 hours and had no recurrence.

Vignette 14

HS is a 62-year-old physician who visits your clinic because he "hasn't had a physical examination for the past 10 years." He has a history of mild hypertension, treated intermittently with diuretics. He has no complaints other than some nocturia, urinary hesitancy, and a feeling that his bladder is not emptying completely. These symptoms seem to be made worse by coffee and alcohol consumption. When he used a decongestant for the relief of a recent upper respiratory tract infection, his urinary stream was "reduced to a trickle." He has no history of urinary tract infections, urethral manipulation, penile discharge, or sexually transmitted diseases. He has no complaints of back or bone pain.

Physical examination reveals a mildly overweight man with a **blood pressure** of 144/92 mm Hg and **heart rate** of 78 beats/min. His general physical examination findings are normal. **Rectal** examination reveals normal rectal tone. The **prostate** is nontender but enlarged 2+ to 3+, with a small, hard nodule on the left posterior lobe. **Inguinal nodes** are not palpable.

Vignette Objective

1. What are the symptoms and signs of benign prostatic hypertrophy (BPH) and prostate cancer?

Prostate Hypertrophy and Cancer

The androgen-mediated growth of the prostate gland continues as men age, and more than 80% of men over age 80 have BPH. The prostate gland surrounds the urethra, and enlargement results in compression of the urethra in this site. Digital rectal examination usually detects prostate enlargement, but because palpation only evaluates one side of the gland, a normal-sized prostate does not necessarily exclude BPH. That is, hypertrophy of the anterior gland can cause obstruction, even though the gland feels normal to palpation. Carcinomas usually are indurated and appreciated as either a single, discrete nodule or an irregular nodular area. Palpable nodules require biopsy, because benign processes cannot be distinguished from cancer on the basis of physical examination findings. Ten to thirty percent of biopsied nodules are found to be malignant.

In men, prostate cancer is the second most common cancer and the third most common cause of cancer death. Prostate cancer occasionally presents with symptoms of urinary outflow obstruction, but it often is asymptomatic, especially in its early stages. Digital palpation is the best way to detect prostate cancer (with the exception of Stage A cancer, which, by definition, is a cancer not detectable by digital examination).

Prostate cancer spreads by contiguous, lymphatic, and hematogenous dissemination. Common sites of bony metastasis include the pelvis, vertebrae, ribs, skull, and long bones. Bone involvement can cause pain or be asymptomatic until pathologic fracture or spinal cord compression occurs.

Vignette Follow-up

Dr. S is found to have an elevated PSA level, and an ultrasound-guided needle biopsy specimen shows prostate cancer. He has no evidence of distant metastasis or local spread from the prostate capsule. A radical prostatectomy is performed, and he continues to do well 2 years after treatment. His PSA level remains normal.

Objectives Review

1. What communication strategies are useful when talking with patients about a treatment plan? What strategies improve patients' adherence to treatment plans?
2. What history and physical examination findings are associated with end-stage renal disease?
3. What aspects of a patient's evaluation are most important for establishing the cause of oliguria or a low urine output?
4. How do the findings differ in patients with lower extremity edema due to congestive heart failure, cirrhosis, nephrotic syndrome, and venous obstruction?
5. What are the most frequent causes of nephrotic syndrome and how does the assessment differ for each?
6. Describe how patient assessment allows determining the cause of hyponatremia.
7. List the manifestations of hypercalcemia that are independent of its cause.
8. How do the history and physical examination findings relate to the different causes of hypercalcemia?
9. How can you obtain information about continence? What additional information would help establish the problem's cause?
10. How do the history and physical examination findings relate to possible causes of "red urine"?
11. What are the symptoms of a kidney stone and renal colic?
12. How do the findings of renal colic differ from those with an "acute abdomen"?
13. How do the history and physical examination findings help differentiate among potential diagnoses in a patient with dysuria?
14. How do the list of diagnoses differ for women and men with dysuria?
15. How do the history and physical examination findings help differentiate among the causes of vaginitis?
16. What are common causes of a ureteral discharge and which aspects of the history and physical examination can help identify the cause?
17. What are causes of acute scrotal pain and how can the history and physical examination findings differentiate among the conditions causing acute scrotal pain?

18. What are the symptoms and signs of benign prostatic hypertrophy and prostate cancer?

Suggested Reading

Berg AO, Soman MP. Lower genitourinary infections in women. *J Fam Pract* 1986;23: 61–7.
The authors review the topics of vaginitis, cystitis, urethral syndrome, urethritis, and cervicitis; typical findings and a management algorithm are presented.

Berger RE. Acute epididymitis: etiology and therapy. *Semin Urol* 1991;9:28–31.
Discussion of epididymitis among children and heterosexual and homosexual men; author points out that scrotal pain of epididymitis is accompanied by pyuria, especially in first 50 ml of voided urine; torsion can be evaluated with ultrasound and technetium scanning; one of four men with a testicular tumor has pain, and if pain and mass do not resolve, patients require surgical exploration.

Bilezikian JP. Management of acute hypercalcemia. *N Engl J Med* 1992;326:1196–1202.
The author addresses the management of patients hospitalized with severe hypercalcemia; differential diagnosis is discussed briefly; most of the text focuses on therapeutic options.

Chauveau D, Knebelmann B, Grünfeld J-P. Inherited kidney diseases: polycystic kidney disease and Alport's syndrome. *Adv Intern Med* 1995;40:303–39.
The authors present a thorough review of both conditions, including new information about genetics and prenatal/presymptomatic screening.

Edelstein H, McCabe RE. Perinephric abscess. Modern diagnosis and treatment in 47 cases. *Medicine* 1988;67:118–31.
Authors present data on patients collected over 30 years at U.C.S.F.; abscesses were associated with nephrolithiasis, genitourinary surgery, and diabetes; CT scans were useful for diagnosis.

Garnick MB. Prostate cancer: screening, diagnosis, and management. *Ann Intern Med* 1993;118:804–18.
Review article in which the author synthesizes information on the screening, presentation, staging, and treatment [including newer managements of prostate cancer].

Johnson JR, Stamm WE. Urinary tract infections in women: diagnosis and treatment. *Ann Intern Med* 1989;11:906–17.
The authors present a thorough review of women's urinary tract infections, including a discussion of the choice of antibiotics and duration of therapy.

Raghavan D, Shipley WU, Garnick MB, Russell PJ, Richie JP. Biology and management of bladder cancer. *N Engl J Med* 1990;322:1129–36.
Review that includes information on the malignancy's biologic characteristics and newer managements; authors point out that risks for bladder cancer include tobacco use, phenacetin use, coffee consumption, schistosomiasis, and exposure to aniline dyes.

Resnick NM, Yalla SV. Management of urinary incontinence in the elderly. *N Engl J Med* 1985;313:800–4.
Brief review article in which the DDIAPERS mnemonic is presented.

Schaat VM, Perez-Stable EJ, Borchardt K. The limited value of symptom and signs in the diagnosis of vaginal infections. *JAMA* 1990;150:1929–33.
Although certain findings can characterize vaginal infections—vaginosis (foul-smelling discharge), candidiasis (pruritus), and trichomoniasis (copious purulent discharge)—the symptoms and signs are not discriminatory; despite appropriate evaluation, no definite cause is established for many women's symptoms.

Stamm WE, Hooton TM. Management of urinary tract infections in adults. *N Engl J Med* 1993;329:1328–34.
Authors highlight recent treatment advances for young women with cystitis, those with recurrent cystitis and pyelonephritis, adults with asymptomatic bacteriuria, and patients with complicated infections (due to anatomic abnormalities or unusual organism); useful tables and a management algorithm are presented.

Stephenson BJ, Rowe BH, Haynes RB, Macharia WM, Leon G. The rational clinical examination: is this patient taking the treatment as prescribed? *JAMA* 1993;269:2779–81.
Careful questioning identifies about half of patients not adhering to recommendations; nonadherence is more likely among those who miss appointments and for whom therapy is not working.

Sutton JM. Evaluation of hematuria in adults. *JAMA* 1990;263:2475–80.
The author discusses microscopic and gross hematuria; much information is contained in this brief review, including a tabulation of causes and specific recommendations for evaluation.

Williams ME, Pannill FC III. Urinary incontinence in the elderly: physiology, pathophysiology, diagnosis, and treatment. *Ann Intern Med* 1982;97:895–907.
The authors review the topics of bladder physiology and incontinence management; they classify incontinence as detrusor instability, overflow incontinence, sphincter insufficiency, functional, and iatrogenic.

Woods DR, Bender BS. Long-term urinary tract catheterization. *Med Clin North Am* 1989;73:1441–53.
The authors present indications for chronic catheterization, management of bacteriuria and urinary sepsis treatment, and appropriate catheter care.

6 Hematologic and Oncologic Problems

Objectives

Discuss appropriate ways of delivering bad news and list history and physical examination findings for the following problems:

- Adenopathy
- Anemia
- Bleeding disorders
- Breast cancer
- Cancer screening
- Colon cancer
- Erythrocytosis (increased RBC mass)
- Fever and neutropenia
- HIV disease progression
- Hodgkin's disease
- Lymphoma
- Monoclonal gammopathy
- Myeloma
- Myeloproliferative disorders
- Paraneoplastic syndromes
- Paraproteinemias
- Pernicious anemia
- Polycythemia (elevated hematocrit)
- Prostate cancer
- Pseudoclaudication
- Spinal cord compression
- Superior vena cava syndrome
- Thrombocytopenia
- Thrombocytosis
- Unintentional weight loss
- Vitamin B_{12} deficiency

Pertinent Points

History

History of anemia?
- When, how discovered?
- What caused it?
- Treatment and duration of therapy
- Last hemoglobin or hematocrit
- Symptoms of anemia, such as exertional dyspnea, chest pain, light-headedness

If iron deficiency:
- Diet (meat, tea)
- Pica
- Menses, pregnancy
- Blood donation
- Gastrointestinal (GI) blood loss (melena, hematochezia, use of barrier breakers such as aspirin or NSAIDs, alcohol consumption, history of ulcer or colitis, change in bowel habits)

If macrocytic anemia:
- Alcohol consumption
- Cold intolerance, skin or hair changes
- Memory, balance, family history, ethnicity
- Prior GI problems
- Exposure to parasites
- Diet
- Drugs

If other types of anemia:
- Chronic illnesses
- Family history, ethnicity
- Exposure to marrow toxins, drugs

If polycythemia:
- smoking history, symptoms of chronic pulmonary disease
- weight loss
- heart murmur, cardiac problems
- family history
- bleeding problems or arterial thrombosis
- kidney disease
- pruritus (effect of hot showers)

History of tumors?
- What, when?
- How diagnosed?
- Benign versus malignant
- Available records
- Treatment, follow-up
- Family history of malignancy

Bleeding problems?
- Bleeding with dental work, at surgery or childbirth, menorrhagia
- Bleeding into joints
- Family history of coagulopathies or connective tissue disorders
- Use of aspirin, NSAIDs, other medications
- Liver or renal disease, malabsorption

Swollen glands (lymph nodes)?
- Where, onset, progression
- Fever, tenderness of nodes
- Cutaneous disorders, rash
- Kitten exposure
- Weight loss
- HIV risk factors, prior HIV test

Is your weight stable? For evaluation of unintentional weight loss:
- Other evidence of weight loss (records, pictures, clothing)
- Appetite, intake, food access
- Poor-fitting dentures, problems chewing
- Nausea, vomiting, dysphagia
- Mood, anhedonia, sleep disorder
- Fever, sweats
- Change in stools
- Polyuria, polydipsia
- Heat intolerance, palpitations, tremor

Prior health maintenance procedures?
- Breast self-exam, mammogram, cervical cytology (Pap smear)
- Occult-blood, sigmoidoscopy
- Rectal exam, prostate-specific antigen (PSA)

Physical Examination

Weight, height

Inspection
- for nutritional state

Vital signs
- Blood pressure and heart rate (orthostatic changes if concern about recent blood loss)
- Temperature

Skin and mucous membranes
- Petechiae, purpura, ecchymoses
- Cutaneous signs of malignancy

HEENT
- Plethora, facial edema
- Conjunctival pallor
- Fundi
- Glossitis

Chest
- Percussion and auscultation, evidence of chronic obstructive pulmonary disease (COPD) (erythrocytosis)

Breast
- Mass, tenderness, discharge
- Review breast self-examination

Cardiac
- Jugular venous pressure (JVP)
- Point of maximal impulse (PMI)
- S_1, S_2, additional sounds

Abdominal
- Hepatic size, splenomegaly, mass
- Ascites
- Occult-blood in stool
- Digital prostate exam, anal sphincter tone

Nodes
- Cervical, supraclavicular, axillary, inguinal

Back
- Inspection
- Range of motion
- Paraspinal muscle spasm
- Percussion tenderness of spine

Extremities
- Cyanosis, pallor, petechiae
- Clubbing
- Edema

Mental status
- Orientation, affect, memory, concentration, judgment

Motor
- Proximal and distal muscle strength and symmetry

Reflexes
- Symmetry, pathologic reflexes

Sensory
- Distal vibratory and position sense
- Perineal sensation

Vignettes 1 and 2

Cyanosis: bluish discoloration resulting from deoxygenation of hemoglobin. Peripheral cyanosis is confined to the distal extremities and nail bed capillaries. Central cyanosis involves the areas affected with peripheral cyanosis, as well as the lips and mucous membranes; its presence indicates hypoxemia.

PM is a 62-year-old man being seen in the clinic for several problems, including peripheral vascular disease, long-standing hypertension, alcoholism, and chronic bronchitis. He has a 75 pack year history of smoking cigarettes and continues to smoke. Despite his problems, he generally feels well and is active. He was seen last week because of an exacerbation of his bronchitis. His condition is now improving. A complete blood cell count (CBC) obtained last week revealed a hematocrit of 52%.

BJ is a 59-year-old man who was diagnosed as having polycythemia rubra vera (PRV) 10 years ago. The diagnosis was established on the basis of the findings of erythrocytosis (hematocrit, 53% to 57%), thrombocytosis (platelet count, approximately 900,000/mm^3), and splenomegaly. His CBC is checked at regular intervals, and the hematocrit has never been greater than 57%. He has not required either phlebotomy or myelosuppressive agents. Over the past few years, his hematocrit and platelet count gradually have decreased. Currently his only complaint is pruritus after warm showers. His weight is stable, and he denies a history of headache, neurologic symptoms, abdominal pain, bleeding of thromboembolic problems. He exercises without difficulty five times each week, by swimming or using an exercycle.

Physical examination reveals a well-appearing man. Vital signs: **blood pressure** of 146/80 mm Hg and **heart rate** of 76 beats/min. **Skin:** no rash, excoriations, petechiae, or ecchymoses. **HEENT:** fundi show normal vessels; neck is supple without thyromegaly or adenopathy. **Cardiac:** no jugular venous distention (JVD); nondisplaced PMI; normal S_1 and S_2, without other sounds. **Chest:** clear to auscultation. **Abdomen:** liver span is 10 cm to percussion; spleen is markedly enlarged, nontender, and palpable 11 cm below the left costal margin. **Extremities:** no edema, cyanosis, or clubbing. **Motor:** strength and reflexes are normal and symmetrical.

The patient's CBC includes a white blood count (WBC) of 11,700/mm^3, hemoglobin level of 14.4 gm/dl, and platelet count of 368,000/mm^3; teardrop-shaped red blood cells and an occasional giant platelet are seen on a blood smear. A bone marrow biopsy specimen shows granulocyte hyperplasia, erythroid hypoplasia, and marrow fibrosis. Culture of blood mononuclear cells demonstrates erythroid colonies without erythropoietin stimulation.

Vignette Objectives

1. List the history and physical examination findings relevant to the causes of polycythemia and erythrocytosis.
2. Explain why cyanosis is not a sensitive indicator of hypoxemia, and describe the significance of central and peripheral cyanosis.

Elevation of Hemoglobin and Hematocrit

Polycythemia versus Erythrocytosis

An increased hemoglobin level and hematocrit value (polycythemia) can result from either an increased red blood cell (RBC) mass or reduced plasma volume ("relative" erythrocytosis). A nuclear medicine RBC mass study can distinguish between these disorders and determine whether an elevated hematocrit is due to an increased RBC mass or a decreased plasma volume. The latter disorder is called *Gaisböck's syndrome* (stress or relative erythrocytosis). Gaisböck's syndrome usually affects obese, middle-aged men who smoke. Their hematocrit is rarely greater than 60%. Besides cigarette smoking, they often have other cardiac risk factors, including hypertension and a sedentary life-style. Although relative erythrocytosis does not progress, these patients have a cardiovascular morbidity that is approximately sixfold greater than normal. Management is directed toward reducing the risk factors. Diuretics, which can further increase the hematocrit, are avoided as therapy for their hypertension.

Erythrocytosis

True or absolute erythrocytosis is often separated into either PRV, a myeloproliferative disorder with autonomous RBC production, and secondary causes, in which the marrow is responding to erythropoietin. Most of those with erythrocytosis have the latter problem, although the likelihood of PRV increases with higher hematocrit values. The various causes of erythrocytosis and features of the conditions that result in an elevated hematocrit are listed in Table 6-1.

Hypoxia and Cyanosis

Cyanosis is due to the deoxygenation of hemoglobin and, as already noted, is characterized as being central or peripheral in nature. Approximately 5 gms/dl of deoxygenated hemoglobin are needed for central cyanosis to be seen. However, not all patients with hypoxemia have cyanosis. That is, a patient could be hypoxic, but because of his or her anemia, the deoxygenated hemoglobin could be insufficient for cyanosis to be apparent. Conversely, a patient with an elevated hematocrit would be more likely to show cyanosis with hypoxemia.

Polycythemia Rubra Vera

PRV should be considered whenever the hematocrit is consistently greater than 55% (men) or 50% (women). PRV is one of the myeloproliferative diseases. Depending on the clone of stem cells involved, a myeloproliferative disorder can manifest as PRV, chronic myelogenous leukemia, essential thrombocytosis, or myeloid metaplasia with myelofibrosis. Thrombocytosis usually is due to causes other than a myeloproliferative disorder. The causes of an elevated platelet count and the features of these disorders are listed in Table 6-2.

The findings of PRV result from hypermetabolism (weight loss, increased serum uric acid level, and gout), sludging as the result of the increased blood viscosity (headache), and abnormalities affecting the other cell lines. An increase in the number of basophils is often seen, and patients' pruritus probably relates to this abnormality. This symptom is not a feature of secondary erythrocytosis, in which basophilia does not occur. A predisposition for arterial thrombosis relates to both the degree of hyperviscosity and the degree of thrombocytosis. Splenomegaly is present in approximately three quarters of patients with PRV, but it is not found among those with an elevated hematocrit from other causes.

Phlebotomy is the primary therapy for PRV, because the development of iron deficiency stabilizes the hematocrit at a lower level. H_2-blockers can reduce pruritus, and those with significant thrombocytosis can be treated with aspirin or dipyridamole to prevent platelet aggregation. Marrow suppression therapy increases the long-term risk of malignancy (leukemia, lymphoma) and usually is reserved for older patients.

Table 6-1. Causes of erythrocytosis

Cause	Diagnosis	History	Physical examination
Autonomous RBC production	Polycythemia rubra vera	Headache, pruritus (especially after a hot bath or shower), weight loss, thrombotic events	Facial plethora, engorged retinal veins, suffusion of conjunctiva (blood-shot appearance); splenomegaly
Hypoxia causing appropriate erythropoietin production (compensatory increase in erythropoietin production occurs with PaO_2 <65 mm Hg [saturation <90%])	Pulmonary disease; excess carboxy-hemoglobin level (normal level <0.5%; it increases 0.9% per cigarette, with half-life of 4 hours; smokers can have levels of up to 20%); obstructive sleep apnea (see Table 4-17); high altitude	Smoker (90% of smokers with increased hematocrit have it secondary to smoking–COPD); cough, sputum production, dyspnea on exertion, leg swelling	Central cyanosis; abnormal chest examination findings, if right ventricular failure (due to hypoxia causing pulmonary hypertension), elevated JVP and peripheral edema
	Cyanotic congenital heart disease	History of a murmur	Clubbing, central cyanosis, abnormal cardiac findings
Inappropriate erythropoietin production (elevated erythropoietin with a normal PaO_2 and carboxyhemoglobin level)	Malignancy (usually renal, hepatic, or lung tumors)	Weight loss; lung tumors associated with smoking; hepatomas usually associated with preexisting liver disease, right upper quadrant pain; renal tumors associated with flank pain, hematuria	Lung malignancy often has no signs (see discussion of findings with lung cancer p. 114, in Chapter 4); hepatomas can be accompanied by stigmata of chronic liver disease or by hepatic bruit or rub; renal tumors can have palpable mass
	Benign tumors (cerebellar hemangioma)	Headache; ataxia; hemangiomas can be component of phakomatosis (von Hippel-Lindau disease, autosomal dominant inheritance)	Cerebellar ataxia; with von Hippel-Lindau disease, patient also can have retinal hemangiomas
	Uterine fibroid	Symptoms can be menorrhagia or effects of the mass	Pelvic mass
	Renal cysts and hydronephrosis	Family history of polycystic kidney disease	Palpable kidneys

Table 6-2. Causes of thrombocytosis

Disorder	Findings
Iron deficiency	Peripheral smear shows microcytic and hypochromic RBCs (low mean corpuscular volume and hemoglobin concentration) and elevated platelet count; with iron therapy, platelet count decreases before the hematocrit increases
Post splenectomy	Immediately after surgery, platelets can be >1,000,000/mm³; platelet count is slightly greater than normal levels after several months
"Reactive" thrombocytosis due to inflammatory disorders (rheumatoid arthritis, polyarteritis nodosa), post-operative and acute bleeding	Findings of the underlying inflammatory disorder; history of recent surgery or blood loss
Myeloproliferative disorders	Can be the only abnormality (essential thrombocytosis) or associated with PRV or chronic myelogenous leukemia; increase in number of platelets is related to an increased risk of thrombosis (thrombotic events can include digital ischemia, cerebrovascular accidents, coronary ischemia, and Budd-Chiari syndrome)

Vignette Follow-ups

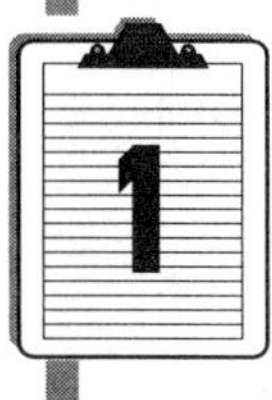

Mr. M's arterial blood gases while breathing room air are as follows: PaO_2, 54 mm Hg, $PaCO_2$, 46 mm Hg, and pH, 7.38. Physical limitations imposed by his other problems perhaps have prevented Mr. M from being more aware of exertional dyspnea. Mr. M is treated with home oxygen therapy and he limits himself to smoking two cigarettes per day. Both these measures cause his erythrocytosis to resolve.

Mr. J is thought to have postpolycythemia myeloid metaplasia, associated with massive splenomegaly and myelofibrosis. He has teardrop-shaped poikilocytosis and extramedullary hematopoiesis.

Vignettes 3 and 4

Pallor: paleness of the skin in areas that usually are pink, an appearance produced by visible capillary vasculature. It is best assessed in the palpebral conjunctivae and palmar creases. However, because of individual variability in skin pigmentation, pallor is not a sensitive indicator of anemia.

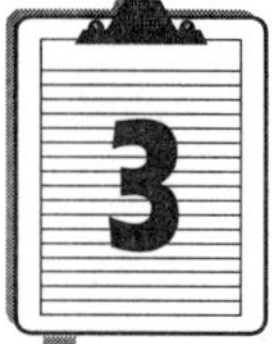

Mrs. S is a 64-year-old woman who has been seen in the clinic for several years. She is in good health and has no chronic problems, except for degenerative joint disease in her hips, which necessitated right hip replacement 2 years ago. This is a routine annual visit to update her health maintenance, but she also has a new concern. She had a blood count done at a local health fair and was told to see her medical care provider because of the finding of anemia. She has felt well and specifically denies fatigue, weight loss, epigastric pain, a change in her bowel habits, blood in her stool, or easy bruising. She eats a "regular diet," that includes red meat every other week. She has donated blood every 6 months for many years. She last donated about 6 months ago and was not told about anemia at that time. Her family history reveals that her mother died of colon cancer.

Her past medical history is significant for the hip surgery and an episode of depression 20 years ago, treated with amitriptyline but not requiring hospitalization. Her only medication is an occasional aspirin. She stopped smoking in 1982 and rarely consumes alcohol. She has been married 43 years and has three grown children, all of whom are alive and well. She and her husband have retired and now live in an isolated area, about 90 minutes from clinic.

Mrs. S is a healthy-appearing woman. Her **blood pressure** is 140/92 mm Hg, and her **heart rate** is 96 beats/min. **Skin:** a few scattered seborrheic keratoses are noted. **HEENT:** normal funduscopic exam findings; the oropharynx is clear; no thyromegaly or adenopathy. Carotids are 2+ without bruits. **Lymph nodes:** none palpable. **Chest:** clear to auscultation. **Cardiac:** no JVD; normal PMI; normal S_1 and S_2, no murmur or gallops. **Breasts:** without masses. **Abdomen:** soft, without organomegaly or mass. **Genitourinary** exam: normal postmenopausal cervical and vaginal mucosa; bimanual exam reveals a normal uterus and no palpable adnexa. Stool is occult-blood negative. **Extremities:** no cyanosis, clubbing, or edema. Her **neurologic** exam findings are normal. Reflexes are symmetrical and 2+, and vibratory sense is intact.

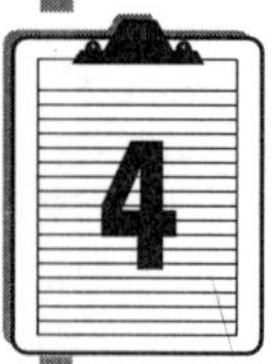

GT is an 86-year-old man who comes to clinic with the complaint of dyspnea on exertion. He has enjoyed good health and has not "needed" a physician in 8 years. Mr. T is extremely active, but this summer he noted shortness of breath while cleaning his house's gutters. He takes no medications and neither smokes nor drinks alcohol. Review of systems does not disclose any general or organ-specific complaints. He is a "confirmed" bachelor and a retired mechanic. Mr. T's physical examination findings are remarkable only for a resting **tachycardia** of 92 beats/min. After an hematocrit value of 18% is unexpectedly found, a repeat assessment reveals pallor, occult-blood negative stool, and absent vibratory sense at his toes and malleoli.

Vignette Objectives

1. Describe a systematic evaluation of a person who has anemia.
2. What are the common causes of iron deficiency?
3. What findings are typical of pernicious anemia?

Anemia

The assessment of anemic individuals involves categorizing the anemia according to the reticulocyte count, RBC morphology, and the presence of other cell line abnormalities (Fig. 6-1). After this initial differentiation, the history, physical examination, and laboratory tests are used to define specific causes. The more frequent types of anemia and their features are listed in Table 6-3.

Table 6-3. Findings associated with commonly acquired anemias

Disorder	Findings
IRON DEFICIENCY	
Dietary Blood loss (menstrual loss, GI loss, blood donation) Reduced iron absorption (celiac disease post gastrectomy)	History and / or reason for blood loss (menorrhagia, peptic ulcer disease); occult-blood positive stool; occasionally splenomegaly; manifestations of Plummer-Vinson's syndrome include pica (craving for ice, cornstarch, olives, or clay), dysphagia, glossitis, koilonychia, and esophageal web
ANEMIA OF CHRONIC DISEASE	
Inflammatory disorders, renal disease (due to reduced erythropoietin production), and noninflammatory chronic illnesses	Inflammatory disorder (chronic infections, chronic immunologic-autoimmune illness); malignancy; chronic illness (long-standing diabetes, congestive heart failure)
B_{12} DEFICIENCY	
Pernicious anemia Post gastrectomy Ileal resections Stagnant loop of bowel with bacteria overgrowth Parasites	Glossitis; decreased vibratory and position sense; ataxia; mental status can be normal or patient can demonstrate mild confusion to moderate dementia; B_{12} level can be normal, and if symptoms indicate the diagnosis, other tests may be needed (e.g., serum methylmalonic acid and total homocysteine levels)
MULTIFACTORIAL ANEMIA OF ALCOHOLISM	
Inadequate diet (folate deficiency) GI blood loss Alcohol–induced suppression of marrow function	Alcoholism, inadequate diet, stigmata of chronic liver disease, occult-blood positive stool

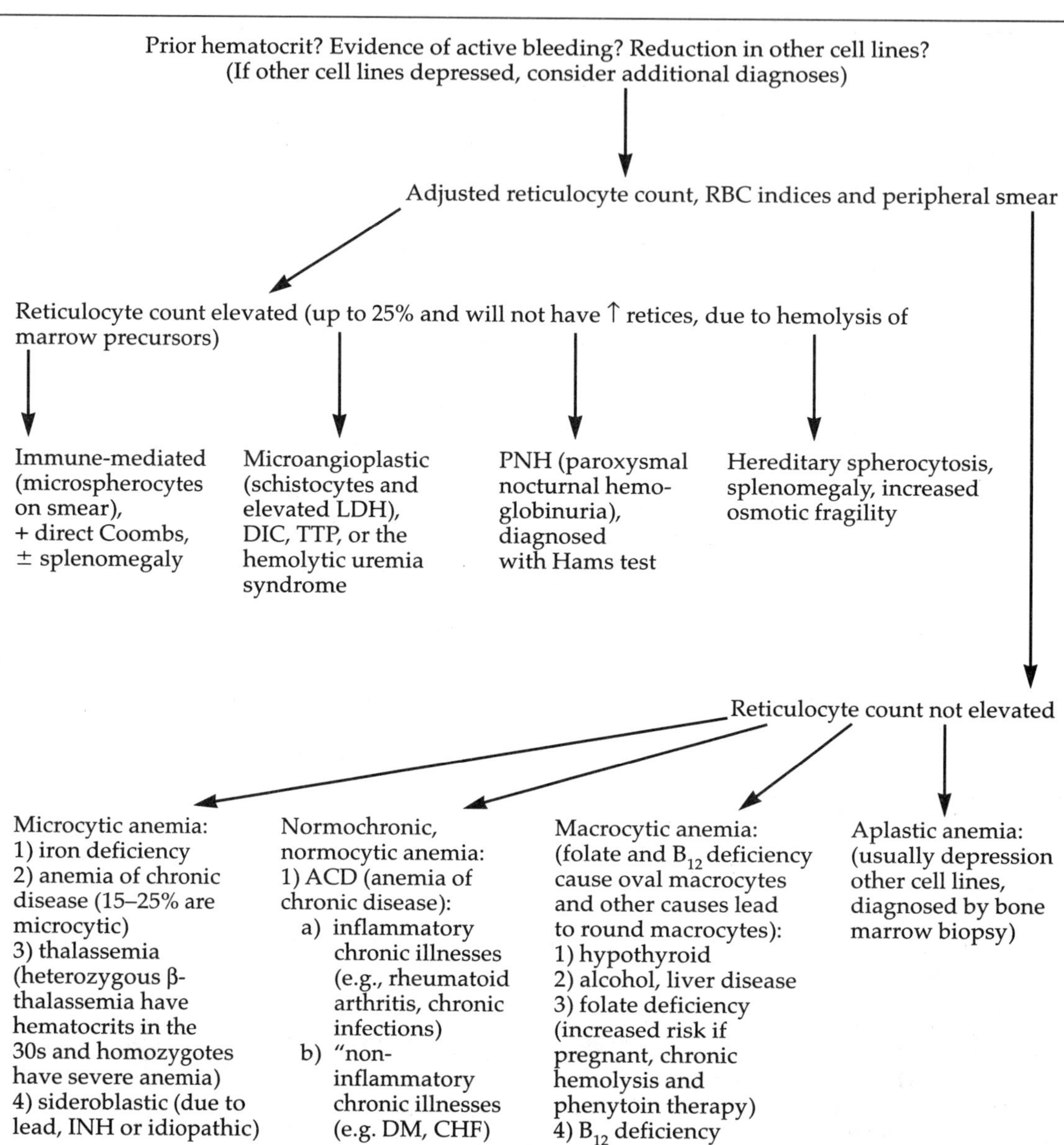

Figure 6-1. Evaluating a patient's anemia is simplified by recognizing major branch points that depend on the adjusted reticulocyte count, RBC indices, and appearance of the peripheral smear. (*LDH* = lactic dehydrogenase; *DIC* = disseminated intravascular coagulation; *TTP* = thrombotic thrombocytopenic purpura; *DM* = diabetes mellitus; *COPD* = chronic obstructive pulmonary disease; *CHF* = congestive heart failure.)

Vignette Follow-ups

No additional studies are performed to confirm Ms. S's iron deficiency anemia. She is begun on oral iron therapy. Although Ms. S is postmenopausal, her frequent blood donation was resulting in a significant iron loss. The iron loss from a three-times-per-year donation is roughly equivalent to that from a year of normal menses. However, concern about the potential for an occult gastrointestinal (GI) blood loss contributing to her iron deficiency is discussed with Ms. S. The family history of colon cancer and its implications are also presented. After reviewing the options, Ms. S undergoes flexible sigmoidoscopy and an air-contrast barium enema. The findings from both studies are normal. Her hematocrit value becomes normal in response to the iron therapy, and iron deficiency has not recurred during 4 years of follow-up.

The Leser-Trélat sign is a marked increase in the number of seborrheic keratoses, that occurs in association with GI and other malignancies. It is not present, as more keratoses than those Ms. S has would have been necessary for the sign to be present.

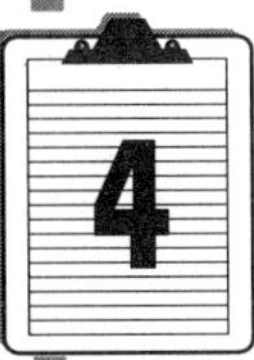

Mr. T's WBC and platelet count are normal. However, the polymorphonuclear leukocytes (PMNs) are noted to be hypersegmented (≥six lobes per PMN or >5% PMNs with five lobes). An electrocardiogram is normal, without evidence of ischemia. Vitamin B_{12} and folate levels are measured, thyroid function is assessed, and a reticulocyte count is done. On the basis of his clinical presentation, he is begun on therapy consisting of daily B_{12} injections and oral folate. His potassium level, which can decrease acutely while B_{12} therapy is being initiated for the treatment of pernicious anemia, is followed closely and remains normal. After 1 week of daily injections, he is given an injection every other week. His hematocrit value increases, and the dyspnea resolves. He is presumed to have pernicious anemia, and no additional studies are obtained.

Vignettes 5 and 6

Ecchymosis: bruising, "black and blue" discoloration of the skin.

Petechiae: tiny, pinpoint-sized, erythematous, nonraised, nonblanching macules visible in the dermis.

Purpura: multiple coalescing petechial and ecchymotic lesions that are greater than 1 cm in diameter, resulting from bleeding into the dermis.

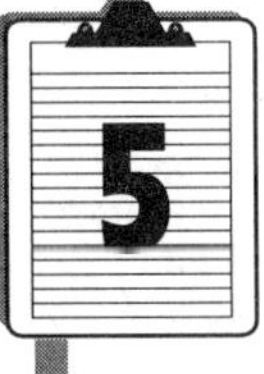

SG is a 38-year-old woman who is seen before a planned hysterectomy for a large uterine fibroid. She has told the anesthesiologist that she bruises easily and is referred for evaluation of a "bleeding disorder." She reports that she always has bruised easily after minor trauma. However, she had her wisdom teeth extracted and has had two normal vaginal deliveries without bleeding problems. Her parents and three siblings are well, without bleeding problems. Ms. G eats a normal diet and takes no medications, including no aspirin. A preoperative CBC is normal.

WH is a 52-year-old man who has had a runny nose and cough and has felt "feverish." Three days after the onset of these symptoms, he noticed a "rash" on his ankles, and while brushing his teeth, he noticed that his gums began to bleed. Mr. H has no risk factors for HIV infection and has not been exposed to any particular medications or toxins. Because of the gum bleeding, he saw his dentist, who noticed "small red spots" on his palate. His dentist recommended that he see his physician.

Vignette Objectives

1. What clues in the history and physical examination are helpful in detecting and characterizing a bleeding disorder?
2. What preoperative evaluation is needed to rule out a bleeding disorder?
3. What are the causes of thrombocytopenia and how would the findings differ for patients suspected of having these disorders?

Bleeding Disorders

There are several types of bleeding disorders, and these can be broadly classified as abnormalities of (1) platelets, (2) plasma coagulation, (3) blood vessels, or a combination of these abnormalities. The findings that can be of assistance in distinguishing among those disorders are listed in Table 6-4. Causes of thrombocytopenia and associated findings are listed in Table 6-5. Often, pe-

Table 6-4. Assessment of "bleeding disorders"

	Disorders with abnormal platelet number or function	Disorders affecting plasma coagulation factors	Disorders with vascular abnormalities
Causes	Von Willebrand's disease (autosomal dominant), thrombocytopenia, uremia	Hemophilia A (sex-linked recessive), vitamin K deficiency, disseminated intravascular coagulopathy	Vitamin C deficiency, vasculitis, Rocky Mountain spotted fever, hereditary connective tissue diseases
History	Menorrhagia, delayed bleeding about 12 hours after tooth extraction, aspirin* or NSAID use, family history	Cirrhosis, malabsorption, prior hemarthrosis or soft-tissue bleeding, family history	Inadequate diet (vitamin C deficiency); arthralgias, mononeuritis, hypertension (vasculitis); fever, tick exposure (Rocky Mountain spotted fever); family history
Physical examination	Petechiae of palate or dependent areas (ankles), ecchymosis	Stigmata of cirrhosis, ecchymosis—extensive purpura, arthritis (acute hemarthrosis or due to prior joint hemorrhage)	Corkscrew hairs, perifollicular hemorrhage (scurvy); hypertension, palpable purpura, fever, rash (vasculitis); increased joint laxity

*Irreversibly affects platelet function and prolongs bleeding time slightly, but usually not to times greater than normal.

Table 6-5. Causes of thrombocytopenia

Disorder	Findings
Marrow suppression (due to chemotherapy, radiation, malignant infiltration, or infection)	History of chemotherapy, radiation treatment, or therapy with drugs affecting the marrow (such as chloramphenicol, gold compounds, phenylbutazone, phenytoin, quinidine, sulfonamides); pallor (when RBC line involved); petechiae; weight loss and cachexia (when tumor infiltration has occurred)
Hypersplenism due to portal hypertension	History of alcoholism or hepatitis, stigmata of cirrhosis (splenomegaly, ascites, spider angiomas, palmar erythema)
Idiopathic thrombocytopenia purpura (ITP)	History of "viral illness" 1 to 3 weeks before onset; easy bruising, petechiae, epistaxis, gingival bleeding, menorrhagia; female > male; peak onset, ages 20 to 30 years
Non–ITP immune-mediated thrombocytopenia (viral syndrome [such as mononucleosis] or HIV associated)	History of HIV risks or illness; symptoms of viral illness; thrombocytopenia with viral infections usually mild
Thrombotic thrombocytopenic purpura	Syndrome of (1) fever (without infectious cause), (2) fluctuating CNS abnormalities, (3) thrombocytopenia, (4) microangiopathic hemolytic anemia, (5) renal dysfunction, and (6) normal coagulation studies
Hemolytic uremic syndrome	Occurs in infancy and early childhood; fever, hypertension, and renal failure; often prior febrile illness; associated with certain GI pathogens
Heparin-associated thrombocytopenia	Usually in first 2 weeks of use; paradoxically, causes thrombosis; this potential is the reason for monitoring every-other-day platelet count in patient receiving heparin therapy; measure HAT (heparin-associated thrombocytopenia) antibody if diagnosis suspected
Disseminated intravascular coagulopathy	Consequence of many conditions: infections (gram-negative sepsis, meningococcemia), malignancy, abruptio placentae, hemolytic transfusion reactions; microangiopathic smear; other laboratory indices include prolonged prothrombin and partial thromboplastic times, increased fibrin monomers
Preeclampsia	More than 15 weeks pregnant, hypertension, edema, proteineuria, hyperreflexia

techiae develop in patients with thrombocytopenia when a tourniquet is placed on their arm. Similar to the way in which petechiae form in dependent areas, the tourniquet causes increased venous hydrostatic pressure, capillary leak, and a petechial "rash."

It is not routinely necessary to measure prothrombin and partial thromboplastin times preoperatively, if a careful history and physical examination do not identify features indicating a higher risk of bleeding. High risk is defined by (1) a personal or family history of a bleeding disorder, (2) prolonged bleeding after dental work or surgery, (3) current use of broad-spectrum antibiotics, (4) liver disease or malabsorption, (5) Ashkenazic Jewish heritage (the prevalence of factor IX deficiency is increased in this ethnic group), or (6) evidence of petechiae, ecchymosis, or hematoma.

Vignette Follow-ups

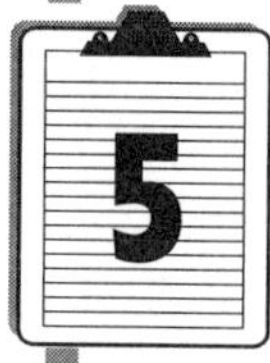

"Easy bruisibility" is a nonspecific complaint. Ms. G's history is not indicative of a bleeding disorder. She does well during and after surgery.

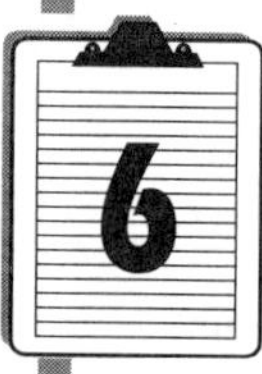

Mr. H is found to have a platelet count of 12,000/mm^3, with a normal WBC and hemoglobin level. An urgently obtained bone marrow biopsy specimen shows abundant megakaryocytes, findings characteristic of idiopathic thrombocytopenic purpura. He is begun on corticosteroid therapy that day. Hepatitis serology and HIV antibody test results are negative.

Vignette 7

TM is an 82-year-old man who is seen because of a complaint of "trouble with my mouth," which lasted about 2 hours and gradually resolved. Upon further questioning, he describes the symptoms of a transient dysarthria. He did not note palpitations, faintness, diplopia, motor symptoms, or dyesthesias. He was in good general health until a year ago, when weight loss and decreased visual acuity developed. At that time, he had a hematocrit of 26%. A bone marrow specimen showed an increase in the number of plasmacytoid lymph cells, and this and laboratory study findings established the diagnosis of Waldenström's macroglobulinemia. His serum viscosity was 5 (normal is 1.5 to 1.9; levels greater than 3 are associated with symptoms of hyperviscosity), and a paraprotein level of 1.2 gm/dl was measured.

On physical examination, Mr. M is found to be an elderly man who is in no acute distress. His **blood pressure** is 120/70 mm Hg, and **heart rate** is 60 beats/min. **HEENT:** findings are unchanged from previous exams. **Chest:** clear except for a few scattered wheezes in the right upper lobe. **Cardiac:** no JVD; carotids are 2+, symmetrical, and without bruits; S_1 and S_2 are normal, and no additional sounds are heard. **Abdominal:** liver is palpable three finger breadths below the right costal margin, with a span of 14 cm. No masses are present, and stool is occult-blood negative. On **neurologic** exam his speech is found to be fluent and no dysarthria is detectable. His reflexes are 1+ and symmetrical, and toes are downgoing. He has symmetrical motor tone, without pronator drift.

Vignette Objective

1. List the different illnesses caused by a monoclonal increase in serum immunoglobulins and the history and physical examination findings associated with each.

Paraproteinemias

A monoclonal increase in serum proteins can cause several types of problems, depending on the type of immunoglobulin involved. The characteristics of paraproteinemias are presented in Table 6-6.

Table 6-6. Paraproteinemias

Diagnosis	Findings
Monoclonal gammopathy of unknown significance ("benign gammopathy")	Elderly; incidentally detected; patients usually are asymptomatic; can be associated with neuropathy; no proteinuria; no bone lesions; <5% plasma cells in marrow; myeloma likely if IgG > 2 mg/dl; IgA > 1 gm/dl, or IgM > 2 gm/dl; rare progression to myeloma
Myeloma	Patients usually >60 year old; 60% are anemic; 20%–95% of marrow is plasma cells; 70% have lytic bone lesions, 15% have osteoporosis, and 15% have normal bones; abnormal serum electrophoresis; 50% have light-chain (Bence Jones) proteinuria; hypogammaglobulinemia results in bacterial infections; multifactorial renal dysfunction
Waldenström's macroglobulinemia (IgM)	Elderly; men > women; symptoms result from hyperviscosity, such as CHF and encephalopathy; normal viscosity = 1.5–1.9, symptoms occur when viscosity >3.0; viscosity increases exponentially as IgM increases; bone lesions uncommon; slight hepatosplenomegaly and diffuse adenopathy; bleeding due to platelet dysfunction; marrow contains lymphocytoid plasma cells
Amyloid (light-chain deposition) (this is one of several types of amyloid)	Symptoms vary with organ involvement; manifestations include cardiomyopathy, cardiac conduction defects, malabsorption, increased capillary fragility, hepatomegaly, nephrotic syndrome, and neuropathy; usually marrow plasma cells are not increased

Vignette Follow-up

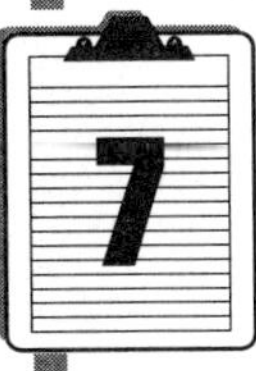

Mr. M's serum viscosity is elevated at 4.2, which is thought to have caused his transient symptoms. However, Mr. M has a history of first-degree atrioventricular block, so 24-hour Holter monitoring is also done, which does not reveal an arrhythmia. He is treated with plasmapheresis and low-dose chlorambucil.

Vignette 8

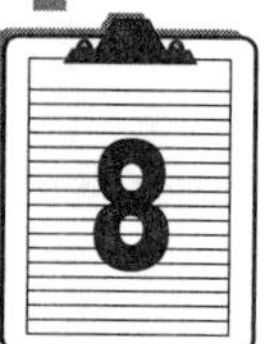

CG is a 71-year-old man who is seen in the emergency room for the treatment of a finger laceration. He is brought in by his neighbor, who has been "worried about the old guy." Mr. G also complains of trouble walking and "problems with my thinking." His history is significant for a left lower lung lobectomy performed for removal of a squamous cell carcinoma almost 2 years ago. The emergency room physician has noticed that Mr. G has had no follow-up medical care since his surgery.

Physical examination reveals a disheveled elderly man who is not oriented to time or place. Vital signs: **blood pressure** is 150/94 mm Hg, and **heart rate** is 82 beats/min. Pertinent findings include those from the **chest** exam, which demonstrates percussion dullness in the left base. **Cardiac:** JVP is estimated at 8 cm H_2O. S_1 and S_2 are normal, and an early peaking 2/6 systolic ejection murmur is heard in the aortic area. **Neurologic** exam: in addition to disorientation, Mr. G's gait is ataxic and visual field confrontation reveals a left homonymous hemianopia. The abnormal mental status and neurologic findings raise concerns about an emergent problem related to his prior malignancy.

Vignette Objectives

1. List the history and physical examination findings encountered in the following oncologic emergencies: brain metastasis, malignant pericardial effusion, and superior vena cava (SVC) obstruction.
2. List four categories of paraneoplastic syndromes and an example of a specific disorder in each.

Oncologic Emergencies

Brain Metastases

Brain metastases represent a major cause of morbidity in patients with metastatic malignancies and are found at autopsy in 15% to 20% of patients with terminal cancer. Lung cancer is the most common malignancy resulting in brain metastases and accounts for 40% to 80% of cases of metastasis to the brain. Other neoplasms with a propensity to metastasize to the brain include breast cancer, melanoma, and hypernephroma.

The neurologic findings vary according to the location of the metastasis in the central nervous system, the extent of the surrounding edema, and the intracranial pressure. Headache, motor weakness, and impaired mentation are common presenting features. Seizures, cranial nerve deficits, and cerebellar dysfunction also can occur.

Malignant Pericardial Effusion

Malignancy involving the pericardium occurs in approximately 8% of patients dying from cancer. Lung cancer is the most common tumor associated with pericardial involvement, accounting for one third of all cases. Breast cancer and hematologic malignancies each account for approximately 20% of the total number of cases.

The clinical manifestations of the effusion depend on the rate of fluid accumulation and the pericardium's compliance. When effusions accumulate slowly, large volumes can be tolerated without a clinically observed effect on cardiac function. However, tamponade can result if a small volume of fluid accumulates within a noncompliant pericardium, such as occurs when the pericardium is fibrotic as the result of radiation therapy or as occurs in the setting of pericardial tumor infiltration.

The topic of cardiac tamponade is reviewed in Chapter 3. Its most common symptoms are nonspecific and include dyspnea and cough. The classic physical examination findings encountered in patients with tamponade are tachycardia, an elevated JVP, Kussmaul's sign, and pulsus paradoxus.

Superior Vena Cava Obstruction

The SVC is surrounded by lymph nodes that drain the right thoracic cavity, and node enlargement can cause SVC compression. Malignancies cause approximately 85% of SVC obstructions. Three quarters of these are lung cancers, with lymphomas and other metastatic neoplasms accounting for approximately 10% each.

In most cases, SVC obstruction develops slowly over several weeks. Symptoms include headache, facial and neck swelling, chest pain, cough, and orthopnea. Characteristic physical findings are distention of the neck veins and cutaneous vessels of the face (plethora) and upper chest, with edema of the face and upper extremities. The diagnosis is established on the basis of these clinical findings and the findings of a superior mediastinal mass on a chest radiograph.

Paraneoplastic Syndromes

Paraneoplastic syndromes are due to the remote effects of malignancies. There are four general categories of disorders, and these can be remembered by the mnemonic BEND (Table 6-7). (See also Chapter 8 for additional information on paraneoplastic neurologic problems.)

Table 6-7. Paraneoplastic syndromes: BEND

General category	Specific manifestations
Blood disorders	**Hypercoagulability** resulting in recurrent deep venous thrombosis, migratory superficial thrombophlebitis, or marantic endocarditis (especially due to mucin-producing adenocarcinomas) **Erythrocytosis** due to erythropoietin production (hypernephroma, hepatoma, lung cancer) **Thrombocytosis**
Endocrine effects	**Cushing's syndrome** from ectopic production ACTH, usually associated with small-cell lung carcinoma **SIADH** from (squamous cell carcinoma of the lung or oropharynx and transitional cell carcinoma of the bladder) **Hypercalcemia** can be due to ectopic parathyroid hormone, osteoclast-activating factors [multiple myeloma], prostaglandins [breast cancer], and direct skeletal involvement
Neurologic sequelae	**Eaton-Lambert** syndrome or reverse myasthenia (see Chapter 8, p. 273) **Cerebellar degeneration** **Limbic encephalitis** resulting in dementia
Dermatologic problems (skin also can be involved directly or with metastases)	**Skin changes** due to a malignancy's hormone/protein products (such as occurs with carcinoid, amyloid deposition, glucagonoma) **Acanthosis nigricans** **Multiple seborrheic keratosis** (Leser-Trélat sign, p. 165) **Hypertrichosis lanuginosa acquisita** or lanugo

Vignette Follow-up

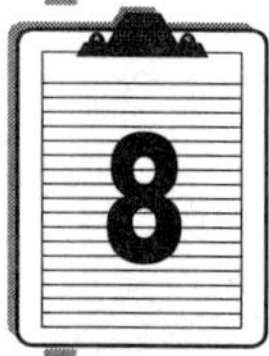

CG is found to have a single right posterior occipital metastasis, with surrounding cerebral edema. The mass is treated acutely with high-dose steroids and subsequently with surgery (for the purpose of tissue diagnosis) and radiation therapy. His mental status clears once his cerebral edema resolves, although his visual field deficit persists. Remarkably, he remains free of disease 5 years after therapy.

Vignette 9

JB is a 76-year-old man who has received a cycle of chemotherapy for lymphoma 4 days ago. He was doing well, but his wife calls to say that he awoke this evening from a nap feeling "unwell." He now has a fever (103°F [39.4°C] orally) and seems "confused." She relates that he tried to get in the car while in his pajamas. He is not complaining of anything in the way of specific complaints or localizing symptoms. What would you advise?

Vignette Objective

1. Explain how the history and physical examination findings can be used to evaluate patients with fever and neutropenia.

Malignancy and Fever

Most tumors do not cause fever unless there is a secondary problem. Exceptions are the lymphomas and, occasionally, a solid tumor, such as hypernephroma. Usually, when fever is associated with malignancy, it is due to disrupted anatomy, obstructed drainage, and a bacterial infection. For example, tumor obstruction of the biliary tract, urinary tract, and bronchi can cause cholangitis, pyelonephritis, and pneumonia, respectively.

Neutropenia and Fever

Patients with neutropenia resulting from their malignancy, its treatment, or both, pose additional concerns if fever develops. The assessment of patients with fever and granulocytopenia (an absolute granulocyte count of less than 500/mm^3) requires special care, because the lack of WBCs limits the usual inflammatory response and the symptoms and signs of infection therefore may not be present. For example, a patient with pneumonia may not have a productive cough or findings of consolidation on pulmonary examination. In one series of neutropenic patients with pneumonia, one third had normal chest radiograph and one third had no cough. Clinical problems and their manifestations are listed in Table 6-8. Because of the potential for rapid deterioration in a neutropenic patient with an untreated infection, empiric antibiotics should be administered after a thorough examination and while culture results are pending.

Vignette Follow-up

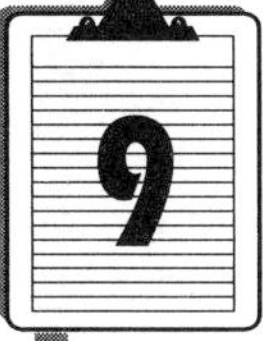

JB is brought to the emergency room, where he is found to be febrile and neutropenic. Although his physical examination does not reveal a site of infection, a chest radiograph shows a new small infiltrate. He is admitted to the hospital, and cultures (sputum, blood, and urine) are obtained. He is begun on empiric broad-spectrum antibiotics. His abnormal mental status clears as his temperature decreases to normal, but a specific organism is never identified. Over 2 days, Mr. B's marrow function recovers, and his WBCs increase. Once his neutropenia resolves, Mr. B is switched to oral antibiotics (for a presumed pneumonia) and is discharged to complete 12 days of antimicrobial therapy.

Table 6-8. Fever and neutropenia

Physical examination component	Common findings	Diagnoses suggested by the findings
Blood pressure	Low blood pressure	Septic shock (can appear flushed, blood pressure will not correct with volume alone); hypovolemia; acute hemorrhage
CNS	Confusion; headache, papilledema, stiff neck; coma	Delirium due to a fever and sepsis meningitis, CNS bleed; metabolic abnormality (e.g., hypoxia, hyponatremia); CSF can be infected without meningeal signs and CSF pleocytosis (decreased glucose will be present)
HEENT	Oral pain or ulcers; plaques of *Candida;* sinus tenderness	Chemotherapy can cause stomatitis Oral candida and herpes simplex infection; sinus infection often requires radiographic diagnosis and procedure to culture fluid
Chest	Tachypnea; findings of pulmonary consolidation can be minimal or absent (such as dullness to percussion, rales, and bronchial breath sounds); acute CHF can be difficult to distinguish from ARDS	Pneumonia (increased alveolar-arterial gradient, infiltrate on chest radiograph can be absent); pulmonary hemorrhage; acute CHF due to cardiotoxic chemotherapy or ischemia
Abdominal	Dysphagia, odynophagia; distention, abdominal pain; diarrhea, hematochezia	Esophagitis due to *Candida* or herpes simplex; necrotizing enterocolitis; pseudomembranous colitis; perirectal abscess
Rectal	Rectal pain, induration; rare to find fluctuant mass (due to neutropenia)	
Back	Pain on percussion of costovertebral angles or spine	Vertebral abscess; urinary tract infection; infected retroperitoneal hemorrhage
Skin	Bullae, nodules, ecchymosis; erythema or tenderness at site of venous access	Cellulitis; intravenous line infection

Vignette 10

DP is a 42-year-old man who calls you because of a swelling that has formed under his right arm. He is known to be HIV-positive, with a CD4 count of 480 cells/mm^3 (last checked 3 weeks ago). The current problem began 6 days ago, when he was scratched on his right hand by a kitten. At that time, he was seen in an urgent care clinic and given cephalexin. He took the medication as directed. However, despite that, a painful swelling has developed in his right axilla. Yesterday it was "plum sized," and now it is like a "tennis ball." He reports that his hand shows only mild erythema.

Vignette Objectives

1. What aspects of the history and physical examination are important in determining whether lymphadenopathy is due to an infection or a malignancy?
2. What problems could be associated with a CD4 cell count greater than 500 cells/mm^3, 200 to 500 cells/mm^3, and less than 200 cells/mm^3?

Adenopathy

Regional or generalized adenopathy can be the presenting complaint in a wide variety of underlying illnesses. Adenopathy is characterized by its location, the time course of the enlargement, and the nodes' characteristics, such as soft versus hard, tender versus nontender, and movable versus fixed. In general, nodes caused by a malignancy are firm to hard, nontender, and fixed to surrounding tissues (as the result of tumor infiltration). Suppurative nodes (resulting from infection) are tender, soft, and movable; associated with surrounding cellulitis; and sometimes fluctuant. The diagnostic considerations pertaining to adenopathy in different regions are listed in Table 6-9.

Cat Scratch Fever and Toxoplasmosis

Cat scratch fever causes tender regional adenopathy. The infecting organism is *Rochalimaea henselae,* a Rickettsia-like gram-negative bacillus, and the illness usually is self-limited. Most cases occur among young children. Ninety percent of those affected have a history of cat contact, and a primary inoculation site can be identified in 60% to 70% of patients. The adenopathy develops 1 to 2 weeks after the initial contact. Despite the name *fever,* in one large study, only 30% of patients reported a low-grade fever. This bacteria also causes bacillary angiomatosis and bacillary peliosis hepatis among patients with HIV-induced immunosuppression.

Toxoplasmosis is another pet-associated cause of adenopathy. The house cat is the definitive host of the protozoan intracellular parasite, *Toxoplasma gondii,* which causes toxoplasmosis. After infection resulting from contact with cat feces or the ingestion of undercooked pork or mutton, patients can suffer a mononucleosis-like illness consisting of cervical or generalized adenopathy, low-grade fever, malaise, and hepatosplenomegaly.

Progression of HIV Disease

Knowing the rate of HIV disease progression and the common illnesses associated with each stage allows problems to be anticipated and appropriate

Table 6-9. Assessment of adenopathy

Location of adenopathy	Cause
Preauricular and postauricular	Bacterial or vital conjunctivitis, eyelid infections
Cervical	Bacterial or viral infections of the face or oropharynx; posterior cervical nodes can be due to scalp infections, dermatitis, and occasionally, toxoplasmosis; if smoker, careful head and neck exam to look for squamous cell carcinomas; lymphoma (especially Hodgkin's disease)
Mandibular	Oral infections, lymphoma, head and neck tumors
Supraclavicular (these nodes can hide behind the sternocleidomastoid muscle's clavicular head; having a patient sit up and perform a Valsalva's maneuver can bring out inapparent node)	Most cases associated with malignancy; lymphoma; left supraclavicular node (Virchow's or sentinel node) drains the abdomen, kidney, and pelvis; right node drains the mediastinum, lungs, and esophagus; biopsy usually is required
Axillary	Bacterial infections of the upper extremities, breast cancer, lymphoma, cat scratch disease
Inguinal and femoral (inguinal nodes are along the inguinal ligament, and femoral nodes are inferior to the ligament, along the femoral artery)	Most inguinal nodes caused by sexually transmitted diseases (e.g., syphilis, herpes simplex, lymphogranuloma venereum, and gonorrhea) and lower extremity infections; in rare cases, a lower extremity melanoma, lymphoma, or pelvic malignancy results in isolated inguinal adenopathy
Paraumbilical nodes (Sister Joseph's node)*	Abdominal and pelvic neoplasms
Generalized adenopathy	Causes are divided into categories: (1) infections (including secondary syphilis, HIV infection, toxoplasmosis, mononucleosis, and other viral infections); (2) malignancy (lymphoma, leukemia); (3) dermopathies (diffuse skin conditions); and (4) hypersensitivity reactions (drug reaction); HIV-associated adenopathy most often involves the cervical, axillary, and occipital nodes

*Sister Joseph was Dr. William Halsted's scrub nurse. She felt this node while prepping a patient's abdomen before surgery. This node often is incorrectly called *Sister Mary Joseph's nodule,* perhaps because Sister Joseph was the superintendent at St. Mary's hospital.

Table 6-10. Risks relating to different CD4 counts in HIV-positive patients*

CD4 counts (per mm^3)	Risks	Management
>500	Little immediate risk of progression to AIDS; <10% risk for AIDS-defining illness in next 18 months	Patient education; baseline laboratory studies; CD4 count every 3 to 6 months
200–500	Potential for pneumococcal disease and herpes zoster; low risk for PCP; 10% to 35% risk for AIDS-defining illness in next 18 months	May begin antiviral treatment and PCP prophylaxis
<200	High risk for PCP and other opportunistic infections	Antiviral therapy, PCP prophylaxis, consider other prophylactic treatments

PCP = *Pneumocystis earinii* pneumonia.
*These risks and recommendations may antedate new drug combination treatment, protease inhibitors and early, aggressive prophylaxis of opportunistic organisms.

prophylactic interventions to be instituted. In general, CD4 cell counts change relatively slowly, with an average reduction of approximately 30 to 60 cells each year. Table 6-10 provides information on HIV progression and the appropriate interventions for patients with different CD4 counts.

Vignette Follow-up

Mr. P is believed to have cat scratch fever and is treated with oral ciprofloxacin. His adenopathy slowly resolves over 2 months.

Vignette 11

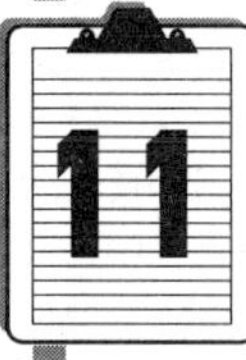

TF is 38-year-old woman who is seen in clinic for an annual cervical cytology (Pap smear). Her history is notable for Hodgkin's disease at age 24. At that time, left supraclavicular adenopathy developed, and a biopsy specimen showed nodular, sclerosing Hodgkin's disease. She had no fever or weight loss, and a staging laparotomy, splenectomy, and liver biopsy specimen showed no evidence of disease beyond the supraclavicular area. She underwent mantle irradiation as her only treatment.

Over the subsequent 14 years, she has done well, without evidence of recurrent disease. She has had three normal pregnancies, and her sons are healthy. She takes no medication. In addition to routine health maintenance, she has received pneumovax, because of her splenectomy. Because of her prior mantle radiation therapy, her thyroid function is assessed annually. Her **physical examination** findings are entirely normal. Because of her exposure to radiation, she asks whether she needs a mammogram.

Vignette Objectives

1. List the symptoms and signs of Hodgkin's disease and other lymphomas.
2. What are the late sequelae of treatment for malignancies?

Hodgkin's Disease and Lymphomas

Lymphomas can be composed of a variety of cell types and exhibit a wide spectrum of clinical manifestations. The staging system for lymphomas is shown in Table 6-11. Hodgkin's disease is a malignant lymphoma, distinguished by the

Table 6-11. Lymphoma staging

Stage	Clinical involvement
I	Single lymph node region or extralymphatic site
II	Two or more lymph node regions (includes extralymphatic site) on the same side of the diaphragm
III	Nodes, extralymphatic site and/or spleen involvement on both sides of diaphragm
IV	Diffuse disease of one or more extralymphatic organs (e.g., bone marrow, liver, lungs)

presence of multinucleate, giant (Reed-Sternberg) cells. Its manifestations and high potential for cure are unique among the lymphomas. The incidence of Hodgkin's disease has two peaks: it occurs in young adults (early 20s) and older people (60 to 70 years old). The illness often is manifested as a unilateral cervical adenopathy.

The stage of the disease, determined before therapy, defines the extent of disease, which in turn dictates its management. The designation A signifies no systemic symptoms or weight loss; the designation B signifies the occurrence of symptoms that include fever, night sweats, and loss of more than 10% of body weight. Approximately 30% of patients with Hodgkin's disease have systemic symptoms, and their occurrence is associated with a worse prognosis. The fever can be of the Pel-Ebstein variety, in which several days of fever alternate with days without fever. The presence of pruritus and alcohol-induced lymph node pain do not alter prognosis. Splenic enlargement usually indicates hepatic involvement.

Hodgkin's disease often is localized, with asymptomatic cervical and/or supraclavicular adenopathy being the most common feature. The overall cure rate in affected patients is more than 75%. Non-Hodgkin's lymphomas usually are not localized and frequently involve the bone marrow and noncontiguous viscera. Their overall cure rate in affected patients is less than 50%. However, response rates vary greatly and are influenced by the lymphoma's histology and cellular markers. The treatment of lymphomas and other malignancies can have several late sequelae, and these are listed in Table 6-12.

Vignette Follow-up

Ms. F is at risk for several sequelae from her treatment of Hodgkin's disease. Because of an increased risk for breast cancer, she undergoes mammography.

Table 6-12. Late consequences of Hodgkin's disease treatment

Treatment	Late consequences
Splenectomy	Encapsulated organisms (especially pneumococcal infections) can cause an overwhelming infection, with disseminated intravascular coagulopathy and a mortality >30%; pneumococcal vaccine administration is important, but it does not uniformly prevent pneumococcal infection
Mantle radiation therapy (mediastinum and supraclavicular areas)	Thyroid dysfunction leading to hypothyroidism in up to 50%, especially if patient subsequently receives an iodine load (such as with contrast used for IVP); can occur more than 5 years after treatment
	Increased risk of thyroid cancer
	Pneumonitis can occur immediately to 5 years after radiation therapy
	Accelerated coronary artery disease; pericarditis 5 to 9 months after radiation therapy
	Fourfold increased risk of breast cancer
	Increased risk of malignancy (lung, head, and neck)
Chemotherapy	Permanent azoospermia develops in 90% of males; occasionally low testosterone level
	If older than age 25 when treated with radiotherapy plus chemotherapy, premature ovarian failure in >90%; less risk if younger than age 25 when treated; oophoropexy at laparotomy can reduce radiotherapy exposure
	Slightly increased risk for leukemia, but no increased risk for solid tumors
	Certain agents (bleomycin, nitroureas, procarbazine) are associated with pulmonary toxicity
	Prior treatment is not linked with increase in fetal wastage, congenital abnormalities, or problems with fetal development

Vignette 12

WW is a 52-year-old woman whom you are seeing for a "check-up." She has no insurance and has not seen a physician in over 10 years. However, her children insisted that she make a doctor's appointment, and she finally agreed to do so. She takes no medications and smokes cigarettes (one pack per day for 30 years). Her past history is noncontributory. Her **general physical examination** findings are normal. She wants to know which blood work and general health maintenance screening procedures are "really needed."

Vignette Objective

1. What general health maintenance procedures are suggested for people in different age groups?

Screening for Malignancies

Different expert groups (e.g., the U.S. Preventive Services Task Force, American College of Physicians, American Cancer Society, and Canadian Task Force on the Periodic Physical Examination) have made recommendations concerning appropriate assessments for the early detection of malignancies. These recommendations have been made despite the fact that only a few large, randomized controlled studies on specific cancers have been conducted that could be used as the basis for such recommendations. Tables 6-13 and 6-14 provide information on the cost and benefits of different medical interventions. (Additional discussion of the "screening" examination is presented in Chapter 1, p. 5.)

Table 6-13. Cost-effectiveness of medical intervention[a]

Strategy	Approximate dollar cost per year of life saved
Smoking-cessation counseling[b]	6,500
Renal dialysis[c]	46,000
Coronary artery bypass surgery (triple-vessel disease, 55-year-old man)	115,000
Screening mammography for women under 50 years of age[d]	170,000

[a]Data as reported in the medical literature, with dollars inflated to 1989 dollars using the Medicare medical inflator.
[b]Data apply to counseling a 45- to 49-year-old man, with a 1% rate of quitting and a 50% relapse rate.
[c]Data based on gross costs of in-center dialysis.
[d]Data apply to screening in women less than 50-years-old.
Source: Schulman KA, Lynn LA, Glick HA, Eisenberg JM. Cost effectiveness of low-dose zidovudine therapy for asymptomatic patients with human immunodeficiency virus (HIV) infection. *Ann Intern Med* 1991;114:798–802.

Table 6-14. Suggested routine examinations at different ages

Age (yr)	Annually	Every other year	Every 3 years	Every 5 years	Every 10 years
20–39	—	Blood pressure	Pap test*	Interim history and physical examination as appropriate, cholesterol	Tetanus-diphtheria booster
40–49	Breast exam	Blood pressure, mammography, stool for occult-blood	Interim history and physical exam, as appropriate; height and weight; Pap test*	Cholesterol	Tetanus-diphtheria booster
50–59	Breast exam, mammography, stool for occult-blood	Blood pressure, interim history and physical exam, as appropriate	Pap test,* height and weight	Cholesterol	Tetanus-diphtheria booster
Older than 59	Interim history and physical exam, as appropriate; blood pressure; height and weight; visual acuity; hearing; oral examination; mammography; stool for occult-blood; influenza vaccine	—	Pap test*	Cholesterol, pneumococcal vaccine	Tetanus-diphtheria booster

*Cervical cytology (Papanicolaou smear) can be done at 3-year intervals after two cervical cytologies done 1 year apart have been normal.

Vignette Follow-up

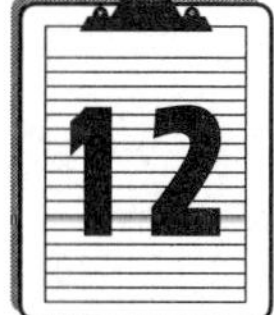

WW is counseled about her smoking, and she has her cholesterol level measured, and a mammogram, cervical cytology, and stool occult-blood testing performed. All results are normal.

Vignettes 13, 14, and 15

GB is an 82-year-old woman whose past history is significant for mastectomies for breast cancer approximately 6 and 8 years ago. Both times the nodes were negative, and she has had no additional therapy or evidence of recurrence. Her active medical problems are essential hypertension and an "anxiety disorder." When seeing the nurse for a routine blood pressure check, Ms. B reports that she experienced the onset of "low back pain" 2 weeks ago. She describes the pain as an ache in her low back that is worse when she is upright. The pain does not radiate to her legs, and she has not experienced lower extremity dysesthesia or weakness.

RS is a 76-year-old man who has experienced low back pain for the past month. He believes it resulted from lifting a heavy rock while working in his yard. He describes the pain as a dull ache, which is made worse by twisting and bending. He had back pain many years ago and relates having undergone lumbar laminectomy for a "trapped nerve" 10 years ago, with subsequent resolution of the back pain. He has had no change in his bowel or urinary habits. His history also is significant for prostate cancer, treated with local irradiation 5 years ago. At that time, his pretreatment prostate-specific antigen (PSA) level was 13 ng/ml (normal, less than 4 ng/ml) and it decreased to 2 ng/ml by 8 weeks after therapy. Mr. S.'s **physical examination** findings are remarkable only for loss of the left patellar reflex, a finding noted on prior examinations. There are no sensory abnormalities, pathologic reflexes, or spinal tenderness.

MD is an 85-year-old woman admitted through the emergency room with a chief complaint of "back pain." Her history is notable for an abdominal perineal resection for colon carcinoma 21 years ago. Nine years ago, she had a left radical mastectomy for infiltrating ductal carcinoma, with 17 of 17 nodes negative for metastatic disease. She received no additional therapy. For 2 months, Ms. D has noted low back pain, with radiation to the inside of her left thigh. Ms. D has been widowed for 12 years and lives alone in a housing development for senior citizens.

On physical examination, she is found to be a slender woman in mild distress. Vital signs: **blood pressure,** 134/80 mm Hg; **heart rate,** 80 beats/min. **Findings** include bilateral **carotid bruits** and a well-functioning colostomy. **Deep abdominal palpation** revealed a nontender aorta, estimated to be 3 cm in diameter. Her **spine** is nontender to direct percussion; **motor** exam reveals that lower extremity tone, muscle mass, and strength are normal; her **reflexes** are 1+ and symmetrical. **Perineal sensation** is normal. Radiographs show osteolytic-blastic lesions at L-3 and L-4.

Vignette Objectives

1. What historical features are typical of musculoskeletal low back pain? What aspects of the examination detect neurologic involvement? Which findings indicate the need for radiographs early in the diagnostic evaluation?

2. What is the likelihood and timing of breast cancer recurrence?
3. What is the natural history of prostate cancer? What is the pattern of metastasis?

Back Pain and Cancer

Musculoskeletal back pain and malignancies are both common disorders, but when they occur in the same setting, spinal cord compression becomes a concern. Early diagnosis is critical for preventing irreversible neurologic damage. Back pain is the initial symptom in more than 90% of patients with spinal cord compression resulting from malignancy. In most cases, metastatic tumors reach the epidural space by direct extension from adjacent vertebrae. Accordingly, spinal cord compression usually is associated with the development of skeletal malignancies (such as multiple myeloma) or neoplasms that frequently metastasize to bone (e.g., lung, breast, prostate, kidney, and thyroid cancers).

Although the characteristics of the back pain related to metastatic disease can differ from the characteristics of musculoskeletal back pain, they are not specific enough to differentiate malignant from musculoskeletal disease. Musculoskeletal pain characteristically is intermittent and less intense when the patient is supine. However, in the setting of malignancies, the pain often is constant, worsens when the patient is lying down, and awakens the patient at night. Radicular symptoms are present in 50% of patients with thoracic lesions and in more than 75% of those with cervical or lumbar involvement.

Normal neurologic findings do not exclude spinal cord compression, however, in that more than 40% of patients with spinal cord compression have normal findings. The signs of cord compression include (1) direct spine tenderness in response to gentle percussion, (2) bilateral lower extremity weakness (paraparesis), (3) sensory abnormalities (especially loss of sacral sensation), (4) decreased anal sphincter tone, (5) urinary retention, and (6) lower extremity hyperreflexia. Because the physical examination findings can be normal in the setting of impending cord compression, patients with a history of cancer and back pain must undergo additional studies to rule out or confirm metastatic disease as the cause of the complaint. The appropriate assessment of individuals with back pain is discussed further in Chapter 10, p. 347.

Breast Cancer

Breast cancer is the most common malignant disease among women of the western world. Six to twelve percent of U.S. women will be affected during their lifetime, and approximately 4 percent of all women will die from the disease. At the time of detection, the average size of primary lesions is 2.5 cm and about half will have metastasized to the lymph nodes. Screening programs can detect smaller breast tumors. Seventy-five to eighty percent of patients whose cancers are detected by screening have negative axillary lymph nodes, and approximately 40% have no mass detectable with a clinical breast examination. At this earlier stage, the likelihood of cure is greater.

The clinical breast examination and mammography complement each other in the early detection of breast cancer, as borne out by the fact that programs combining these techniques have been found to bring about a decreased mortality from breast cancer. The evidence for the benefits of screening mammography is strongest for women aged 50 to 59 years. For this group, the combination of mammography and clinical breast exam has been observed to reduce mortality by about one third to one half. Because breast cancer can exist despite normal mammogram findings, any suspicious mass should be biopsied; any suspicious findings on mammography should also be cause for having a biopsy done. The ratio of nonmalignant to malignant findings for breast biopsy specimens varies with age, from 16:1 for women aged 35 to 39 to 3:1 for women 70 to 74 years-old.

A woman's prognosis for cure depends on the number of axillary lymph nodes involved, the tumor's nuclear grade, and, to a lesser extent, the primary tumor size. However, a relapse rate as high as 20% is observed, even among patients with no axillary lymph node involvement. Among patients with one to three involved axillary lymph nodes, more than 60% will suffer relapse within 10 years of diagnosis. The relapse rates in those with more than three involved axillary lymph nodes are greater than 85% by 10 years.

Relapse occurs on average 3 to 4 years after diagnosis in women with one to three involved nodes and 1 to 2 years after diagnosis in patients with more than three involved nodes. Unlike most malignancies, however, a long disease-free interval does not signify cure, in that a breast cancer patient is at risk for recurrence for up to 20 years after the initial diagnosis.

Prostate Cancer

Prostate cancer is the second most common malignancy among men, with approximately 100,000 new cases diagnosed annually in the United States. It is uncommon before age 50. Its natural history is variable, in that it can be an aggressive tumor or asymptomatic and slow growing. Symptomatic men can ex-

Vignette Follow-ups

On examination, GB's back pain is localized to an area of tenderness along the lateral eleventh rib. Plain radiographs of the ribs are normal, and her condition improves in response to symptomatic treatment.

A lumbosacral spine radiograph is obtained in RS, which shows abnormal findings initially interpreted to be old changes resulting from his prior surgery. However, his PSA level is 8 ng/ml (greater than normal) and additional studies are ob-

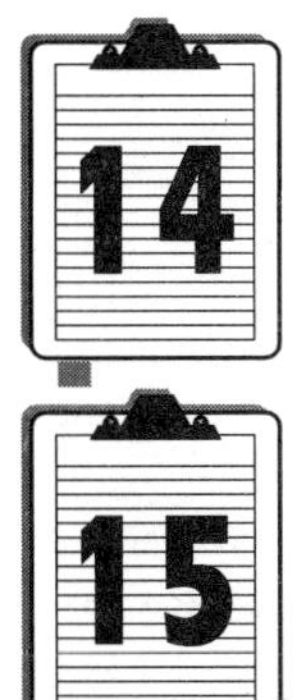

tained. A techetium 99m bone scan shows multiple abnormalities in the lumbar spine and ribs, indicating new metastatic disease. An MRI scan shows no evidence of spinal cord compression. Radiation therapy is begun, with subsequent resolution of his back pain. He remains pain free 10 months after therapy.

Abnormal bone scan findings are present in the region of the L-5 vertebra, the L2-3 pedicle, and the right occipital region of the calvarium. Chest radiograph, liver scan, and head CT findings are normal, as are the results from serum protein electrophoresis (assessing for myeloma). Consultants consider the risk from a biopsy greater than that from treatment for presumed metastatic breast cancer. Ms. D is therefore begun on radiation treatment.

perience pain on voiding, hematuria, and obstructed urinary flow (resulting in reduced force of stream and hesitancy).

Stage A carcinoma is not palpable by rectal examination and usually is diagnosed on the basis of biopsy findings or detected as an incidental finding during a transurethral prostate resection. Stage B is detectable as a firm nodule, during the digital rectal examination and confined to the prostate. Stage C involves extension beyond the prostate, without metastatic disease. Stage D involves metastasis to pelvic nodes only (D1) or distant metastasis (D2), with the latter affecting bone more than other organs, most commonly the pelvis and lumbar vertebrae.

PSA is a glycoprotein that is produced only by the prostate. It can be a marker for prostate cancer and may be elevated in patients with localized disease. However, an elevation is not specific to prostate cancer. Greater than 50% of men with PSA levels above 10 ng/mL and approximately 25% with levels between 4 and 10 ng/mL will be found to have prostate cancer. Although some advocate levels as an annual screening procedure for men older than age 50, it is unknown whether PSA testing will lead to a reduction in the mortality associated with the malignancy.

Vignette 16

EW is a 54-year-old woman who you saw last week when she came in for her annual exam. At that time, you did not detect any breast masses and ordered an annual "screening" mammogram. Clusters of microcalcifications are seen on the mammogram, and these are interpreted as suspicious for malignancy. How would you contact Ms. W with this "bad news" and what information should be provided?

Vignette Objective

1. Outline the communication principles used to deliver bad news effectively.

Delivering Bad News

When relating bad news to patients, it is important that there be high degree of certainty about the diagnosis, such as that provided by a tissue findings or a "gold-standard" laboratory test result. In the absence of such certainty, the emphasis is on telling the patient about the potential for diseases and explaining the steps needed to establish a definite diagnosis.

There is no one "right" way to relate bad news, but there are a few basic principles that can be applied. The means of communication (phone versus in person) depends on many factors, such as the gravity of the diagnosis and its prognosis, insights about the patient, whether the information is expected, and the inconvenience and expense to the patient of returning to the office. Considerations pertaining to the delivery of bad news are listed in Table 6-15. Skill in communicating has a bearing on subsequent patient hopefulness. That is, patients are more hopeful when they believe their physician has expertise and offers ongoing emotional support. Patients are less hopeful when information is delivered over the phone and their physician seems sad or unsure of how to proceed.

Table 6-15. Guidelines for delivering bad news

1. Understand the patient's support system (e.g., family, friends, church), beliefs, and knowledge of the disorder.
2. Know the condition's natural history and management options.
3. Identify a private setting and a time when interruptions can be avoided.
4. Avoid using technical terms and medical jargon.
5. Anticipate that the patient's recall of facts will be limited.
6. Arrange specific follow-up and subsequent actions.

Vignette Follow-up:

The biopsy specimen shows a benign fibroadenoma.

Vignette 17

Life context of an illness: this is the interaction between a person's medical problem and its impact on his or her life. Sometimes patients spontaneously relate their feelings about an illness' effect. At other times, questions such as "How has it affected your ability to work?," "Was that disrupting to your usual routine?," or "How have you had to change things?" are needed to draw out people's feelings about their illness.

Attributes: a patient's perception about what is causing symptoms and why he or she thinks that they have the current problem. Sometimes people spontaneously say, "I was worried it might be. . . ." At other times asking a question such as "Are you concerned about anything in particular?" elicits a patient's description of the attributes of their problem.

AP is a 56-year-old man with a complaint of weight loss. He reports an unintentional loss of 15 pounds (6.75 kg) over the past 4 to 6 weeks. He is concerned that "this might be something serious." He has been a two–pack-per-day smoker for the past 30 years and has a chronic cough, expectorating "phlegm" most mornings. He believes that his food intake has been about the same, although his appetite may be is a little less than usual. He complains that he has not felt as "peppy" over the past few weeks. He has not experienced nausea or vomiting, and his bowel habits have been normal. Since marrying 25 years ago, he has been monogamous. He has no history of intravenous drug use or transfusions. He relates that his work as a tax preparer is stressful. He has been busy, working 12- to 14-hour days, even on weekends.

Vignette Objectives

1. What historical and physical examination aspects are most relevant when evaluating unintentional weight loss?
2. Define "attributes" as they relate to a patient's medical history.

Weight Loss

Before evaluating weight loss, it is useful to confirm a reported loss with objective measures, such as with recorded weights, pictures of the patients, and changes in clothes sizes. A careful history and physical examination usually will identify the causes of weight loss, or at least indicate what further studies need to be done. Although cancer is an important consideration, several diagnoses are possible. The findings associated with specific diagnoses are given in Table 6-16.

Table 6-16. Assessment of unintentional weight loss

Etiology	History	Physical findings
Malignancies		
Gastric or esophageal	Early satiety, dysphagia, epigastric pain	Occult-blood positive stool, supraclavicular adenopathy
Pancreatic	Epigastric or back pain, decreased food intake, smoking, alcoholism, depression	Jaundice (painless)
Lung	Smoker, asbestos or radiation exposure, cough, hemoptysis	Clubbing
Lymphoma	Fever, sweats; pruritus; alcohol-induced lymph node pain	Adenopathy, splenomegaly, hepatomegaly
Depression	Anhedonia, depressed mood, sleep disturbance, anorexia	Sad facies, tearful, increased latency for verbal responses
Malabsorption	Diarrhea, floating and foul-smelling stool	Evidence of fat-soluble vitamin deficiencies (such as easy bruising due to vitamin K deficiency)
Metabolic		
Diabetes	Polyuria, polydypsia (weight loss due to loss of body mass and dehydration)	
Hyperthyroid	Sweating, heat intolerance, palpitations, hyperdefecation	Goiter; tachycardia; warm, sweaty, moist skin; brisk reflexes; tremor; "stare", proptosis, lid lag
Infection	Fever, risks for tuberculosis or HIV infection	Depends on site of infection
Social	Low income; limitations to food access; social isolation	—
Oral disorders	Difficulty chewing	Absence of teeth, ill-fitting dentures

Vignette Follow-up

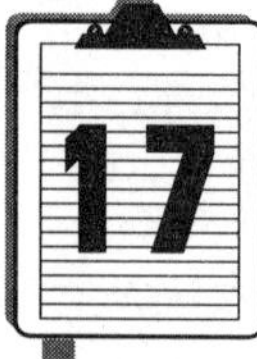

Because of Mr. P's smoking history and cough, a chest radiograph is obtained, which is normal. On further interview, Mr. P admits he has been feeling depressed, experiencing a reduced libido, and not sleeping well. He relates that he "almost hoped it was cancer, so I can retreat from my life." His condition and outlook improve with antidepressant treatment and psychotherapy.

Vignette 18

ST is a 66-year-old man with a history of abdominal discomfort and an increasing reliance on laxatives to maintain regular bowel movements. He smoked for several years but quit at age 35. He has a family history of breast cancer (mother and sister) but no other known heritable illnesses. He is married and retired and likes to travel. He has just returned from an ocean cruise and believes the rich food he ate while on the cruise is responsible for many of his symptoms. Physical examination reveals a cooperative older man, whose examination findings are normal, except for nonspecific **lower abdominal tenderness** noted during deep palpation and **occult-blood positive** stool.

Vignette Objectives

1. What are the symptoms and physical examination findings indicative of colorectal cancer?
2. How do the clinical presentations of right- and left-sided colon cancer differ?

Colon Cancer

Abdominal discomfort and constipation are nonspecific symptoms, but when these complaints are of recent onset, they indicate the possibility of a colonic tumor, especially if the patient is an older adult. The symptoms and signs of colonic malignancies vary with the site (Table 6-17). Right-sided colorectal cancers often are asymptomatic, and they are more likely to have metastasized by the time of diagnosis because of the attendant delay in the diagnosis. Because left-sided lesions obstruct the passage of more formed stools, they become symptomatic earlier than right-sided lesions.

The pathologic stage and grade are prognostic factors in colon cancer. Stage A disease, which is limited to the mucosa, is associated with a 75% to 100% 5-year survival; stage D disease, which involves distant metastasis, is associated with a less than a 5% 5-year survival. Well-differentiated carcinomas are associated with greater survival than poorly differentiated malignancies.

Unexplained iron-deficiency anemia in a man or a nonmenstruating woman is strongly suggestive of GI tract diseases, such as ulcers, benign and malignant

Table 6-17. Symptoms and signs of colon cancer

Symptom/sign	Right colon	Left colon
Bowel habits	No change	Reduced stool caliber
Abdominal pain	None or minimal	Nonspecific, lower abdominal or "gas" pain, symptoms of obstruction
Blood loss	Long duration of symptoms leads to iron deficiency	Earlier obstructive symptoms result in less total GI blood loss
Metastasis	Third of cases at diagnosis	Variable

tumors, an inflammatory process, or diverticula. This finding always necessitates a thorough GI tract evaluation.

Polyps and Familial Colon Cancers

Most colonic polyps are hyperplastic and do not have a malignant potential. However, adenomatous polyps are at risk for becoming malignant, especially if (1) they are greater than 2 cm in diameter, (2) they are multiple in number, or (3) they have a villous morphology. Colorectal malignancies usually begin as polyps; therefore removal of adenomatous polyps can reduce the risk of colon cancer.

Certain hereditary polyposis syndromes are associated with an increased risk for malignancy. One of these syndromes is familial polyposis, which is an autosomal dominant disorder that begins with the formation of polyps during adolescence. The probability of malignant transformation in patients with this disorder greatly increases after age 30. Other syndromes with a malignant potential include Turcot's syndrome (autosomal recessive, associated with glioblastoma and medulloblastoma), Gardner's syndrome (autosomal dominant, associated with many other benign and malignant tumors), and the rare Cronkhite-Canada syndrome (associated with alopecia, atrophy of the fingernails, and malabsorption).

There are also familial colon cancers, with affected members manifesting cancer as early as age 30 years of age. The risk of colorectal cancer is increased in patients who have parents or siblings who have had breast, ovarian, or endometrial malignancies. In addition, people with a history of ulcerative colitis are at increased risk for colon cancer. These patients require close monitoring and sometimes are treated prophylactically with colectomy.

The tumor marker carcinoembryonic antigen (CEA) can be elevated in patients with colorectal cancer. However, an elevation in the CEA level can also result from smoking, chronic lung disease, and inflammatory bowel disease; therefore measurement of the CEA level is not a cost-effective screening test.

Vignette Follow-up

Mr. T has normal liver enzyme levels and a normal hematocrit. Because of the occult-blood positive stool and the change in bowel habits, flexible sigmoidoscopy and an air-contrast barium enema are performed. The radiograph shows a narrowed lumen near the splenic flexure, and biopsy specimen findings confirm adenocarcinoma. A metastatic workup, which includes liver and bone imaging, is negative. A large resection is performed, and Mr. T does well for about 10 months, after which he begins to have abdominal cramping and his abdominal girth increases. A CT scan of his abdomen reveals metastases of the adenocarcinoma, with peritoneal extension and colonic obstruction. Palliative surgery is performed, and he is treated with an experimental chemotherapy. Mr. T dies 9 months after his second surgery.

CEA measurement is used best as part of an overall evaluation to assess those at high risk for tumor, to monitor the completeness of resection, and to use in surveillance for recurrences.

Objectives Review

1. List the history and physical examination findings relevant to the causes of polycythemia and erythrocytosis.
2. Explain why cyanosis is not a sensitive indicator of hypoxemia, and describe the significance of central and peripheral cyanosis.
3. Describe a systematic evaluation of a person who has anemia.
4. What are the common causes of iron deficiency?
5. What findings are typical of pernicious anemia?
6. What clues in the history and physical examination are helpful in detecting and characterizing a bleeding disorder?
7. What preoperative evaluation is needed to rule out a bleeding disorder?
8. What are the causes of thrombocytopenia and how would the assessment findings differ for patients suspected of having these disorders?
9. List the different illnesses caused by a monoclonal increase in serum immunoglobulins and the history and physical examination findings associated with each.
10. List the history and physical examination findings encountered in the following oncologic emergencies: brain metastasis, malignant pericardial effusion, and superior vena cava (SVC) obstruction.
11. List four categories of paraneoplastic syndromes and an example of a specific disorder in each.
12. Explain how the history and physical examination findings can be used to evaluate patients with fever and neutropenia.
13. What aspects of the history and physical examination are important in determining whether lymphadenopathy is due to an infection or a malignancy?
14. What problems could be associated with a CD4 cell count greater than 500 cells/mm^3, 200 to 500 cells/mm^3, and less than 200 cells/min^3?
15. List the symptoms and signs of Hodgkin's disease and other lymphomas.
16. What are the late sequelae of treatment for malignancies?
17. What general health maintenance procedures are suggested for people in different age groups?
18. What historical features are typical of musculoskeletal low back pain? What aspects of the examination detect neurologic involvement? Which findings indicate the need for radiographs early in the diagnostic evaluation?
19. What is the likelihood and timing of breast cancer recurrence?
20. What is the natural history of prostate cancer? What is the pattern of metastasis?
21. Outline the communication principles used to deliver bad news effectively.
22. What historical and physical examination aspects are most relevant when evaluating unintentional weight loss?
23. Define "attributes" as they relate to a patient's medical history.

24. What are the symptoms and physical examination findings indicative of colorectal cancer?
25. How do the clinical presentations of right- and left-sided colon cancer differ?

Suggested Reading

Aisenberg AC. The staging and treatment of Hodgkin's disease. *N Engl J Med* 1978;299: 1228–32.
The author presents a concise summary of the staging scheme for Hodgkin's disease.

Bookman MA, Longo DL, Young RC. Late complications of curative treatment in Hodgkin's disease. *JAMA* 1988;260:680–3.
The authors review the effects of treatment for Hodgkin's disease, including risks of splenotomy, thyroid dysfunction, pulmonary toxicity, pericarditis, accelerated coronary atherosclerotic disease, gonadal dysfunction, and secondary malignancies.

Brett AS. The mammography and prostate-specific antigen controversies: implications for patient-physician encounters and public policy. *J Gen Intern Med* 1995;10:266–70.
Recent discussion of whom to screen.

Byrne TN. Spinal cord compression from epidural metastases. *N Engl J Med* 1992;327: 614–9.
The author presents a succinct discussion of the pathophysiology, clinical presentation, imaging procedures, and management pertinent to this disorder.

Elliot DL, Tolle SW, Goldberg L, Miller JB. Pet-associated illness. *N Engl J Med* 1985;313: 985–95.
The authors present a scholarly review of illnesses acquired from pets.

George JN, El-Harake MA, Raskob GE. Chronic idiopathic thrombocytopenic purpura. *N Engl J Med* 1994;331:1207–12.
A brief review article that presents the clinical features, differential diagnosis, natural history, and management of this disorder.

Hancock SL, Tucker MA, Hoppe RT. Breast cancer after treatment of Hodgkin's disease. *J Natl Cancer Inst* 1993;85:25–31.
Women who receive radiation treatment before age 30 have up to a fourfold increase in breast cancer risk.

Harris JR, Lippman ME, Veronesi U, Willett W. Breast cancer (parts I, II, and III). *N Engl J Med* 1992;327:319–28, 390–8, and 473–80.
The authors present a three-part review, covering the epidemiology, primary treatment, and adjuvant therapy of breast cancer.

Karim A, Cockerell CJ, Petri WA. Cat scratch disease, bacillary angiomatosis, and other infections due to *Rochalimaea. N Engl J Med* 1994;330:1509–15.
Only in the past few years have these disorders' pathogen been identified.

Miranda J, Brody RV. Communicating bad news. *West J Med* 1992;156:83–5.
Brief review and summary of principles for delivering bad news; text includes sample dialogues.

Nachman RL, Silverstein R. Hypercoagulable states. *Ann Intern Med* 1993;119:819–27.
Literature review that focuses on primary inherited disorders and secondary conditions, such as drug effects, malignancy, the antiphospholipid syndrome, heparin-associated thrombopathy, and myeloproliferative disorders.

Pizzo PA. Management of fever in patients with cancer and treatment-induced neutropenia. *N Engl J Med* 1991;328:1323–32.

The author discusses empiric therapy, antibiotics, potential infections, and management other than antibiotics in patients with cancer treatment–induced neutropenia.

Reife CM. Involuntary weight loss: significance of involuntary weight loss. *Med Clin North Am* 1995;79:299–313.
Recent concise review article.

Rosenthal DS. Clinical aspects of chronic myeloproliferative diseases. *Am J Med Sci* 1992;302:109–24.
The author reviews the myeloproliferative disorders, including the differential diagnoses pertaining to cell line elevations, the criteria for diagnosis, different clinical presentations, and options for management.

Sardell AN, Trierweiler SJ. Disclosing the cancer diagnosis. *Cancer* 1993;72:3355–65.
Patients were more hopeful if the provider exhibited expertise and up-to-date technical abilities and provided ongoing involvement and emotional support; conversely, hopefulness was decreased when physicians were nervous or sad, diagnoses were given over the phone, and the information provided was limited.

Schwartzman WA. Infections due to *Rochalimaea:* the expanding clinical spectrum. *Clin Infect Dis* 1992;15:893–900.
Interesting review article that presents the "story" of how a bacteria was linked with cat scratch disease and bacillary angiomatosis.

Sickles EA, Greene WH, Wiernik PH. Clinical presentation of infection in granulocytopenic patients. *Arch Intern Med* 1975;135:715–9.
Granulocytopenic patients become febrile with infections; however, other signs of infection (exudate, fluctuant, local heat, edema, and regional adenopathy) were less common; erythema and tenderness can be the only findings indicating a localized infection.

Slap GB, Connor JL, Wigton RS, Schwartz S. Validation of a model to identify young patients for lymph node biopsy. *JAMA* 1986;255:2768–73.
The authors validated a model that identifies the nodes of 9 to 25 year olds as being either malignant or granulomatous; components were +5 for an abnormal chest radiograph, +3 for node >2 cm in diameter, and −3 for ENT symptoms; positive scores indicated malignancy, and negative scores indicated nonmalignant disease.

Sox HC. Screening mammography in women younger than 50 years of age. *Ann Intern Med* 1995;122:550–2.
This commentary responded to two articles in the issue, each reaching a different conclusion concerning the need for mammography among women 40 to 49 years old; as is true for many screening maneuvers, the data about the cost efficacy of mammography are incomplete.

Stabler SP, Allan RH, Savage DG, Lindenbaum J. Clinical spectrum and diagnosis of cobalamin deficiency. *Blood* 1990;76:871–81.
Over one third of those responding to cobalamin treatment had a normal hematocrit and mean corpuscular volume; the authors concluded that vitamin B_{12} deficiency should be sought in those with unexplained neuropsychiatric abnormalities; measurements of the serum methyl malonic acid and total homocysteine levels were useful laboratory studies.

Stolinsky DC. Paraneoplastic syndromes (Medical Progress). *West J Med* 1980;132:189–208.
The author discusses the remote effects of malignancies; such effects can occur in the setting of endocrine disorders (e.g., Cushing's syndrome, SIADH, and hypercalcemia), hematologic problems (e.g., polycythemia and thrombocytosis), coagulopathies, and neurologic syndromes.

Strobach SR, Anderson SK, Doll DC, Ringenberg SQ. The value of the physical examination in the diagnosis of anemia; correlation of the physical findings and the hemoglobin concentration. *Arch Intern Med* 1988;831–2.

Although pallor can be used to detect moderate anemia (hematocrit, <30%), it is not a sensitive finding.

U.S. Preventive Services Task Force. *Guide to clinical preventive services, 2nd ed.* Baltimore: Williams & Wilkins; 1996.
Extensive review of the evidence for and against various history findings, physical examination components, and laboratory studies.

Wallach PM, Flannery MT, Stewart JM. Paraneoplastic syndromes for the primary care physician. *Prim Care* 1992;19:727–43.
Review article on this topic.

7 Gastrointestinal Problems

Objectives

List history and physical examination findings for the following problems:

- "Acute abdomen"
- Acute diarrhea
- Alcoholism
- Appendicitis
- Cholecystitis
- Chronic diarrhea
- Cirrhosis
- Dyspepsia
- Gastroesophageal reflux
- Hepatic encephalopathy
- Hepatitis
- Inflammatory bowel disease
- Irritable bowel syndrome
- Jaundice
- Lower GI tract hemorrhage
- Malabsorption
- Occult-blood testing
- Pancreatitis
- Peptic ulcer disease
- Upper GI tract hemorrhage

Pertinent Points

History

Any problems with your GI tract?
Any abdominal operations?
Ever think you had an ulcer?
- Character and location of discomfort
- Nocturnal pain
- What lessens and worsens symptoms
- Effect of meals, antacids, H_2-blockers, omeprazole
- Early satiety, nausea, vomiting
- Hematemesis, melena
- Barrier breakers (e.g., aspirin, NSAIDs, alcohol)
- Family history of ulcers

History of heartburn?
- Acid taste in mouth
- Retrosternal discomfort
- Dysphagia for liquids and solids
- Intensification of symptoms after meals or when supine
- Effect of antacids

Any change in bowel habits?
- Caliber of stools, frequency
- Rectal bleeding
- Family history of colon cancer
- Abdominal pain, weight loss

When evaluating abdominal pain:
- History of GI tract problems or operations
- Location, radiation
- Severity (1 to 10 scale)
- Duration and quality of pain (e.g., sharp, dull, crampy)
- What lessens and worsens symptoms
- Associated symptoms (e.g., anorexia, nausea, vomiting, change in bowel habits)
- Associated GU tract symptoms
- Menstrual history, possibility of pregnancy

When evaluating a patient with suspected pancreatitis:
- Location, radiation
- Onset, quality, severity of pain
- Effect of position
- Nausea, vomiting, effect of food
- Assessment for potential causes: alcohol use, history of gallstones, abdominal trauma, hyperlipidemia, hypercalcemia, medications, symptoms of peptic ulcer disease

When evaluating a person who is jaundiced:
- Onset and progression
- Change in color of urine and stool
- Prior liver disease
- History of alcohol use
- Risks and exposures (contacts, travel, IV drug use, sexual activity, drugs, hepatotoxins)
- Associated symptoms (fever, malaise, weight loss, abdominal pain, change in abdominal girth, arthralgias)
- Family history of liver disease

When evaluating a person with worsening hepatic encephalopathy:
- Dietary protein
- Recent symptoms or signs of GI tract bleeding
- Medications, recent alcohol ingestion
- Abdominal pain, fever

When evaluating a person with diarrhea of recent onset:
- Number, character of stools (volume, watery, formed, blood)
- Abdominal cramps, tenesmus
- Associated symptoms (e.g., fever, nausea, vomiting, myalgias, rash)
- Risks and exposures (travel, recent antibiotics treatment, ingestion of undercooked meat or poultry, consumption of shellfish or picnic food, new medications, sexual activity)

When evaluating hematemesis or melena:
- Quantify bleeding
- Light-headedness
- Prior GI tract bleeding
- Heartburn or symptoms of peptic ulcer disease
- Barrier breakers (aspirin, NSAIDs, alcohol)
- Vomiting or retching before hematemesis
- History of liver disease
- Pepto-Bismol or iron ingestion

When evaluating hematochezia:
- Quantify bleeding (number of stools, volume of blood)
- Light-headedness
- Prior GI tract bleeding
- Symptoms of peptic ulcer disease or barrier breakers
- Hemorrhoids, rectal pain, itching
- History of diverticular disease
- Change in stool caliber or bowel habits
- Fever, arthritis, rash

Physical Examination

Vital signs Blood pressure, heart rate, temperature, respiratory rate, orthostatic change in blood pressure and heart rate

Inspection
- Nutritional state
- Jaundice, scleral icterus
- Palmar erythema, spider angiomas
- Gynecomastia, testicular atrophy
- Abnormal pigmentation, telangiectasia
- Petechiae, bruising

Abdominal examination
- Contour of abdomen (scaphoid, flat, distended)
- Venous pattern on abdominal wall
- Bowel sounds
- Bruits
- Ascites (bulging flanks, fluid wave, shifting dullness)
- Percussion of upper and lower liver borders of liver
- Percussion of left upper quadrant during inspiration (sphlenic enlargement)
- Percussion four abdominal quadrants (tympany with increased gas, dullness mass)
- Palpation of liver edge, tenderness, nodularity
- Light and deep palpation for tenderness, organomegaly, abdominal aorta, masses, rebound
- Pelvic examination
- Digital rectal examination (mass, fissure, hemorrhoids)
- Stool for occult-blood

Signs relating to specific abnormalities
- Murphy sign: cholecystitis
- Courvoisier's law: palpable gallbladder + obstructive jaundice = malignancy
- Sister Joseph's node: paraumbilical lymph node
- Psoas sign: hip extension increases pain
- Obturator sign: external rotation of flexed hip increases pain
- Chandelier sign: intense pain made worse by palpation (so that the patient jumps for the chandelier)

Extremities
- Arterial bruits, peripheral pulses
- Palmar erythema
- "Tracks" or venous scarring

Neurologic
- Mental status
- Cranial nerves: extraocular movements inspection of cornea (Kayser-Fleischer ring seen with slit-lamp)
- Motor: atrophy, strength, muscle tenderness, asterixis
- Sensory
- Reflexes
- Gait

Vignette 1

Acute abdomen: an abdominal problem that may necessitate emergent surgery; often characterized by severe abdominal pain, peritoneal irritation, and an ileus.

CAGE questions: mnemonic used to remember the four questions used to screen for alcoholism.

Ileus: loss of normal GI peristalsis.

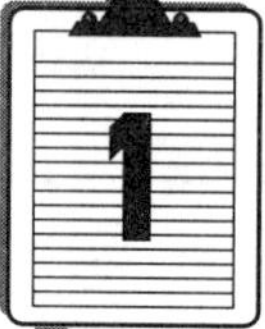

EW is a 41-year-old man admitted to the ward with "abdominal pain." For 5 days before admission, Mr. W experienced constant abdominal discomfort, localized in the epigastrium and radiating to his midback and associated with nausea and occasional vomiting. He has been able to drink liquids but has not been able to tolerate solid foods. He has experienced no diarrhea or lower abdominal pain. Because a friend advised him that he might have appendicitis, EW came to the emergency room. Additional history reveals a similar pain occurring approximately 1 year ago that lasted for 3 days, but he did not seek care for that episode. He has no other history of abdominal pain, GI tract illnesses, or abdominal surgery.

The patient has a 20-year history of alcohol consumption. Recently he has been drinking one to two fifths of whiskey a day. He has a history of "black outs," early-morning drinking, and hallucinations when he stops drinking. He has never successfully stopped drinking for more than a few weeks, and he has never enrolled in any structured alcohol rehabilitation program. For the past 5 days, he has felt "shaky" and experienced some visual hallucinations (seeing "bugs" on his body), but these have resolved by the time of admission. He currently lives with his mother and is employed part-time in low-skilled jobs.

Physical examination reveals a disheveled man who is lying on his side and curled up on the gurney. Vital signs: **supine blood pressure** is 130/100 mm Hg, with a **heart rate** of 100 beats/min. His **standing blood pressure** is 130/105 mm Hg, with a **heart rate** of 120 beats/min. **Skin** examination reveals palmar erythema but no spider angiomas. **HEENT:** full extraocular movements, normal fundi; clear oropharynx. His neck is supple, without thyromegaly or adenopathy. **Chest:** clear to auscultation. **Cardiac:** no jugular venous distention (JVD); normal point of maximal impulse (PMI); normal S_1 and S_2, no murmurs or gallops. **Abdomen:** mild distention; bowel sounds are present but reduced (only two are heard in 90 seconds). His abdomen is soft, with tenderness in his epigastrium. The liver span is 15 cm to percussion, with the edge three finger breadths below the right costal margin, mildly tender, and smooth. No spleen is percussed or palpated. No masses are palpable. **Rectal** exam: light yellow, formed, occult-blood–negative stool. **Extremities:** no cyanosis, clubbing, or edema. **Reflexes:** absent Achilles tendon reflexes; decreased vibratory sense in his feet; no asterixis. Laboratory studies show a white blood cell count of 9,800/mm^3; hematocrit is 39%, with macrocytic indices (mean corpuscular volume, >100 μm^3) and low platelet count (96,000/mm^3).

Vignette Objectives

1. What history and physical examination findings are most important when prioritizing potential causes of abdominal pain?
2. What are the findings of a patient with an "acute abdomen"?
3. What aspects of the history and physical examination are important when evaluating a patient for alcoholism?

Abdominal Pain

Acute Abdomen

The differential diagnosis of abdominal pain is extensive. The initial assessment is used to narrow the number of diagnoses and determine whether the patient has an acute condition requiring surgical intervention. Several conditions can be cause for surgical intervention, the most life-threatening ones being perforation or rupture of a viscus, bowel obstruction, and necrosis of the intestinal tract. Overall, a diagnosis determined on the basis of the clinical assessment findings is correct in approximately half of patients; diagnostic accuracy is increased by about 10% when findings from serial observations are added to the initial assessment.

Findings characteristic of an acute abdomen include peritoneal irritation, manifested by involuntary guarding, severe localized or diffuse pain, rebound tenderness, and a "quiet" abdomen, with absent bowel sounds. Involuntary guarding is due to parietal peritoneum inflammation, causing the abdominal wall muscles to spasm. Unlike involuntary guarding (which causes a rigid abdomen), voluntary guarding is under the patient's control and results from the anticipation of pain with palpation. Rebound tenderness is assessed by pressing gently on the abdomen, followed by quick release of the pressure. If pain is worsened upon release of the pressure, the patient has rebound tenderness, and this is caused by peritoneal irritation at the point of pain. Normal bowel sounds usually occur every few seconds, but their frequency is highly variable. The examiner must therefore listen for at least 2 minutes before concluding that they are absent.

Among the elderly and those taking corticosteroids, abdominal pain can be mild, despite the presence of perforation or peritoneal inflammation. Accordingly, one should not underestimate the seriousness of mild abdominal pain in an elderly patient, especially if it is associated with confusion, fever, and leukocytosis. Potential causes of abdominal pain, including those leading to an "acute abdomen," are listed in Table 7-1. Gynecologic and obstetric problems are additional considerations in women, and these disorders are discussed in Chapter 9.

Bowel obstruction often necessitates surgical intervention. The supine and upright abdominal radiograph (sometimes referred to as a *KUB study* because it visualizes the kidneys, ureters, and bladder) can show the presence and dis-

Table 7-1. Causes of acute abdominal pain

Condition	History	Physical exam
Peritonitis	Patient has sterile transudative ascites (portal hypertension or nephrotic syndrome) that becomes infected, with onset of abdominal pain and fever (spontaneous bacterial peritonitis); also caused by condition resulting in diffuse peritoneal inflammation, such as bowel infarction or perforation	Generalized tenderness and involuntary guarding; rebound tenderness; hypoactive or absent bowel sounds; findings of ascites, if spontaneous bacterial peritonitis
Appendicitis	Peak age 10–20 years; 10% of cases occur among elderly; males > females; initially anorexia, nausea, and vomiting (if patient is hungry, think of another diagnosis); subsequent localized right lower quadrant pain; similar history to that of appendicitis can be caused by mesenteric adenitis, pelvic inflammatory disease, and diverticulitis	>90% of patients have right lower quadrant tenderness, guarding, and rebound; discrete tenderness at McBurney's point; two thirds of patients have rebound tenderness; retrocecal location can be associated with less localized findings; perforation more likely among elderly
Acute cholecystitis	Despite being called *biliary colic,* cholecystitis usually causes constant pain; typically pain is in right upper quadrant and can radiate to scapula	Right upper quadrant tenderness and guarding; Murphy's sign; patient can be febrile
Small bowel and colonic obstruction	Epigastric or periumbilical pain, vomiting; no flatus or bowel movements	Distention; hyperactive high-pitched bowel sounds, progressing to absent bowel sounds; distention greater with distal colonic obstruction
Bowel infarction	Risks for atherosclerotic disease or embolus	Periumbilical or lower quadrant abdominal pain; initially pain >> tenderness; rectal bleeding, if venous thrombosis
Ruptured abdominal aortic aneurysm	Back pain; elderly individuals with risk atherosclerotic vascular disease	Hypotension; pulsatile tender mass; asymmetry of lower extremity pulses
Pancreatitis	Steady, severe, left upper quadrant and epigastric pain, radiating to the back; pain reduced when sitting forward; can be history of alcoholism, gallstones, abdominal trauma, hyperlipidemia, drug use, or viral infection	Decreased bowel sounds; diffuse abdominal tenderness; hypotension due to decreased intake and transudation of fluid due to retroperitoneal inflammation
Diverticulitis	Left lower quadrant pain (left colon to right colon location, 3 : 1); prior similar symptom (recurrence rate is approximately 50%)	Fever; left lower quadrant tenderness; localized rebound and guarding; possible tender mass on digital rectal exam
Acute toxic megacolon	History of ulcerative colitis or other cause for diffuse colonic inflammation (e.g., pseudomembranous colitis)	Diffuse abdominal pain; reduced bowel sounds; tympany due to colonic dilatation
Perforating ulcer	Symptoms of peptic ulcer; acute epigastric pain which can radiate to shoulders or neck (due to diaphragmatic irritation)	Absent bowel sounds; diffuse tenderness; free air can result in percussion tympany over the liver (free air visible on upright KUB in about 25% of perforations)

tribution of bowel gas and help differentiate an ileus, resulting from a mechanical obstruction, from an adynamic ileus, resulting from metabolic or inflammatory disorders (Table 7-2). In addition, upright abdominal radiographs can show subdiaphragmatic air, and calcium in the pancreas, biliary system (15% of gallstones are calcified), and genitourinary (GU) tract may be visualized.

A markedly dilated colon and absent bowel sounds are suggestive of an adynamic ileus referred to as Ogilvie's syndrome or intestinal pseudoobstruction. The amount of dilatation can be shown by a KUB study. The overall risk of colon perforation is about 15%, and if the cecum is more than 11 cm in diameter, the likelihood of this complication increases. The disorder usually occurs among elderly people with an acute infection or metabolic abnormality, and management is directed at correcting the underlying disorder, use of nasogastric suction, minimizing further dilatation, and close serial follow-ups.

Onset, Location, and Progression

Abdominal pain that begins abruptly often is caused by perforation of a viscus, such as that resulting from a perforated peptic ulcer or colonic diverticulum. Inflammation of a viscus (e.g., diverticulitis, cholecystitis, or appendicitis) has a more gradual onset. The term *colic* refers to intermittent wavelike, crampy pain, and it usually is caused by intestinal distention, with intermittent peristalsis accentuating the pain.

The location of the abdominal pain reflects the embryonic origin of the structures involved and the site of any parietal peritoneal involvement. Abdominal discomfort originating from the small bowel and colon sometimes is referred to as *visceral pain,* and it typically is felt diffusely. Somatic pain is localized to the site of parietal peritoneum inflammation. In addition, because of shared innervation, pain can be referred to areas distant to involved structures. For example, left neck

Table 7-2. Mechanical versus paralytic ileus

Type of ileus	Intestinal gas pattern on upright KUB	Air-fluid levels on upright KUB
Mechanical obstruction (due to adhesions, incarcerated hernia, volvulus, tumor, diverticulitis)	Only proximal to obstruction, no rectal air	Air-fluid levels at end of loops are at different levels
Paralytic ileus (due to metabolic abnormality, sepsis, pancreatitis, peritonitis, after abdominal surgery, and in late stages of mechanical obstruction)	Scattered throughout small and large intestine	Air-fluid levels at ends of loops are at same level (U-shaped)

or shoulder pain can be due to irritation of the left hemidiaphragm and referred pain in a C_5, C_6, and C_7 distribution (phrenic nerve).

Serial observations can help identify a certain disorder by revealing its characteristic progression. For example, the first manifestations of appendicitis are diffuse abdominal pain, anorexia, nausea, and vomiting—visceral symptoms similar to the discomfort associated with gastroenteritis. However, as the inflammation progresses to involve the adjacent peritoneum, the pain localizes in the right lower quadrant, which the pain of viral gastroenteritis does not do.

Occasionally, problems involving the abdominal wall simulate an intraabdominal process. Bleeding into the rectus sheath, which can occur among anticoagulated individuals, can cause pain and tenderness. Such abdominal wall tenderness is worsened by tensing the abdominal muscles unlike intraabdominal problems, which are associated with less tenderness and with voluntary guarding. In addition, radicular pain due to nerve root irritation with herpes zoster or from diabetic radiculopathy can cause abdominal wall pain in a nerve root distribution. This type of neuropathic pain often is elicited by gentle palpation and can be accompanied by cutaneous hyperesthesia.

Abdominal Aortic Aneurysm

An aneurysm of the abdominal aorta is a disorder that affects approximately 10% of elderly people with atherosclerotic vascular disease. The typical findings in patients with aortic rupture are back pain or flank discomfort (15% to 50% of patients) or a pulsatile, tender abdominal mass and shock. Other less common symptoms include hip pain, rupture into the duodenum with GI tract bleeding, and the signs and symptoms of embolic events distal to the aorta (e.g., lower extremity arterial occlusion and the "blue toe syndrome").

Although aortic rupture usually is not confused with intraabdominal problems, it is considered here because the aorta is assessed during the abdominal examination. However, the ability to detect an aneurysm varies with the patient's body habitus. It is easier to palpate the lateral margins of the aorta and estimate its diameter in slender people; in these patients, physical examination is more than 90% sensitive in detecting an aneurysm. Its sensitivity decreases to 50% or less in obese patients. Aortic size tends to be overestimated during physical examination. An abdominal ultrasound can accurately assess the size when enlargement is suspected. Aneurysms 5 cm or more in diameter have a 25% to 40% chance of rupturing in the next 5 years, and elective surgery is recommended to prevent this complication.

Assessment for Alcohol Abuse

Alcoholism is an illness with a wide spectrum of manifestations, and many studies have documented that the illness often goes unrecognized by physicians. Because most people with alcoholism do not fit the stereotype of a disheveled person, questions concerning alcohol use and abuse are appropriate for all patients. Some patients can be easily identified as "alcoholic," however, and these severely affected people are overrepresented in the population of hospitalized patients.

History of Alcohol Use

The quantification of alcohol consumption is unreliable, because many regular alcohol users underreport their intake. However, if a person says that he or she drinks heavily (e.g., "a fifth a night"), the patient probably does drink excessively. The concern is that many who drink heavily do not admit their intake. A strategy for eliciting an alcohol history using the CAGE questions is shown in Figure 7-1.

Medical Concerns in Patients with Alcoholism

A mnemonic to remember the potential clinical complications that can occur in hospitalized patients with alcoholism is **WINO** (Table 7-3).

Alcohol Withdrawal Syndromes

Alcohol withdrawal's initial syndrome ("the shakes") is associated with increased adrenergic activity, causing nausea, tremulousness, tachycardia, and

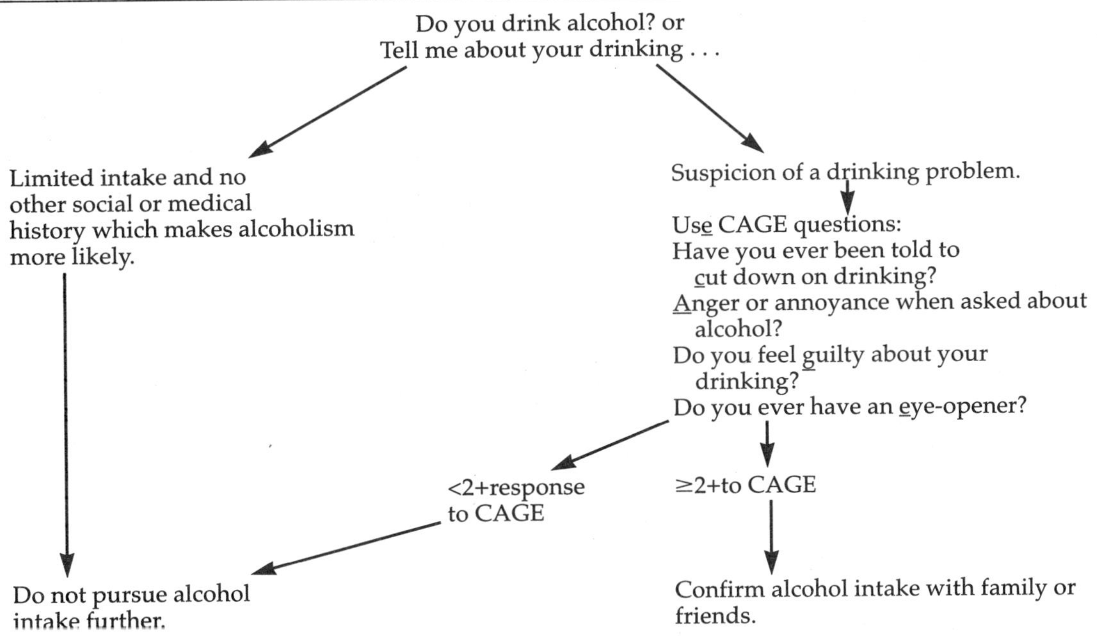

Figure 7-1. A social or medical history suggesting alcohol abuse or more than infrequent use of alcohol should prompt use of CAGE questions to assess for alcoholism. A positive response to two or more CAGE questions is 90% sensitive and 80% specific for a diagnosis of alcoholism.

Table 7-3. Clinical complications of alcohol abuse

W = withdrawal	All heavy drinkers are at risk for withdrawal. It is a severe disorder and can result in autonomic overactivity (tachycardia, hypertension, agitation), seizures ("rum fits"), hallucinations ("pink elephants"), and delirium ("DT's") (Table 7-5).
I = ions	Metabolic and electrolyte problems are common among alcoholics. Specific abnormal laboratory findings include hypokalemia, hypophosphatemia, hypomagnesemia, and acid-base disorders. If rhabdomyolysis occurs, hyperphosphatemia, hyperuricemia, and hypocalcemia can accompany renal dysfunction.
N = nutrition	Nutritional deficiencies are common. Thiamine, folate, and multivitamins should routinely be administered in alcoholic patients. Thiamine deficiency causes Wernicke's syndrome, which manifests as ataxia, nystagmus or ophthalmoplegia, and confusion, findings that might be confused with being "drunk." If intravenous glucose is administered (as when starting intravenous fluids) to a patient deficient in thiamine, this can exacerbate the thiamine deficiency and lead to Korsakoff's psychosis, which is a confabulating dementia resulting from permanent central nervous system (CNS) damage.
O = other organs	Alcoholism can have manifestations in any organ system (Table 7-4).

hypertension. The characteristics of this and the other stages of alcohol withdrawal are summarized in Table 7-5. Withdrawal seizures occur approximately 12 hours after a marked decrease in or discontinuance of alcohol intake. Seizures typically are generalized, single (40% of cases), and not associated with localizing symptoms or signs. If more than one seizure occurs, they are confined to an 8-hour interval. Delirium resulting from alcohol withdrawal occurs 12 or more hours after the last drink. It is associated with a high morbidity and mortality, because the altered mental status and sedation required can result in aspiration and other medical problems that go unrecognized.

Table 7-4. Alcohol's effects on organ systems

Organ system	Potential adverse consequences
Neurologic	Withdrawal seizures, delirium tremens, head trauma, Wernicke's and Korsakoff's syndromes, cerebellar degeneration, peripheral neuropathy
Cardiac	Arrhythmias, cardiomyopathy
Pulmonary	Aspiration pneumonia
Hepatic	Fatty liver, hepatitis, cirrhosis
GI tract	Gastritis, malabsorption, pancreatitis, varices if cirrhosis and portal hypertension present
Musculoskeletal	Myopathy, rhabdomyolysis, osteoporosis, aseptic necrosis, trauma
Renal	Electrolyte abnormalities, effects of rhabdomyolysis
Endocrine	Hypogonadism, hypercortisolism (pseudo-Cushing's syndrome)
Other	Fetal alcohol syndrome

Table 7-5. Alcohol withdrawal syndromes

Stage	Time since last drink	Duration of stage	Symptoms and signs
"Shakes"	6 to 8 hours	Up to 14 days	Nausea, anxiety, insomnia, tachycardia, tremor, hypertension
Hallucinations	24 hours	Up to 6 days	Hallucinations (auditory > visual); otherwise sensorium clear
"Seizures"	6 to 48 hours	<6 hours	Generalized tonic-clonic (overall risk 3%–15%; risk greater if prior withdrawal seizures)
"DTs"	2 to 3 days	≤3 days	Delirium, agitation, fever, tachycardia (mortality up to 15%)

Pancreatitis

Pancreatitis can vary in severity from a mild illness to a severe life-threatening disorder. It is associated with an overall mortality of approximately 10%. About half of the episodes are related to gallstone disease, and alcohol-related pancreatitis is a close second.

It requires several years of alcohol abuse for pancreatitis to occur, and the reason why the problem develops in only a small percentage (approximately 5%) of alcoholics is not known. Alcohol-associated pancreatitis is a chronic condition, with episodes of more severe disease producing symptoms. Biliary disease is discussed further in Vignette 2. There are many other causes of pancreatitis, however, and these include therapy with certain drugs (valproic acid, pentamidine, sulfonamides, azathioprine, prednisone, hydrochlorothiazide), abdominal trauma, hypercalcemia, hypertriglyceridemia, viral infections, and vasculitis.

Patients with pancreatitis typically experience epigastric or supraumbilical abdominal pain which radiates to the back, and they usually feel better sitting forward. Inflammation of adjacent bowel can result in abdominal tenderness and distention. The peritoneal inflammation causes an ileus and decreased bowel sounds. A sentinel loop is a characteristic feature of pancreatitis seen on KUB studies and is a dilated loop of bowel that overlies pancreatic inflammation. An ileus is a marker for more severe disease. Additional clinical features suggestive of more severe illness are fever of 101°F (38.3°C) or more, intravascular volume depletion, and diffuse abdominal pain. Hemorrhagic pancreatitis can result in flank ecchymosis (Grey Turner's sign).

However, physical findings alone are unreliable in identifying patients with severe pancreatitis. Adding results of laboratory tests on admission and during the following 48 hours provides a severity ranking that can predict the likelihood of complications and mortality (Table 7-6).

Table 7-6. Ranson's criteria for prognosis of pancreatitis

CRITERIA ASSESSED ON ADMISSION
Age, >50 years
WBC, >16,000/mm³
Glucose, >200 mg/dl
LDH, >350 IU/L
AST (SGOT), >250 IU/L

CRITERIA DEVELOPING IN THE FIRST 48 HOURS
Hematocrit decrease, >10%
BUN increase, >5 mg/dl
Calcium decrease, to <8 mg/dl
PO_2, <60 mm Hg
Estimated fluid sequestration, >6 L
Base deficit, >4 mEq/L

Number of criteria	Mortality
0–2	1%
3–4	16%
5–6	40%
7–8	100%

Vignette Follow-up

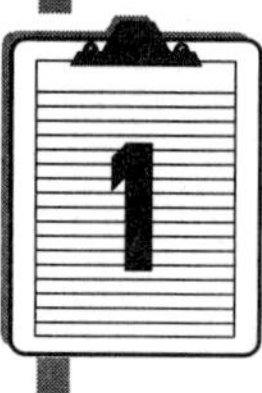

EW is thought to have chronic relapsing pancreatitis, associated with alcoholism. An abdominal ultrasound study shows edema of the pancreas and a possible pseudocyst, without evidence of cholelithiasis. After nasogastric suction and bowel rest, Mr. W's abdominal pain lessens, his serum amylase level decreases, and he is discharged to undergo a follow-up ultrasound scanning as an outpatient. He declines rehabilitation for his alcohol use.

Vignette 2

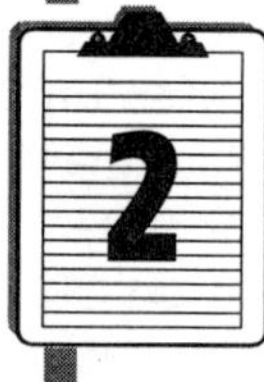

SH is a 75-year-old minister who is in good health, other than having stable coronary artery disease. His son calls and relates that Mr. H is experiencing dull abdominal and chest pain, especially after eating. The last episode was 3 days ago, and his discomfort lasted approximately 4 hours. Now, the pain is persistent and extends to his right shoulder. Mr. H has felt nauseated and vomited once. Although he has not taken his temperature, he has felt warm. There is no history of GI surgery, peptic ulcer disease, lipid abnormality, or abdominal trauma. He denies alcohol intake, which his family confirms. His only medications are enteric-coated aspirin and nitroglycerin, as needed.

Physical examination reveals an elderly, cooperative man in moderate distress. Vital signs: **blood pressure** is 130/85 mm Hg, **heart rate** is 72 beats/min, and oral **temperature** is 38.0°C. **HEENT:** sclerae are anicteric (no icterus).

Chest: clear to auscultation. **Cardiac:** no JVD; PMI is not palpable; chest wall is nontender; S_1 and S_2 are normal, without gallop or murmur. **Abdomen:** hypoactive bowels sounds; tender epigastrium and right upper quadrant; when palpating the right upper quadrant, inspiration dramatically increases the pain (Murphy's sign). There is no rebound tenderness or involuntary guarding. **Rectal** exam: nontender; occult-blood negative stool.

Vignette Objective

1. List the history and physical examination findings that indicate acute cholecystitis.

Cholecystitis

Acute cholecystitis is a common cause of abdominal pain. It results from obstruction of the cystic duct by a stone, which in turn results in biliary colic. Prolonged obstruction leads to edema, gallbladder inflammation, and infection. If the obstruction is distal to the cystic duct and involves pancreatic drainage, pancreatitis can occur; if it also obstructs hepatic drainage, jaundice, fever, and pain can occur (Charcot's triad).

Traditionally, the characteristics of those in whom gallstones are likely to develop are remembered by the letter "F": *f*emale, *f*air (fair-skinned, Caucasians), *f*orty (age >than 40 years), *f*ertile (prior pregnancies), and *f*at (obese). The physical findings in patients with acute cholecystitis can include fever and right upper quadrant tenderness.

Studies of patients with gallstones have shown that the symptoms often linked to cholecystitis (bloating, nausea, and fatty food intolerance) are not specific to gallbladder disease. Although over two thirds of patients describe the onset of pain in response to eating, with the discomfort beginning more than an hour after meals, pain can be associated with the consumption of any food (not predominantly fatty foods). The pain usually is located in the right upper quadrant, but it also can be in the midline or retrosternal area. Despite the fact that the pain is called *biliary colic,* the pain is characteristically dull and constant, not crampy or colicky, and lasts for over an hour.

At autopsy, a significant percentage of people are found to have asymptomatic gallstones, and their presence may not be sufficient to diagnose acute cholecystitis. Nuclear medicine testing is as sensitive and more specific in making the diagnosis.

Vignette Follow-up

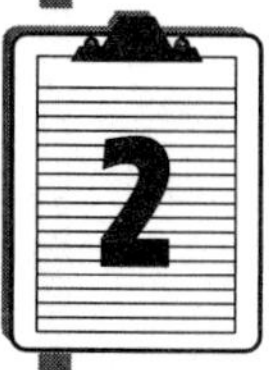

An abdominal radiograph reveals the presence of radiopaque material in the right upper quadrant, a finding consistent with calcium containing gallstones. SH's amylase level and white blood cell count are elevated, and a nuclear medicine (hepatoiminodiacetic acid scan with technicium—99m—labeled HIDA [lidofenin study]) shows cystic duct obstruction, as the hepatic and common bile ducts, but not the gallbladder, are seen. Mr. H is taken to the operating room, where a cholecystectomy is performed, followed by an uneventful recovery.

Vignette 3

Asterixis: rhythmic, jerking movements interrupting sustained muscular contraction; it usually indicates the existence of a metabolic problem affecting CNS function. It is assessed by observing the movement associated with sustained wrist hyperextension; the jerking or waving motion of asterixis is referred to as a *liver flap.*

Carotenemia: condition resembling jaundice; it is due to the excessive ingestion of carotene-containing vegetables; in carotenemia, although the skin is yellow-orange, the sclerae are not discolored.

Jaundice: yellow pigmentation of the sclerae and skin, which becomes visible when the bilirubin level exceeds 2.5 mg/dl (normal, 0.3–1.0 mg/dl).

Palmar erythema: erythema of palms due to vasodilatation produced by increased estrogen levels; often seen in patients with liver disease or pregnant women.

Scleral icterus: yellow pigmentation of the sclerae due to an elevated bilirubin level.

"Spider" angiomas: cutaneous arteriovenous malformations that characteristically fill from the center (the spider's body) and radiate outward.

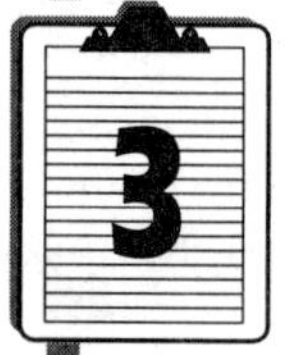

AD is a 32-year-old man who is seen in the clinic because of weight loss, fatigue, and abdominal pain. He states that he became ill several weeks ago, when loss of appetite and generalized muscle aches developed. He has no rash or joint complaints. His stool has become lighter in color, and his urine has become "darker." He believes his weight loss is due to his anorexia. He relates that he is homosexual and practices safe sex, except for one time "a couple of months ago." He lost contact with that individual and does not know about his former partner's health. The patient was tested for HIV disease 6 months ago, and the result was "negative." Mr. D takes no medications, drinks little alcohol, and was an avid exerciser prior to his current complaints.

Physical examination reveals a slender man (6 feet, 2 inches tall [1.85 m], weight, 175 pounds [79 kg]), who does not appear acutely ill. Vital signs: **blood pressure** is 112/76 mm Hg, and **heart rate** is 78 beats/min. **HEENT:** icteric sclerae, funduscopic exam findings are normal. Neck is without adenopathy or thyromegaly. **Chest:** clear to auscultation. **Cardiac:** normal S_1 and S_2; no murmurs or rub. **Abdomen:** flat with normal bowel sounds; liver percussion span is 14 cm, and the edge is tender and smooth; no other masses are felt. **Genitourinary** exam: normal male genitalia. **Rectal** exam: light yellow stool, occult-blood negative. **Extremities:** no joint deformities, rash, or edema. There is no bruising or cutaneous stigmata of chronic liver disease. **Neurologic** exam findings are normal, without localizing signs or asterixis.

Vignette Objectives

1. List causes of a palpable but not enlarged liver.
2. How do the history and physical examination findings relate to the potential causes of jaundice?

Liver Disease

Assessing Liver Size

Liver size and consistency assist in the categorization of hepatic disease. Percussing the span of liver dullness determines whether hepatomegaly is present, and palpation can delineate the lower border and determine hepatic consistency and whether there is tenderness. All palpable livers are not enlarged, however, in that downward displacement can cause a liver to be palpable. Percussing the upper and lower borders to define the liver span in the midclavicular line avoids mistaking a palpable, nonenlarged liver for an enlarged one.

Causes of a palpable, nonenlarged liver include chronic obstructive pulmonary disease (due to a depressed diaphragm), a subdiaphragmatic problem (e.g., a subdiaphragmatic abscess), and an aberrant lobe (an enlarged right lobe [Riedel's lobe]is a normal anatomic variant).

The spleen is normally not palpable and must be enlarged two to three times to be felt. Even with deep inspiration, the left upper quadrant superior to the costal border should be resonant-tympanic. The finding of dullness would prompt a careful palpation for an enlarged spleen.

Table 7-7. Jaundice in an adult

INTRAHEPATIC CHOLESTASIS
Hepatocellular liver function abnormalities[a]
Hepatitis: viral (A, B, C, E-B, CMV, delta agent), alcoholic, chronic active, drug-induced (e.g., INH, tetracycline, acetaminophen), hepatotoxins (e.g., carbon tetrachloride)
Wilson's disease
Alpha$_1$-antitrypsin deficiency
Hemochromatosis
Cholestatic liver function abnormalities[b]
Drugs (e.g., chlorpromazine, haloperidol, oral anabolic steroids)
Primary biliary cirrhosis
Liver metastasis
EXTRAHEPATIC OBSTRUCTION
Gallstones (choledocholithiasis)
Carcinoma of the hepatic duct, ampulla, or pancreas
Hepatic duct stricture
Duct inflammation (sclerosing cholangitis)

[a]AST (SGOT) elevation > alkaline phosphatase elevation.
[b]Alkaline phosphatase elevation > AST (SGOT elevation).

Assessing Jaundiced People

Jaundice occurs in the setting of many illnesses, and the two major categories and specific diagnoses to consider are listed in Table 7-7. Viral hepatitis and alcohol-associated liver disease are the most common causes of jaundice, but it is important to consider other causes, especially in the event of new-onset jaundice or when previously stable disease worsens. Relevant historical items are listed in Table 7-8, and physical examination findings and their implications are presented in Table 7-9.

Additional Information about Conditions Causing Jaundice

Primary biliary cirrhosis is an illness affecting more women than men, with a ratio of 9 : 1. The usual initial symptoms are fatigue and pruritus. Although the alkaline phosphatase level is elevated, affected patients usually are not jaundiced and the icteric phase develops a few months to several years later. Other patients may come to attention as the result of the malabsorption caused by the cholestasis. The disorder is associated with several autoimmune problems,

Table 7-8. Historical findings and the etiology of liver disease

Questions	Diagnostic possibility being evaluated
SYMPTOMS BEFORE ONSET OF JAUNDICE:	
Flu-like illness?	Viral hepatitis
Prior liver function tests?	Duration and progression of liver disease
Weight loss?	Cancer
Arthralgias, polyarthritis?	Prodrome of hepatitis B
Right upper quadrant pain	Biliary disease, hepatomegaly stretching the liver capsule
SYMPTOMS ASSOCIATED WITH JAUNDICE:	
Fever, chills?	Viral hepatitis, biliary obstruction with cholangitis
Arthralgias, rash, alopecia?	Autoimmune chronic active hepatitis ("lupoid" hepatitis)
Abdominal swelling?	Ascites, tumor
Pruritus?	Obstructive jaundice
Dark urine, light stools?	Confirms jaundice
HISTORY ASSESSING THE CAUSE OF JAUNDICE:	
Alcohol use?	Alcoholic hepatitis / cirrhosis
IV drug use? sexual preference? occupational exposure to transfusions? blood or blood products?	Viral hepatitis, hemolysis
Prior biliary tract surgery?	Extrahepatic obstruction
Medication use?	Drug-induced liver disease
Family history?	Inherited disorder (Wilson's disease, hemochromatosis, $alpha_1$-antitrypsin deficiency)
Occupation?	Toxin or blood product exposure

Table 7-9. Physical examination findings and the etiology and complications of liver disease

Examination	Findings	Implication
General	Age	Inherited problems are more likely if patient is young; cancer more likely among older patients
	Female versus male	Chronic active liver disease and primary biliary cirrhosis more common in women; sclerosing cholangitis more common in men
Vital signs	Orthostasis	Can be indication of acute bleeding
	Low body temperature	Hypothermia can be seen in severe liver disease (liver metabolism generates much of body heat)
	Increased respiratory rate	Hyperventilation due to hepatic encephalopathy
Skin	Icterus	Present when bilirubin >2.5 mg/dl
	Bronze color	Hemochromatosis
	Spider angiomas, telangiectasia, palmar erythema, gynecomastia	Stigmata of chronic liver disease
	Ecchymosis	Malabsorption of vitamin K or inability to synthesize clotting factors due to cirrhosis
	Xanthoma	Primary biliary cirrhosis
HEENT	Normocephalic, atraumatic	Trauma common among alcoholics
	Scleral icterus	Any cause of jaundice (elevated bilirubin >3 mg/dl)
	Kayser-Fleischer rings	Wilson's disease
	Extraocular movements impaired	Thiamine deficiency (alcoholism)
Cardiac	Jugular venous distention	Cirrhosis can be due to long-standing passive liver congestion from chronic CHF
Lung	Reduced chest expansion and decreased breath sounds	COPD can result in a palpable liver due to its downward displacement, when no hepatomegaly is present; ascites can result in reduced diaphragmatic excursion and/or pleural effusion
Abdomen	Distended, bulging flanks, shifting dullness, fluid wave (findings of ascites)	Portal hypertension (e.g., as with hepatic vein thrombosis, cirrhosis) or exudative ascites (e.g., malignancy) (see Table 7-11)
	Dilated venous pattern	Portal hypertension or inferior vena cava thrombosis (venous flow toward umbilicus in portal hypertension and cephalad in inferior vena cava thrombosis)
	Bruit over the liver	Hepatoma
	Hepatic span/palpitation for size, consistency, tenderness	In malignancy, enlarged, firm and nodular; in hepatitis, enlarged and tender; in cirrhosis, often small; in infiltrative liver disease (e.g., amyloidosis, hemochromatosis), enlarged and firm
	Palpable gallbladder	Malignancy of cystic or hepatic duct
	Splenomegaly	Portal hypertension
	Rectal examination and stool occult-blood	Malignant ascites can be associated with palpable metastatic disease; GI blood loss with varices
Genitourinary	Reduced volume of testes	Hypogonadism with alcohol use
Neurologic	Asterixis	Hepatic encephalopathy
	Decreased vibratory sense	Neuropathy with alcoholism
	Ataxia	Cerebellar degeneration with alcoholism and Wernicke's syndrome
	Incoordination, tremor, dysarthria	Wilson's disease
	Confusion-coma	Hepatic encephalopathy

Table 7-10. Comparison of types of viral hepatitis*

	Hepatitis A	Hepatitis B	Hepatitis C
Transmission route	Fecal-oral (RNA virus)	Blood borne: IV drug use, transfusion, sexual exposure, perinatal transmission (DNA virus)	20% community acquired acute viral hepatitis; transfusion related; risk for other forms of blood-borne transmission not established (probably similar to hepatitis B) (RNA virus)
Incubation	2–6 weeks	6–20 weeks	3–20 weeks
Infectious period	During late incubation and early clinical phase (2–3 weeks)	Greatest during HBs Ag positivity, 4 weeks+	Not known
Symptoms	Anorexia, nausea, vomiting, fever; 50% develop jaundice, usually 2 weeks after onset of symptoms	Arthralgias, nausea, vomiting; 35% develop jaundice, usually 2 weeks after onset of symptoms	Milder than other hepatitis viruses; similar to those of hepatitis B, except arthralgias less common; infrequently other manifestations (e.g., porphyria cutanea tarda, cryoglobulinemia)
Outcome	>99% recover	90% recover, 5% become carrier; chronic active chronic persistent hepatitis, in 3%; fulminant hepatic failure in 2%; risk for future hepatocellular carcinoma	80% chronic hepatitis, 25% develop cirrhosis; most common cause end-stage liver disease requiring transplantation; risk for future hepatocellular carcinoma

*Other less frequent viral hepatitis include E (causing epidemic hepatitis in developing countries), D (only affects patients with concomitant hepatitis B), Epstein-Barr, and cytomegalovirus

cholestasis. The disorder is associated with several autoimmune problems, such as rheumatoid arthritis, sicca syndrome, and thyroiditis.

Primary sclerosing cholangitis is an illness usually affecting young men. It is caused by inflammation of the intrahepatic and extrahepatic bile ducts. Over half of patients also have ulcerative colitis. The course consists of progressive obstruction, recurrent infections, and hepatic dysfunction resulting from the cholestasis.

Several viruses cause hepatitis, including cytomegalovirus, Epstein-Barr virus, and delta agent. The most common causes of viral hepatitis (hepatitis A, B, and C) are compared in Table 7-10. Hepatitis A is transmitted by the fecal-oral route, and infection often occurs as the result of the ingestion of water or food in geographic locations where sanitation is poor. There is no carrier state or long-term adverse sequelae. Hepatitis B is transmitted by needles, blood or blood products, and contact with bodily secretions. Hepatitis B infection can result in five different outcomes: resolution, fulminant hepatitis with liver failure, chronic active hepatitis, chronic persistent hepatitis, and an asymptomatic carrier state. The presenting features of hepatitis C are often similar to those of hepatitis B.

Wilson's disease is inherited as an autosomal recessive trait and involves abnormal copper deposition. Its manifestations include hepatitis, neurologic disorders (tremor, dystonia, psychiatric manifestations), and a hemolytic anemia. Adolescents and young adults are more likely to have the hepatic dysfunction, and older patients more commonly have the neurologic problems. A unique finding among symptomatic patients is a Kayser-Fleischer ring (copper deposition in the cornea). It appears as a brown discoloration among fair people and a greenish gray ring in those whose eyes are brown.

Hemochromatosis is a hereditary disorder that results in an iron overload that causes damage to tissues. Deposition can lead to cardiac dysfunction, polyglandular disorders (hypogonadism, diabetes, hypopituitarism), hepatic dysfunction, and arthritis (due to synovial deposition). The accumulation of hemosiderin in the skin can lead to a bronze or blue-gray discoloration. Because of menstrual blood loss, a woman's manifestations develop approximately 10 years later than a man's illness.

Gilbert's syndrome is a benign condition of indirect hyperbilirubinemia. It is inherited as an autosomal dominant disorder, with variable penetrance. Bilirubin levels seldom are greater than 5 mg/dl, and higher levels are associated with low caloric intake, (as when patients come in fasting for blood tests).

Assessment of Liver Disease Severity

The severity of liver disease is evidenced by the degree of metabolic and synthetic dysfunction and whether there are signs of portal hypertension, not necessarily by liver size or the degree of jaundice. Impaired synthetic function results in reduced clotting factor levels, a prolonged prothrombin time, and easy bruising. Because vitamin K malabsorption can accompany cholestasis, parenteral vitamin K administration is required to rule out malabsorption before attributing clotting abnormalities to hepatic synthetic function.

Metabolic sequelae include an increased metabolism of androgens to weak estrogens, leading to the findings of feminization, such as cutaneous vascular angiomas, palmar erythema, and gynecomastia. Hepatic encephalopathy also is a metabolic consequence of severe liver disease. It is manifested by mental

Vignette Follow-up

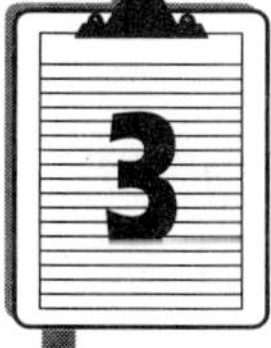

AD has an SGOT level 25 times normal, with a total bilirubin level of 8.4 mg/dL. His prothrombin time is normal. HIV testing is negative, but testing for hepatitis B surface antigen is positive, and hepatitis B surface antibody is absent. Testing for hepatitis A IgG and IgM antibodies is negative. Over the next few weeks, his hepatic function returns to normal. Hepatitis B surface antibody develops and the hepatitis B surface antigen disappears. He does well during 6 months of follow-up, and no HIV antibody is detected at the end of this period.

Vignette 4

Ascites: fluid that has accumulated between the visceral and parietal abdominal peritoneum.

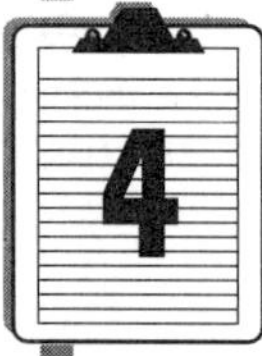

SA is a 50-year-old housewife who comes to the clinic with a complaint of abdominal "swelling." Her children insisted that she see a physician because of her increasing abdominal girth. She reports good health and has not seen a physician over the past 5 years. She relates that her waist size has increased slowly over the previous 3 to 4 months. She has not experienced abdominal pain, although she does note fullness and some decreased appetite. She has altered her clothing to accommodate her increased girth.

Ms. A denies shortness of breath, chest pain, or palpitations. She had jaundice at 12 years of age and was told that she had hepatitis caused by the consumption of contaminated well water. She has had no other episodes of jaundice, exposure to hepatitis, or blood transfusions. There is no family history of liver disease. She is gravida three, para three, and her menses ceased 2 years ago. Her last pelvic examination and Pap smear were done 5 years ago. Ms. A takes no medications. She smokes one pack of cigarettes a day and admits to having three mixed drinks in the evening. Although she occasionally drinks early in the morning, she has never been told to "cut back" on her alcohol intake. She is divorced, works as a legal secretary, and has three grown children.

Physical examination reveals a slender woman, whose **blood pressure** is 92/60 mm Hg and **heart rate** is 80 beats/min, without orthostatic changes. **Skin:** palmar erythema. **HEENT:** normal extraocular movements; scleral icterus; clear oropharynx; no thyromegaly or adenopathy. **Chest:** clear to auscultation. **Breasts:** without masses. **Cardiac:** no JVD; a normal PMI; normal S_1 and S_2, with a 2/6 systolic murmur, loudest at the left upper sternal border. **Abdomen:** protuberant with flank fullness; bowel sounds are present; no bruits. Shifting dullness and a fluid wave are elicited. The liver border cannot be ascertained, and the liver span is estimated to be 6 cm by percussion. No spleen or masses are ballottable. **Pelvic** exam: normal vagina and cervix, but her uterus and adnexa cannot be felt because of the protuberant abdomen. **Rectal** exam: nontender, no masses, stool is occult-blood negative. **Extremities:** trace lower extremity edema; pulses are all present and symmetric; there is bruising on the extensor surface of her forearms. **Neurologic** exam: reflexes 1+ throughout; vibratory sense is diminished in the lower extremities. Cerebellar function is normal. Mental status is normal, and no asterixis is present.

Vignette Objective

1. List the potential causes of ascites and the history and physical examination findings that relate to each?

status changes, ranging from an alteration in the sleep-wake cycle to deep coma. Apraxia (reduced ability to organize items in space, such as constructing a figure with toothpicks) and asterixis are characteristic of hepatic encephalopathy. Evidence of portal hypertension includes splenomegaly, ascites, and dilated abdominal veins. The appearance of the dilated abdominal veins converging at the umbilicus is called *caput medusa.*

Usually an acute worsening of hepatic encephalopathy is precipitated by a secondary problem, and patients should be assessed for a reason for such decompensation. Potential causes are increased dietary protein intake, hemorrhage (resulting in an increased GI absorption of protein), metabolic disorders (such as hypokalemia), spontaneous bacterial peritonitis, and drug ingestion (sedatives or narcotics).

Evaluation of Ascites

Ultrasound scanning is the "gold standard" technique for detecting and quantifying ascites. It can identify fluid when only 100 ml is present. With the advent of ultrasound scanning, the utility of the physical examination in detecting ascites could be studied. Absence of flank dullness was found to constitute good evidence (>90% accurate) against ascites. A fluid wave is more specific (80%),

Table 7-11. Causes of ascites

Disorder	Comments
EXUDATIVE ASCITES (inflammatory and malignant disease)	
Ruptured viscus with peritoneal contamination	Acute diffuse abdominal pain, fever, and peritoneal signs
Spontaneous bacterial peritonitis (from seeding of transudative ascites)	Findings can be subtle, with mild pain, fever, ileus, or exacerbation of hepatic encephalopathy
Pancreatitis	Sequelae of acute pancreatitis, amylase in ascites is elevated
Malignant disease of the peritoneum (mesothelioma, ovarian cancer)	Weight loss, abdominal pain, asbestos exposure (mesothelioma)
TRANSUDATIVE ASCITES	
Elevated central venous pressure (congestive heart failure, constrictive pericarditis)	Elevated JVP; long-standing biventricular congestive heart failure can exhibit few findings pulmonary congestion due to increased pulmonary lymphatic drainage
Obstruction due to thrombosis of the hepatic vein (Budd-Chiari syndrome)	Disorder associated with hypercoagulability
Portal hypertension (cirrhosis, diffuse infiltrative liver disease)	Other stigmata of cirrhosis (palmar erythema, spider angiomas, dilated abdominal veins, splenomegaly), hepatomegaly if infiltrative disease
CHYLOUS ASCITES	
Lymphatic obstruction due to mediastinal tumor	Fever, weight loss, lymphadenopathy
Disruption of lymphatic drainage due to trauma	History of abdominal trauma

but its sensitivity is only 50%. The interpretation of these findings is dependent upon whether liver disease is suspected. When liver disease is suggested because of a prolonged prothrombin time, then these signs (bulging flanks, fluid wave, and shifting dullness) have a high predictive value. However, the same signs would not indicate liver disease if detected while examining a person with obesity and no laboratory evidence of disease.

Ascitic fluid is assessed for its chemical characteristics and cell count. These show whether the fluid is an exudate (resulting from peritoneal inflammation or malignant disease) or a transudate (usually resulting from cirrhosis, nephrotic syndrome, or congestive heart failure). Rarely, ascites can be chylous, which appears milky and contains lipids from the intestinal lymphatics. Table 7-11 presents the findings associated with different causes of ascites.

Other causes of a protruding or distended abdomen (in addition to fluid) include another set of Fs: flatus, fat, feces, fetus, and a full bladder.

Vignette Follow-up

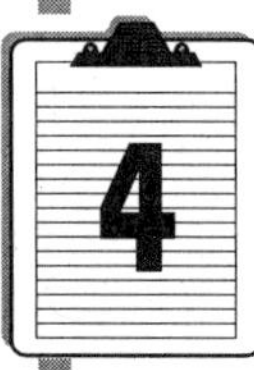

Additional history from the family reveals that Ms. A has been drinking heavily, despite urging from her relatives to quit. Her ascites is a transudate. In addition to her small liver, palmar erythema, bruising, and transudative ascites, other laboratory results indicating a diagnosis of cirrhosis are a prolonged prothrombin time that does not correct with vitamin K administration and a low serum albumin level. An evaluation for other causes of cirrhosis (including hepatitis serology, the antinuclear antibody, $alpha_1$-antitrypsin level, serum ceruloplasmin, and ferritin level) does not indicate a cause other than alcohol intake. It is assumed that her cirrhosis is due to chronic alcohol ingestion.

Vignette 5

Dysphagia: either the sensation of food "sticking" during transit from the mouth to the stomach or difficulty swallowing (solid food, liquids, or both).
Odynophagia: pain experienced during swallowing, localized to either the neck or chest.

ET is a 42-year-old man who is complaining of chest pain of 3 months' duration. He describes the pain as an ache behind the breast bone, which he rates 8 out of 10 in severity at its worst. It does not radiate, and it is not associated with diaphoresis, shortness of breath or palpitations. It occurs randomly and is not associated with exertion. When the pain occurs, he has to stop and take several deep breaths, with the pain resolving after 5 to 10 minutes. On a few occasions, he has had symptoms while eating; he recalls one episode in which he was eating an apple and swallowed it without chewing it well, and this provoked the pain.

He regularly experiences "heartburn," describing it as a burning sensation, which begins in his lower chest and ascends to his mouth, leaving an acid taste. He has "heartburn" three or four times a week, especially when playing sports or when he lies down at night. Antacids somewhat relieve the symptoms. He has no history of a peptic ulcer. He drinks eight to ten cups of coffee a day. He does not take aspirin or other NSAIDs. Cardiac risk factors include a history of smoking one pack per day while he was in his 20s, but he quit at age 29. His father developed coronary artery disease in his 60s. Mr. T has no history of hypertension or diabetes and does not know his cholesterol level. He exercises regularly and plays racquetball three times a week. He is concerned that the pain is due to "heart problems."

Physical examination reveals a healthy-appearing man whose **weight** is 196 pounds (88 kg) and **height** is 70 inches (175 cm). Vital signs: **blood pressure** is 128/80 mm Hg; **heart rate** is 68 beats/min. **HEENT:** normal findings. **Chest:** clear to auscultation. **Cardiac:** no JVD; no PMI palpable; no chest wall tenderness; normal S_1 and physiologically split S_2; pulses are full and symmetrical. **Abdomen:** nontender, without organomegaly or mass. Stool is occult-blood negative. **Extremities:** no edema.

Vignette Objectives

1. What features assist in differentiating between esophageal and cardiac chest pain?
2. When is an electrocardiographic exercise test useful for differentiating between cardiac-related and GI tract pain?

Upper Gastrointestinal Tract Disorders

Esophageal Symptoms

"Heartburn" is the typical symptom of gastroesophageal reflux disease (GERD). It often is described as a burning pain behind the sternum and extending up to the neck. It is a common complaint and occurs monthly among one third of normal people. It can be exacerbated by the consumption of large meals, alcohol, or caffeine-containing beverages, and by the assumption of certain positions, such as reclining supine after eating. Simple GERD usually is not accompanied by dysphagia or odynophagia. These complaints are suggestive of a stricture, motility disorder, or malignancy, and, when they or weight loss, GI blood loss, or long-standing symptoms are present, further studies are indicated.

Chest pain resulting from esophageal spasm can be sharp or squeezing in character. It is located retrosternally and often radiates into the back. These esophageal symptoms can be indistinguishable from angina, and the situation can be confused further by the fact that both angina and esophageal spasm are relieved by nitroglycerin.

Dysphagia often is described as food "sticking" or "holding up" during swallowing. Dysphagia for solids more than liquids indicates the possibility of a structural abnormality and gradual esophageal narrowing, such as that due to a stricture or neoplasm. As the diameter of the esophagus is reduced, symptoms become more frequent and severe. In contrast, dysphagia for both liquids and solids often is associated with esophageal motility disorders.

Odynophagia is the pain experienced during swallowing, and it can be localized to either the throat or chest. Although odynophagia can result from a motility disturbance, it usually is associated with mucosal inflammation.

Test Interpretation (Using Prior Probability, Sensitivity, and Specificity)

No test can be perfectly relied upon, in that normal people can have abnormal test results (false positives) and patients with disease can have normal test results (false negatives). A test is therefore characterized by its *sensitivity,* or the number of positive (or abnormal) test results among 100 patients *with disease,* and *specificity,* which is the number of negative (or normal) tests results among 100 patients *with no disease.* Sensitivity and specificity values are established in people with known disease or a confirmed lack of disease. However, the clinician is not sure whether a patient has the disease and that uncertainty is why the test is being performed. A convenient way to use a test's sensitivity and specificity in the context of a clinician's suspicion of disease (prior probability) is to construct a 2 × 2 contingency table (Table 7-12).

The patient in Vignette 5 describes pain that is likely esophageal in origin. He exercises without pain, has few cardiac risk factors, and relates a history of gastroesophageal reflux. However, coronary artery disease is life-threatening, and it needs to be considered in such a patient, even though it may not be the leading diagnosis. To further assess that possibility, therefore, an electrocardiographic exercise test could be performed. In this patient, for example, assume that, on the basis of the history and examination findings, the chance the patient has angina is approximately 5%. The sensitivity and specificity of an exercise test are both about 80%. The prior probability of disease multiplied by sensitivity (in this example, 5% × 0.8) yields four true positive results, and 5 minus that

Table 7-12. 2 × 2 contingency table

Prior probabilities	Positive test result	Negative test result
5% (if 100 patients had these symptoms, 5 would have cardiac ischemia causing the pain)	4 (with sensitivity of 80%, 0.8 × 5% = 4)	1 (5 − 4 = 1)
95% (95 of 100 patients with these symptoms would not have cardiac ischemia causing the pain)	19 (95 − 76 = 19)	76 (with specificity of 80%, 0.8 × 95% = 76)

Predictive value positive 4/23 = 17% (if the test is positive, the chance of cardiac ischemia has gone from 5% to 17%)
Predictive value negative 76/77 = 99% (if the test is negative, the chance that cardiac ischemia is not present has gone from 95% to 99%)

number (5 − 4) is the number of false negatives. In the same way, 95% multiplied by the specificity (95 × 0.8) yields the true negative. Once the table is completed, the columns are added and the resulting values are used to determine the predictive value of a positive or negative test result. The positive predictive value is the likelihood of disease if the test result is positive and the negative predictive value is the probability of no disease if the test result is negative.

The exercise test is most useful in determining whether coronary artery disease is present, when individuals have an intermediate prior probability of disease. In this patient, the suspicion of angina is low. If the exercise test is positive, your belief that his pain is cardiac in origin moves from 5% to 17%, but that still is low. Patients in whom the suspicion of disease is low will have more false positive than true positive results. In this example, only 4 of 23 (4 + 19) are true positives.

Not all exercise tests are done to establish the presence or absence of coronary artery disease. They can stratify cardiac risk, estimate prognosis, establish safe levels of exertion (e.g., before a patient starts a cardiac rehabilitation program), and determine the effectiveness of treatment.

Vignette Follow-up

ET is reassured that his chest pain probably is not cardiac in origin. However, he remains concerned about cardiac disease and he limits his activity, because he is worried that he is "going to have a heart attack." Despite reassurances, he wants an exercise stress test and undergoes a graded exercise test. Fortunately, the results are normal. His symptoms resolve with 12 weeks of H_2-blockers and reduction in caffeine intake. The H_2-blocker is discontinued, and his chest pain has not been a problem for the past 18 months.

Vignette 6

Dyspepsia: upper abdominal discomfort or pain, not necessarily associated with food intake.

Early satiety: occurs when food intake less than that which typically resulted in feeling "full" causes a sensation of abdominal fullness and loss of appetite.

Hematemesis: vomiting fresh or altered blood; vomited blood that has come in contact with gastric acid and pepsin has the appearance of "coffee grounds."

Melena: black, "tarry" stool, which usually indicates bleeding proximal to the ligament of Treitz; approximately 100 ml of blood loss is necessary for stools to be melenic.

VA is a 58-year-old man admitted to the hospital because of a GI hemorrhage. Three days before admission, the patient relates that he ate prunes because he felt constipated. After this, he noted that his stools became dark and unformed, and nausea and epigastric, crampy pain developed. The pain was intermittent throughout the day, but not severe enough to affect his usual daily routine. Antacids only provided transient relief. Over the weekend, black unformed stools occurred three to four times a day. He denies feeling light headed.

Past history reveals that 10 years ago the patient was told that he had an ulcer, but he does not recall undergoing any diagnostic studies. Currently, he has a daily alcohol intake of two beers. He has been taking one enteric-coated aspirin each day for peripheral vascular disease.

Physical examination reveals an obese man in no distress. Vital signs: **supine blood pressure** is 130/80 mm Hg and **heart rate** is 100 beats/min; when seated, his **blood pressure** decreases to 100 mm Hg by palpation, with a **heart rate** of 120 beats/min. **HEENT:** funduscopic examination shows arterial narrowing; the oropharynx is clear. Neck: supple without thyromegaly; carotids 2+ without bruits. **Chest:** clear to auscultation. **Cardiac:** no JVD, sustained PMI. Normal S_1 and S_2; an S_4 is found and a 2/6 early-peaking systolic ejection murmur is present at the left sternal border. **Abdomen:** mild distention; active bowel sounds; no bruits are heard. The liver span is 12 cm to percussion, with an edge palpable one finger breadth below the right costal margin. The spleen is not palpable, and no masses or tenderness are present. Stool is melenic and occult-blood positive. **Extremities:** no cyanosis or edema. Femoral, popliteal, dorsalis pedis, and posterior tibialis pulses are present and equal. A nasogastric tube is inserted. The aspirate is occult-blood positive and has a coffee grounds appearance. Gastric contents clear with saline lavage.

Vignette Objectives

1. How do the history and physical examination findings help quantify the amount of upper GI tract blood loss and determine the cause of bleeding?
2. What is meant by dyspepsia? What are the typical symptoms of peptic ulcer disease?

Dyspepsia and Symptoms of Peptic Ulcer Disease

The prevalence of gastric and duodenal ulcers are similar. Patients with gastric or duodenal irritation often describe epigastric "burning," "gnawing," or "hunger" pains. The discomfort slowly builds in intensity, remains steady for one half to two hours, and then gradually subsides. Pain usually develops 30 minutes to 4 hours after meals and can awaken the patient from sleep (usually 1 to 2 hours after retiring). The pain of a peptic ulcer is relieved by food or antacids. Gastric ulcers are less predictably relieved by food or antacids, and a meal sometimes can exacerbate the abdominal discomfort.

The management of peptic ulcer has been altered by the recognition that *Helicobacter pylori* infection is the usual underlying cause of the problem. Treatment is now focused on eradicating the infection, with the result that disease persistence and recurrence have been reduced. More than 90% of duodenal ulcers and about one third of gastric ulcers are associated with infection with this organism.

Dyspepsia is used as the diagnosis if the upper GI tract discomfort is not associated with demonstrable disease. The pathogenesis of dyspepsia is not known. Treatment for *H. pylori* does not seem to alleviate the disorder, and dyspepsia probably should be considered as part of the spectrum of functional GI tract disease (p. 227).

Upper Gastrointestinal Tract Bleeding

GI tract bleeding comprises a spectrum of blood loss, from rapid exsanguination to the finding of occult-blood in otherwise normal stools. When the initial assessment indicates significant GI tract blood loss, management is directed at normalizing volume status, correcting any coagulation abnormalities, and locating and treating the bleeding sites. The history and physical examination are important in determining the causes of an upper GI tract hemorrhage (Table 7-13).

Hemodynamic status and bleeding severity (volume lost per time) are evaluated by (1) description of the blood loss (such as the amount of emesis, the number of stools, and the amount of blood in either) and (2) the patient's vital signs, observing for tachycardia, hypotension, and orthostatic changes.

The gastric contents provide information about the location and amount of blood loss. However, absence of blood in a nasogastric aspirate does not exclude active bleeding. If the stomach is free of blood, this may be because the bleeding has stopped or because the active bleeding site is distal to the pylorus. A normal hematocrit also can be misleading. If bleeding is acute, the intravascular volume loss will not be reflected by a similar reduction in the hematocrit, which will decrease only after hydration.

Rectal examination assesses stool color and documents the presence of blood. Blood altered by gastric acid turns black. The occurrence of melena usually indicates a blood loss of at least 100 ml and a bleeding site located proximal to the ligament of Treitz. Passage of red blood or maroon stool often reflects a bleeding site within the colon. However, massive upper GI tract hemorrhage and rapid intestinal transit also can result in red or maroon stool. Black stools also can be present with iron supplementation or use of bismuth products.

Table 7-13. Causes of upper GI tract bleeding

Finding	Bleeding site
Vomited blood or "coffee grounds"; gastric aspirate contains blood	Any upper GI tract bleeding (usually site is proximal to the ligament of Treitz)
Recent or current symptoms of peptic ulcer disease	Duodenal or gastric ulcer
Alcohol intake; barrier breakers, such as aspirin and NSAIDs	Gastritis
History of liver disease or varices, stigmata of cirrhosis	Variceal bleeding (presence of varices does not exclude other bleeding sites, as up to 50% of patients with varices are bleeding from another site)
Vomiting gastric contents and retching, followed by vomiting blood	Mallory-Weiss esophageal tear

Vignette Follow-up

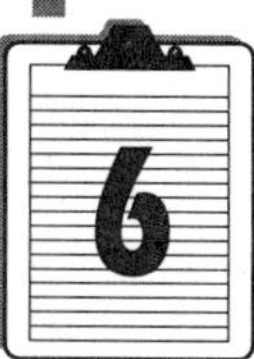

VA is admitted to the hospital and receives a three-unit transfusion. Endoscopy reveals a duodenal ulcer. No rebleeding occurs with medical management, and he has not had recurrent symptoms or evidence of bleeding during one year of follow-up.

Vignette 7

Diverticulosis: herniations of the colonic mucosa through the muscularis mucosae. Most people with diverticula are asymptomatic; complications include diverticulitis and bleeding.

Diverticulitis: acute inflammation of colonic diverticula, which can progress to perforation, abscess formation, and peritonitis. It is characterized by fever, abdominal pain, and peritoneal irritation.

Hematochezia: passage of red blood per rectum; usually results from colonic bleeding.

BC is an 80-year-old retired nursing instructor. Although she has been treated for hypertension for the past 20 years, she has been "doing well" and feeling "fine," until about 5:00 A.M. on the morning of admission when she awoke with mild abdominal cramping and the need to defecate. She went to the bathroom and passed bright red blood, mixed with stool. Over the next 2 hours, she had four bowel movements, each with only bright red blood. She is not sure about the amount, but it was enough to turn the bowl a deep red. She did not feel dizzy or have abdominal pain. She specifically denies epigastric pain, heartburn, and a history of peptic ulcer disease or GI tract bleeding. She has a remote history of "hemorrhoids," manifested by streaks of bright red blood noticed on toilet tissue. She does not drink alcohol and has not noticed easy bruising or bleeding from other sites. Her medications include two aspirins daily for symptoms of degenerative arthritis, atenolol for hypertension, and estrogen replacement therapy.

Physical examination reveals a mildly obese, pleasant elderly woman in no distress. Vital signs: **supine blood pressure** is 174/88 mm Hg and **heart rate** is 88 beats/min; **standing blood pressure** is 150/88 mm Hg, with a **heart rate** of 104 beats/min. **HEENT:** fundi show arterial narrowing and arteriovenous crossing changes; oropharynx is clear, without telangiectasias or petechiae. Her neck is supple, without adenopathy or thyromegaly. Carotids are 2+ without bruits. **Chest:** clear to auscultation. **Cardiac:** sustained, nondisplaced PMI; S_1 is normal, S_2 is physiologically split, and S_4 is present. **Abdomen:** soft with active bowel sounds. Liver percussion span is 9 cm. Spleen and masses are not palpable. Mild tenderness is found in the left lower quadrant. On **rectal** examination, no masses or tenderness are appreciated, and stool appears bloody. No hemorrhoids are seen on anoscopic examination. **Extremities:** no cyanosis or edema. Pulses are present and symmetrical.

Vignette Objectives

1. What findings distinguish an upper from a lower GI tract bleeding site?
2. What are the symptoms of diverticulosis and diverticulitis?
3. What are causes of lower GI tract bleeding and how do the findings for each differ?

Lower Gastrointestinal Tract Disorders

Lower GI Tract Bleeding

Hematochezia is the passage of bright red blood per rectum (often abbreviated as BRBPR). Usually BRBPR indicates a lower GI tract hemorrhage. However, blood in the GI lumen accelerates GI transit, such that upper GI tract hemorrhage can also be the source of BRBPR. Just as with an upper GI tract hemorrhage, initial management consists of replenishing the volume and normalizing hemostatic function. Causes for lower GI tract bleeding are listed in Tables 7-14 and 7-15.

Table 7-14. Evaluation of lower GI tract bleeding in adults

Diagnosis	History and physical examination findings
Hemorrhoids	Usually do not cause hemodynamically significant bleeding; can be history of rectal pain or itching; hemorrhoids can be external or internal (the latter can be seen with anoscopy). Blood usually is mixed with stool or "on the toilet paper."
Diverticular disease	Affects middle-aged or elderly people; history of intermittent crampy lower abdominal pain; bleeding is not associated with inflammation (diverticulitis), and patients are usually pain free at the time of bleeding.
Angiodysplasia	More common in the elderly; possible association with aortic valve stenosis.
Neoplasia (carcinoma and polyps)	Change in bowel habits, weight loss, prior occult-blood positive stool.
Inflammatory bowel disease	Weight loss, abdominal pain, diarrhea; can be systemic manifestations; more common in young people.
Ischemic colitis	Unusual cause of lower GI tract bleeding; abdominal bruits; peripheral vascular disease. "Abdominal angina" is postprandial periumbilical pain due to mesenteric vascular disease.
Infection	Invasive organisms can cause bloody diarrhea (e.g., invasive *E. coli,* amoebiasis, shigellosis, and campylobacteriosis), other features infectious diarrhea (see Table 7-17).

Table 7-15. Causes of lower GI tract bleeding according to age group

Patient age	Common causes
Adolescents	Inflammatory bowel disease Infectious diarrhea Peptic ulcer Polyps
Young adult	Meckel's diverticulum Inflammatory bowel disease Polyps
Adults <60 years old	Diverticulosis Inflammatory bowel disease Polyps Malignancy
Adults >60 years old	Diverticulosis Angiodysplasia Ischemic colitis Polyps Malignancy

Diverticula

Colonic diverticula are a frequent asymptomatic finding in people over 50 years of age and develop more frequently in the descending and sigmoid colon because of the higher intraluminal pressure in these portions of the colon. Diverticulitis develops in approximately 25% of those with diverticula. In general, the symptoms resemble those of appendicitis, with pain localizing to the left lower quadrant ("left-sided appendicitis") and occurring in association with nausea and fever. Physical findings include localized direct and rebound abdominal tenderness, if perforation results in peritonitis, and a tender mass, if a localized abscess results.

Colonic diverticula also can hemorrhage, which occurs in approximately 5% of affected people. This manifestation is associated with noninflamed diverticula (diverticulosis). Although diverticulitis of the left colon is more common, right-sided colonic diverticula are more likely to bleed.

Constipation

Although constipation or a change in bowel habits is promoted as a symptom of colon cancer, it is a nonspecific complaint and can be due to many causes. Other causes for constipation could be the start of therapy with a new medication with anticholinergic effects or ones such as a calcium channel blocker or narcotic analgesic, that affect smooth muscle activity and GI motility. In addition, a change in fiber intake or hydration, and a reduction in physical activity can result in constipation. Identifying potential causes for constipation necessitates inquiring about the prior and current relationship between stress and bowel habits, and the presence of other relevant medical problems (e.g., diabetes, multiple sclerosis, laxative abuse, and Parkinson's disease) and active perianal disease. When a cause is not apparent, the patient is more than 40-years-old, weight loss or occult-blood are present, or symptoms fail to respond to conservative treatment, examination of the colon is needed.

Functional Gastrointestinal Tract Disease

Functional is a term used to refer to GI tract symptoms not associated with identifiable structural abnormalities or pathologic conditions. Other names applied to the condition include *spastic colon, irritable bowel syndrome,* and *mucous colitis.* However, these labels are not meant to suggest that the symptoms are not genuine. For example, GI tract dysmotility and spasm can cause pain, even though laboratory studies and radiographs are normal.

Functional symptoms can relate to any location along the GI tract (Table 7-16). The disorder usually begins in young adulthood, and complaints usually are not associated with weight loss or GI tract blood loss. Symptoms of episodic constipation and diarrhea, with or without cramping, are common lower GI tract complaints. The following psychiatric diagnoses are more common among people with irritable bowel disease: depression, anxiety disorders, somatization disorder, and alcoholism.

Lactose intolerance and giardiasis are problems that are difficult to diagnose and can cause crampy abdominal pain, distention, and flatulence (similar to the symptoms in some patients with irritable bowel disease). Only 50% of patients with chronic giardiasis have cysts or trophozoites identified by stool ova and parasite examination. Empiric treatment of giardiasis and a lactose-free diet can alleviate symptoms in patients with these disorders.

Table 7-16. Functional GI tract disease

Location in GI tract	Findings
Upper GI tract	Symptoms can resemble those of peptic acid disease, but relief with food, antacids, or medications is less likely; nocturnal pain less frequent
Colon (lower GI tract)	Loose, frequent bowel movements alternating with constipation (irregular bowel habits); crampy abdominal pain; relief of pain after defecation; bloating

Vignette Follow-up

Ms. C is admitted to the hospital and given intravenous fluids. Her hematocrit decreases to 21%, and she receives a transfusion of 2 units of packed red blood cells. Her GI tract bleeding spontaneously stops, and she undergoes colonoscopy, which reveals only diverticula. She increased dietary fiber and has done well for the past 14 months, without any further bleeding.

Vignette 8

Tenesmus: rectal urgency and pain with defecation; usually due to inflammation of the rectal mucosa.

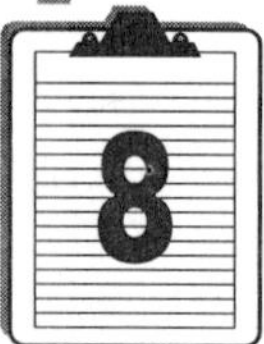

GG is a 39-year-old accountant who calls you because she is having "bloody diarrhea." She was traveling a month ago and spent 2 weeks in Puerto Rico, where she drank the tap water and ate food at local restaurants. She had no problems with diarrhea until she arrived back home. Initially she noticed abdominal bloating and cramps, followed by diarrhea, which became more frequent and was associated with marked tenesmus. The diarrhea was watery but soon progressed to grossly bloody stools. At first she believed the diarrhea was related to her travel and anticipated that it would resolve on its own. She has waited 1 week before seeking medical attention. She relates that she experiences mild nausea at the onset of symptoms but has been able to eat without problems. Her only medication has been an over-the-counter preparation for diarrhea.

She has a history of occasional loose stools associated with stress but has never seen a physician for that problem. There is no history of exposure to people with a diarrhea illness or to sick pets. Her past medical history is remarkable for an absence of other significant problems.

Physical examination reveals a slender woman who appears to be in mild distress. Vital signs: **blood pressure** is 106/80 mm Hg, and **pulse** is 64 beats/min, without orthostatic changes. There is no fever. **HEENT:** no neck rigidity, thyromegaly, or adenopathy. **Chest:** clear to auscultation. **Cardiac:** no JVD; normal PMI, S_1 and S_2; no murmurs. **Abdomen:** no distention; active bowel sounds. Mild diffuse tenderness is elicited with light to moderate palpation. Her liver span is 8 cm to percussion. No liver, spleen, kidneys, or masses are palpable. **Pelvic:** normal vagina, cervix, uterus, and adnexa without tenderness on bimanual exam. **Rectal:** occult-blood positive mucus, without formed stool. **Extremities:** no erythema, rash, evidence of arthritis, edema, or clubbing. Microscopic examination of her stool with methylene blue reveals the presence of many white blood cells.

Vignette Objectives

1. List the history and physical examination findings that relate to the potential causes of acute diarrhea.
2. What aspects of a patient's assessment help establish the presence of inflammatory bowel disease and differential ulcerative colitis and Crohn's disease?

Acute Diarrhea

Acute (less than 3 weeks in duration) diarrhea is a common problem. There are two broad categories of acute diarrhea: secretory (e.g., that resulting from the small bowel effects of food-borne toxins and viral gastroenteritis) and inflammatory (e.g., that resulting from invasive infections or inflammatory colitis).

The former usually is associated with crampy, diffuse abdominal pain and larger but less frequent bowel movements. Colonic inflammation is associated with more pain with defecation (tenesmus) and frequent small stools. The inflammation also causes white blood cells or blood to appear in the stool, often mixed with mucus. The history can provide information about the cause of diarrhea, and important clues are listed in Table 7-17.

Chronic Diarrhea

Chronic diarrhea (lasting more than 3 to 4 weeks) has many causes, and the history and physical examination are important guides in the diagnostic evaluation. Most diarrheas caused by viral and bacterial infections are self-limited and resolve within 2 weeks. However, giardiasis and amoebiasis can continue for many weeks, and certain causes of acute diarrhea can also be causes of chronic diarrhea (Table 7-18). Nocturnal diarrhea, weight loss, the finding of occult-blood in stool, and certain abnormal laboratory findings are indicators of more severe disease and cause for accelerating the evaluation process.

Occasionally, transient lactase deficiency results from viral gastroenteritis and, if an affected patient continues to consume milk or milk products, this can prolong the symptoms. Chronic diarrhea has many potential causes. Important aspects of the history and their implications are listed in Table 7-18. Despite an extensive evaluation, a diagnosis may not be established in some patients.

Table 7-17. Acute diarrhea

History	Potential diagnosis
Exposure to people with diarrhea	Viral gastroenteritis, other infectious diarrhea
Foreign travel	Infectious bacterial diarrhea usually develops 2 to 4 days following exposure and is due to enterotoxigenic *E. coli;* amoebiasis and giardiasis are other infections acquired during travel
Wilderness travel	Giardiasis (half of affected patients have no history of travel or exposure)
New medication	Magnesium-containing agents, antacids, and sorbitol-containing diet foods can cause osmotic diarrhea; quinidine
Recent antibiotic use	Pseudomembranous colitis due to alteration in normal flora and *C. difficile* toxin
Sexual history	Infectious diarrhea, risk for *Chlamydia* and *Neisseria gonorrhoeae,* HIV risk
Ingestion of foods stored without refrigeration (such as at a picnic)	Food-borne toxins (staphylococcal toxin [primarily causes vomiting], *Clostridium perfringens, E. coli, Bacillus cereus*)
Pet exposure	Infectious diarrhea
Raw milk	*Yersinia enterocolitica,*
Seafood, shellfish	*Vibrio parahaemolyticus*
Recent gastroenteritis	Lactase deficiency
Weight loss, progressive change in bowel habits, abdominal pain, systemic symptoms	Inflammatory bowel disease

Table 7-18. Causes of chronic diarrhea

Disorder	Comments
INFECTION	
Giardia lamblia	Incubation of one to three weeks; often asymptomatic; watery, foul-smelling diarrhea, flatulence, abdominal cramps; small bowel pathogen and difficult to identify in stool due to dispersion with feces; more common in hikers exposed to contaminated surface water
Amoebiasis	Usually water or food borne transmission; extent colonic invasion determines symptoms; most asymptomatic; diarrhea can be mild to severe; blood and mucous in stool; can disseminate to other organs and form abscess
HIV associated	Unusual pathogens and persistence of infections that usually are self-limited (e.g., cryptosporidiosis); more than one pathogen can be present; overall, approximately 80% will have an identifiable cause.
INFLAMMATORY	
Inflammatory bowel disease	Abdominal pain, weight loss, occult-blood positive stool
Collagenous colitis	Established by colonic biopsy findings
MECHANICAL	
Partial obstruction	Paradoxically causes diarrhea due to distention and secretory diarrhea proximal to obstruction; due to malignancy, diverticulitis or adhesions
SECRETORY (diarrhea that usually persists when fasting)	
Hormone associated	VIPoma (vasoactive intestinal peptide-secreting tumor); medullary thyroid cancer (calcitonin); carcinoid (serotonin); Zollinger-Ellison syndrome (gastrin)
Stimulant laxatives	Laxative detection in stool; approximately 5% of patients with chronic diarrhea are surreptitious laxative abusers
OSMOTIC	
Ingestion	Sorbitol, milk or milk products when lactase deficiency present
MALABSORPTION AND MALDIGESTION (manifestations can include weight loss, steatorrhea [fatty stools that do not flush well]; may or may not have diarrhea)	
Pancreatic insufficiency	Cystic fibrosis; history of pancreatitis; calcification in area of pancreas on KUB
Bile salt deficiency	Bacterial overgrowth (due to altered small bowel function; e.g., diabetic enteropathy, scleroderma) and deconjugate bile salts
Small-bowel mucosal disease	Gluten-sensitive enteropathy (nontropical sprue), Whipple's disease; Crohn's disease; amyloidosis
Small bowel resection	History of small-bowel resection; amount of bowel resected determines whether it is bile salt induced secretory diarrhea (40 to 100 cm resected) or steatorrhea due to depletion bile salts (>100 cm resected)
MOTILITY DISORDER	
Irritable bowel	Onset usually before age 40, chronic symptoms, no weight loss, no nocturnal diarrhea

Malabsorption has many causes, either reflecting a deficiency in pancreatic enzymes or defect in small bowel absorption (due to local ileal disease or small bowel resection). Effects of malabsorption include weight loss, a reduction in the level of fat-soluble vitamins (e.g., vitamin K deficiency may lead to easy bruising), and often the passage of large, greasy, foul-smelling stools resulting from excessive gas and fat.

Inflammatory Bowel Disease

Inflammatory bowel disease can cause chronic abdominal pain and diarrhea. Ulcerative colitis is a disorder primarily affecting the colon. It usually causes tenesmus and frequent small bloody stools. The other major chronic inflammatory bowel disorder is Crohn's disease, and only half of these patients have colonic involvement. This disorder is associated with more diffuse abdominal pain, fever, and weight loss, in addition to diarrhea. If the small bowel is involved, anorexia, nausea, and vomiting may be present. Loops of bowel can become adherent, resulting in a mass. Table 7-19 shows differences in the two types of chronic inflammatory bowel disease, and their extraintestinal manifestations are listed in Table 7-20.

Table 7-19. Distinguishing features of inflammatory bowel disease

Finding	Ulcerative colitis	Crohn's disease
Rectal involvement	Most patients (rectal involvement in 95%), often frequent passage of small amounts of bloody liquid stool, tenesmus	Rectal involvement and bleeding in 50%; can have perianal ulcerations and fistula
Abdominal pain	Mild to moderate cramps; tenesmus; diffuse colonic involvement can cause severe pain and toxic megacolon	Can be severe; colicky pain due to luminal narrowing; development of fistila or abscess can result in localized abdominal tenderness and mass
Additional findings	Greater likelihood of arthritis, sclerosing cholangitis, thromboembolic events; greater risk of colonic carcinoma	Can involve upper GI tract; malabsorption due to small-bowel involvement; transmural disease can cause fistula, obstruction, and abscess
Sigmoidoscopic findings	Granular mucosa, distal colonic involvement in most patients	Patchy involvement, discrete ulcers with normal intervening mucosa

Table 7-20. Extraintestinal manifestations of inflammatory bowel disease

System	Manifestation
Skin	Erythema nodosum, oral aphthous ulcers, pyoderma gangrenosum
Eyes	Uveitis
Musculoskeletal	Arthritis, enthesopathies (inflammation where tendons attach to bone), spondylitis
Endocrine	Thyroiditis
Gastrointestinal	Crohn's disease can cause granulomatous inflammation anywhere from mouth to anus; malabsorption (due to small-bowel involvement or surgical resection); fistula and abscess formation (overall approximately 85% of patients with Crohn's disease eventually will require surgery)
Liver	Hepatitis, sclerosing cholangitis (approximately 5% of patients with ulcerative colitis), cholelithiasis
Renal	Nephrolithiasis due to dehydration and increased oxalate absorption; right ureter obstruction due to ileal inflammation
Cardiovascular	Thrombophlebitis
Neoplastic	Colonic carcinoma (more likely with long-standing ulcerative colitis; less of a risk with localized proctitis; small bowel lymphoma (associated with Crohn's disease)

Vignette Follow-up

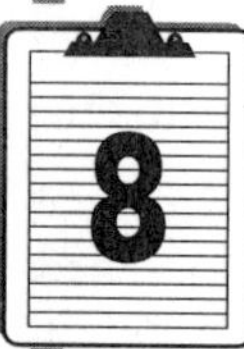

Initial evaluation includes a stool culture, which reveals normal intestinal flora, without evidence of pathogenic *Escherichia coli* or *Campylobacter, Shigella,* or *Salmonella* organisms. Stool examination for amoeba and *Clostridium difficile* toxin is negative. Serologic studies for invasive amoebiasis also are negative. Flexible sigmoidoscopy reveals that the rectal mucosa is inflamed and friable, and biopsy specimens are obtained.

Microscopic evaluation of the mucosa specimens reveals inflammation, crypt abscesses, and a reduced number of goblet cells, consistent with ulcerative colitis. Her symptoms worsen, requiring a 3-day hospitalization for hydration. Oral sulfasalazine therapy, 5-aminosalicylic acid enemas, and a tapering course of oral corticosteroids cause her symptoms to resolve. She has done well for 6 months on oral sulfasalazine therapy.

Occult-Blood Testing

Annual occult-blood testing of the stool is part of general health maintenance beginning at 50 years of age. To avoid false positive results, it is suggested that the patient eat a meat-free, high-residue diet and avoid the consumption of fresh vegetable and fruit peroxidase, (e.g., broccoli, cauliflower, cantaloupe, and horseradish), for three days prior to collecting the specimens. Conversely, vitamin C can cause test results to be falsely negative.

Aspirin and other NSAIDs may result in GI tract blood loss, and to prevent confusion, these drugs should be discontinued for at least a week before specimen collection. Six stool smears are obtained (two from different portions of the stool, from three successive bowel movements). If any one is positive for blood, a further evaluation is indicated.

Overall, occult-blood stool testing is not as sensitive as originally believed, and this is its major limitation as a screening test. Only one half to two thirds of patients with a proven malignancy and about 25% of those with adenomas have positive test results. The combined data from many studies have shown that between 2% and 6% of routine screening tests are positive. Of the positive test results, about half are falsely-positive and no cause for the GI tract blood loss can be identified. Nearly 25% of patients with a positive result will have a polyp or cancer, with the ratio being approximately four polyps to one cancer. Overall, approximately 5% of people with positive test results prove to have a malignancy.

Vignette 9

Occult-blood: blood not visible but detectable by chemical tests.

DB is a 66-year-old woman who undergoes flexible sigmoidoscopy because of the finding of occult-blood–positive stool during a routine physical examination. Her past history is significant for the development of moderate chronic congestive heart failure 1 year ago. She had no symptoms of ischemia, but a resting electrocardiogram showed a left bundle-branch block. Because the cause of her congestive heart failure was unclear, she underwent coronary angiography, which revealed severe triple-vessel coronary artery disease. She underwent coronary artery bypass grafting, and her course was complicated by a perioperative myocardial infarction. Postoperatively, moderate to severe congestive heart failure developed. She has functional class II limitations and is treated with digoxin, captopril, furosemide, and potassium. She lives with her husband, who also is in poor health because of COPD and prostate cancer.

Physical examination reveals a comfortable woman, whose weight is 96 pounds (43 kg) and **height** is 4 feet, 11 inches (1.5 m). Vital signs: **blood pressure** is 140/60 mm Hg, and **heart rate** is 84 beats/min. **HEENT:** no thyromegaly or adenopathy. **Chest:** clear to auscultation. **Cardiac:** JVP is estimated at 8 cm H_2O, with a displaced and dyskinetic PMI; normal S_1, paradoxically split S_2, 2/6 systolic murmur at the left lower sternal border radiating to the apex, no S_3 or S_4 gallop. **Abdomen:** no organomegaly or masses. **Rectal:** no mass palpable, stool was brown and occult-blood positive. **Extremities:** no edema. Her complete blood count is normal. Sigmoidoscopy, performed after antibiotic endocarditis prophylaxis, reveals the existence of a multilobulated mass at 18 cm, which on biopsy proves to be a villous adenoma.

Vignette Objectives

1. What are the indications for occult-blood stool testing?
2. What is the interpretation of occult-blood in stool?

Vignette Follow-up

Initially a surgical resection is planned. However, preoperative pulmonary artery catheterization shows the existence of more severe cardiac dysfunction than anticipated, and surgery is canceled. The tumor is removed successfully by colonoscopy. After 1 year, there has been no evidence of recurrence.

Objectives Review

1. What history and physical examination findings are most important when prioritizing potential causes of abdominal pain?
2. What are the findings of a patient with an "acute abdomen"?
3. What aspects of the history and physical examination are most important when evaluating a patient for alcoholism?
4. List the history and physical examination findings that indicate acute cholecystitis.
5. List causes of a palpable but not enlarged liver.
6. How do the history and physical examination findings relate to the potential causes of jaundice?
7. List the potential causes of ascites and the history and physical examination findings that relate to each.
8. What features assist in differentiating between esophageal and cardiac chest pain?
9. When is an electrocardiographic exercise test useful for differentiating between cardiac-related and GI tract pain?
10. How do the history and physical examination findings help quantify the amount of upper GI tract blood loss and determine the cause of bleeding?
11. What is meant by dyspepsia? What are the typical symptoms of peptic ulcer disease?

12. What findings distinguish an upper from a lower GI tract bleeding site?
13. What are the symptoms of diverticulosis and diverticulitis?
14. What are causes of lower GI tract bleeding and how do the findings for each differ?
15. List the history and physical examination findings that relate to the potential causes of acute diarrhea.
16. What aspects of a patient's assessment help establish the presence of inflammatory bowel disease and differentiate ulcerative colitis and Crohn's disease?
17. What are the indications for occult-blood stool testing?
18. What is the interpretation of occult-blood in stool?

Suggested Reading

Christensen E, Crowe J, Donach D, et al. Clinical pattern and course of disease in primary biliary cirrhosis based on an analysis of 236 patients. *Gastroenterology* 1980;78: 236–46.

Diehl AK, Sugarek NJ, Todd KH. Clinical evaluation for gallstone disease: usefulness of symptoms and signs in diagnosis. *Am J Med* 1990;89:29–33.
Authors compared people with and without gallstones; although a few findings were more indicative of gallstones (pain occurring more than an hour after meals, lasting more than 30 minutes, and steady in quality), the two groups overlapped; several traditional findings did not hold up under study, such as pain with fatty foods.

Donowitz M, Kokke FT, Saidi R. Evaluation of patients with chronic diarrhea. *N Engl J Med* 1995;332:725–9.
Many conditions result in chronic diarrhea; the authors propose that patient assessment and limited laboratory evaluation constitute the initial evaluation, followed by a staged workup; the detection of laxative abuse and the inpatient evaluation for chronic diarrhea are reviewed.

Drossman DA, Thompson WG. The irritable bowel syndrome: review and a graduated multicomponent treatment approach. *Ann Intern Med* 1992;116:1009–16.
Irritable bowel syndrome affects 20% of people from Western countries; authors present a scheme for classifying illness severity and the management measures; palliation rather than cure is the therapeutic objective.

Ernst CB. Abdominal aortic aneurysm. *N Engl J Med* 1993;328:1167–72.
Approximately one third of aneurysms more than 5 cm in diameter will rupture in 5 years; the author discusses ultrasound screening and surgical management.

Gilbert JA, Kamath PS. Spontaneous bacterial peritonitis: an update. *Mayo Clin Proc* 1995;70:365–70.
Review of the pathogenesis, microbiology, differential diagnosis, and management; the authors present an algorithm for therapeutic decisions, based on the PMN count in ascitic fluid.

Greenstein AJ, Janowitz HD, Sachar DB. The extra-intestinal complications of Crohn's disease and ulcerative colitis: a study of 700 patients. *Medicine* 1976;55:401–12.
Large patient data base was used to compile findings regarding the involvement of joints, skin, eye, and kidneys; other GI tract problems, and nonspecific manifestations (e.g., osteoporosis and amyloidosis).

Guerrant RL, Bobak DA. Bacterial and protozoal gastroenteritis. *N Engl J Med* 1991;325: 327–38.

Authors review the gastroenteritis that occurs in several different settings, including travel, food and waterborne, and immunocompromised hosts; pathophysiology and management are presented.

Health and Public Policy Committee, American College of Physicians; Philadelphia, Pennsylvania. Endoscopy in the evaluation of dyspepsia. *Ann Intern Med* 1985;102: 266–9.
Only 20% of patients with dyspepsia have an ulcer; after considering the costs, safety, and efficacy of endoscopy, the committee concluded that initial empiric therapy is indicated; endoscopy is used only if no improvement after 10 days treatment or symptoms persist after 6 to 8 weeks of therapy.

Hickey MS, Kiernan GJ, Weaver KE. Evaluation of abdominal pain. *Emerg Clin North Am* 1989;7:437–51.
This article was written for emergency room physicians, who frequently assess patients with acute abdominal pain; it reviews aspects of the history and physical examination and their relationship to specific causes.

Johnston DE, Kaplan MM. Pathogenesis and treatment of gallstones. *N Engl J Med* 1993; 328:412–21.
This review presents information on management and includes cholecystectomy, oral dissolution, lithotripsy, and laparoscopic cholecystectomy.

Kaplan MM. Primary biliary cirrhosis. *N Engl J Med* 1987;316:521–6.
The author reviews pathogenesis, natural history, and management of primary biliary cirrhosis.

Kirsner JB. The local and systemic complications of inflammatory bowel disease. *JAMA* 1979;242:1177–83.
Local complications include toxic dilatation of the colon, GI tract carcinomas, fistulae, and metabolic consequences; systemic complications are tabulated and briefly presented in the text.

Kitchens JM. Does this patient have an alcohol problem? *JAMA* 1994;272:1782–7.
Part of the Rational Clinical Examination series; men drinking more than four and women drinking more than two drinks per day should be counseled about alcohol's risks, and the CAGE questions are useful for identifying alcoholics.

Marshall BJ. *Helicobacter pylori. Am J Gastroenterol* 1994;89:S116–27.
This paper was the result of a World Congress of Gastroenterology conference; epidemiology, pathogenesis, diagnosis, and therapy are reviewed.

Marshall JB. Acute pancreatitis: a review with an emphasis on new developments. *Arch Intern Med* 1993;153:1185–98.
Author discusses causes and consequences of acute pancreatitis; the newer means to evaluate and manage this problem, such as endoscopic sphincterotomy and CT-guided percutaneous needle aspiration, are reviewed.

Naylor CD. Physical examination of the liver. *JAMA* 1994;271:1859–65.
The author reviews information on liver examination and concludes that if there is a low suspicion of liver disease and the liver edge is not palpable, then there is no hepatomegaly; liver span should be measured in all those in whom liver disease is a concern.

Podolsky DK. Inflammatory bowel disease: part 1 and part 2. *N Engl J Med* 1991;325: 928–35 and 326:1008–14.
The topics of both Crohn's disease and ulcerative colitis are reviewed; part 1 focuses on pathogenesis and natural history, and part 2 focuses on complications and management.

Richter JE, Bradley LA, Castell DO. Esophageal chest pain: current controversies in pathogenesis, diagnosis, and therapy. *Ann Intern Med* 1989;110:66–78.

Review of 117 articles; information is formatted to answer a series of questions about esophageal pain, such as "How can cardiac and esophageal pain be differentiated?," "Do esophageal tests help in evaluating chest pain?," and "What is effective management?"

Steinberg W, Tenner S. Acute pancreatitis. *N Engl J Med* 1994;330:1198–1208.
Authors review all aspects of pancreatitis; especially useful are the discussion of prognostic indices and options for management.

Toribara NW, Sleisenger MH. Screening for colorectal cancer. *N Engl J Med* 1995;332: 861–7.
Discusses risks for colorectal cancer and screening studies consisting of occult-blood testing, flexible sigmoidoscopy, barium enema, and colonoscopy.

Yang JC, Rickman LS, Bosser SK. The clinical diagnosis of splenomegaly. *West J Med* 1991;155:47–52.
The authors review the examination of the spleen and the different percussion methods to detect splenomegaly and conclude that percussion and palpation are complementary; however, neither is sensitive in detecting splenomegaly.

8 Neurologic Problems

Objectives

List history and physical examination findings for the following problems:

- Alzheimer's disease
- Benign positional vertigo
- Brain tumor
- Coma
- Delirium
- Dementia
- Embolic and thrombotic cerebrovascular accidents
- Lacunar infarct
- Meningitis
- Migraine headache
- Multiinfarct dementia
- Multiple sclerosis
- Muscle-contraction headache
- Myopathy
- Parkinson's disease
- Peripheral neuropathy
- Seizure
- Subarachnoid hemorrhage
- Vertigo

Pertinent Points

History

- History of problems with your nervous system?
- Have you ever lost consciousness?
- History of head trauma?
- Headaches?
  - Onset, frequency, duration
  - Location (unilateral, bilateral, frontal) and character of pain (bandlike, throbbing)
  - Warning prior to onset
  - Associated symptoms
  - Family history of migraines
  - Relation to foods, alcohol, menses, or medications
  - History of head trauma
  - What relieves symptoms?
  - Specifics of analgesic and narcotic use
- For those with suspected meningitis:
  - Fever, chills, myalgia, rhinorrhea
  - Progression of symptoms
  - Nausea, vomiting, photophobia, neck stiffness
  - Confusion
  - Rash
  - Exposures, travel
- Patients with coma:
  - Events before onset
  - History of trauma, depression, fever, headache, seizures
  - Medical illnesses
  - Drug use
  - Prior neurologic problems
- For those with numbness and/or paresthesia:
  - Distribution symptoms (e.g., peripheral nerves, dermatome, spinal cord level)
  - Onset, progression
  - History of trauma
  - Relevant illnesses (diabetes, myeloma)
  - Rash (as with herpes zoster)
  - Associated weakness
  - Alcohol, illicit drugs, medications, toxins
- Patients with potential seizure:
  - Prior seizures, evaluation, treatment
  - Observations of witnesses
  - Symptoms before onset (prodrome, aura)
  - Incontinence, postictal weakness or confusion
  - History of head trauma
  - Alcohol, illicit drugs, medications
  - Diabetes (hypoglycemia)
- Trouble with vision?
  - Onset, progression
  - Distribution (field cut, monocular)
  - Eye pain
- "Dizziness," feeling of motion, spinning, or unsteadiness?
  - Onset, duration
  - Circumstances of its occurrence
  - Position and movement effects
  - Tinnitus, hearing loss
  - Associated upper respiratory tract illness
  - History of head trauma
  - Current medications
  - Associated with other neurologic symptoms (e.g., trouble talking, numbness, weakness, headache)
- For those with weakness:
  - Onset, progression
  - Sensory symptoms
  - Distribution of weakness (e.g., proximal, distal, nerve root)
  - Family history
  - Prior symptoms transient ischemic attacks (TIAs)
  - History of alcohol or illicit drug use, thyroid disease, valvular heart disease, atrial fibrillation, recent myocardial infarction, anticoagulation
  - Medications (e.g., corticosteroids, HMG-CoA inhibitors, gemfibrozil), toxins

How is your memory?
- Mood, history of depression
- Examples of deficits
- Short-term, long-term
- Time course

Medications, alcohol, illicit drugs, toxins
History of head trauma
Family history of dementia
Medical problems related to dementia (hypothyroidism, HIV)

Physical Examination

Vital signs
- Blood pressure (both arms, if concern about atherosclerotic vascular disease or aortic dissection), heart rate and rhythm, temperature, and respiratory rate and pattern

HEENT
- Signs of head trauma, tender scalp or temporal arteries, temporomandibular joints, nuchal rigidity

Cardiovascular
- Palpate PMI
- Ausultate precordium
- Palpate pulses, ausultate carotids, subclavian and femoral arteries, aorta

Extremities
- Track marks of IV drug abuse, rash

Mental status (any person over 65 years of age; those with neurologic complaints; and tangential, inconsistent, or inattentive patients)
- Level of alertness
- Orientation to person, place, and time
- Language (ability to follow spoken commands, reading, fluency of speech, naming)
- Memory (registration, short-term recall, long-term recall)
- Affect
- Attention (calculations, spell "world" backwards)
- Judgment and ability to abstract (interpret proverb, problem solve)
- Delusions, hallucinations

Cranial nerves
- Visual acuity
- Extraocular movements
- Visual fields
- Pupil equality, shape, and diameter in millimeters; reaction to light and accommodation
- Funduscopic examination: disk pallor, cup-to-disk ratio, sharpness of disk margin, venous pulsations, arterial width, hemorrhages or exudates
- Facial sensation, muscles of mastication
- Facial symmetry and movement
- Hearing
- Gag reflex, phonation
- Shrug shoulders
- Tongue movement

Motor
- Muscle mass, symmetry, tone (rigid, cogwheeling, flaccid), and strength
- Fine motor movements
- Tremor, abnormal movements

Sensory
- Distal vibratory sensation
- Light touch and pinprick (ability to discriminate between sharp and dull)
- Temperature
- Stereognosis, two-point discrimination, and graphesthesia
- Double simultaneous stimulation

Cerebellar
- Finger to nose
- Heel to shin
- Rapid alternating movements

Reflexes
- Grade 0 to 4+ (with sustained clonus)

Stance and gait
- Symmetry and speed of movement
- Tandem walk (cerebellar)
- Heel-and-toe walk (muscle strength)

Vignette 1

Delirium: acute confusional state characterized by disordered cognition, inattentiveness, and disturbed sleep-wake cycle.

Dementia: memory deficits and problems with orientation, abstract reasoning, and language that interfere with personal or social functioning.

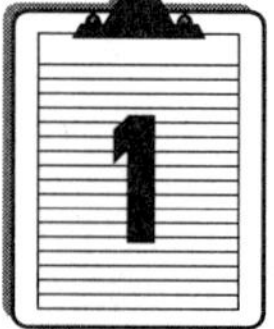

RA is an 81-year-old man who is seen in clinic with the complaint of "a change in my memory." Mr. A has been in good general health. He has a history of mitral valve prolapse and had an episode of herpes zoster in a V_1 distribution 1 year ago. His current problem began 2 days ago when he noticed his writing had changed and he was having "problems with my memory." He noticed his handwriting was different when he was signing about a hundred checks for the tenants' association where he lives. He and his wife also feel that, during the past 2 days, he has seemed more confused and forgetful (not remembering directions). He has not experienced headache, head trauma, loss of consciousness, lateralizing symptoms, palpitations, or chest pain. Mr. A is a retired banker, who lives with his wife in an apartment where he is the treasurer for the residents' organization. He and his wife are active and travel frequently.

Physical examination reveals a spry, elderly man who is in no acute distress. Vital signs: **blood pressure** is 190/88 mm Hg in both arms, **heart rate** is 60 beats/min and regular (clinic notes indicate that his usual blood pressure is approximately 145/75 mm Hg). **HEENT:** atraumatic, normocephalic; fundi show arteriolar narrowing, no crossing changes, no hemorrhages or exudates, disks are sharp; scarring of skin noted in the right V_1 distribution; pharynx is clear; neck is supple; carotids 1+ without bruits; no thyromegaly. **Chest:** clear to auscultation. **Cardiac:** normal S_1, physiologically split S_2, 2/6 late systolic murmur at the apex. **Abdomen:** no bruits, organomegaly, or masses. **Extremities:** no edema, pulses are all present and symmetrical. **Mental status:** speech is fluent; he is unable to write phrases but reading and comprehension appear normal; oriented to time, place, and person; serial 7s starting at 70 are 70, 62, 60; judgment is concrete; remembers two of three objects at 5 minutes (short-term memory testing); no reported depression. **Cranial nerves** II and XII are intact. **Motor** tone is symmetrical, but strength decreased 4+/5 in right (dominant) hand, with decreased ability to manipulate a coin with that hand and mild pronator drift. **Reflexes** are 3+ and symmetrical bilaterally (specifically, no right-sided hyperreflexia), with plantar flexion of his toes; no frontal release signs. **Sensation** is intact to light touch, graphesthesia and two-point discrimination (latter two assess cortical sensation). **Cerebellar:** normal finger-to-nose and heel-to-shin testing. **Gait:** decreased right arm swing.

Vignette Objectives

1. What are the criteria for a diagnosis of dementia? What history and physical examination findings indicate potential diagnoses in a patient with dementia?
2. Describe the typical symptoms and signs observed in patients with Alzheimer's disease and multiinfarct dementia.

3. How would the history and physical examination findings help differentiate among depression, delirium, and dementia?
4. What are the characteristics of a patient who is competent?

Mental Status

Dementia

Dementia is a condition in which memory deficits interfere with personal or social function; there are problems with orientation, abstract reasoning and language, and "higher" cortical functions are impaired (Table 8-1). In addition, primitive reflexes that normally are present in infants can reappear. However, the neurologic examination can be normal, and abnormal reflexes are not required for the diagnosis of dementia.

The observations made in patients over time are more reliable if a standard format for the mental status examination is used. Several instruments have been used to quantify the mental status examination findings (Fig. 8-1). The most common causes of dementia are listed in Table 8-2. Approximately 75% of the cases are due to Alzheimer's disease, and fewer than 5% are due to reversible problems, such as medication effects, metabolic disorders, and depression. The items listed in the history column illustrate the importance of finding out about the onset and progression of symptoms. Because patients' histories often are unreliable, information also should be obtained from family members and housemates. The physical examination is focused on identifying systemic illnesses associated with dementia, and the neurologic examination carefully evaluates for asymmetry. The finding of lateralizing abnormalities increases suspicion that a mass (a rare cause of dementia) is present. In general, head CT scans do not add information to the physical examination, unless (1) the assessment shows focal abnormalities, (2) recent onset of neurologic symptoms, or (3) history of head trauma or malignancy.

Depression, or "pseudodementia," is listed in Table 8-2 as a cause for an abnormal mental status resembling dementia. The features that help distinguish

Table 8-1. Higher cortical functions affected in dementias

1. Memory: short-term recall is impaired more than that of previously established events.
2. Apraxia: inability to organize and carry out complex motor tasks (e.g., unable to dress or draw a complex figure), despite the motor ability to perform the movements.
3. Agnosia: inability to recognize a complex sensory stimulus (e.g., inability to identify a common object).
4. Aphasia: defective verbal understanding or expression.
5. "Primitive" reflexes: with loss of cortical inhibition, reflexes that are normal in infants can reappear; examples are extensor plantar reflexes (upgoing toes) and frontal release signs (snout, suck, palmomental).

Orientation	Maximum Score	Patient's Score
What is the (year), (season), (day of month), (month), (day of week)? (1 point each)	**5**	______
Where are we: (state), (county), (town), (hospital), (floor)? (1 point each)	**5**	______
Registration		
Name 3 objects: 1 second to say each. Then, ask the patient all 3 after you have said them. Give 1 point for each correct answer. Then repeat them until learns all 3. Count trials and record.	**3**	______
Attention and Calculation		
Serials 7's. 1 point for each correct. Stop after 5 answers. Alternatively spell "world" backwards.	**5**	______
Recall		
Ask for the 3 objects repeated above. Give 1 point for each correct	**3**	______
Language	**9**	
Name a pencil and a watch (2 points)		______
Repeat the following: "No ifs, ands, or buts." (1 point)		______
Follow a three-stage command: "Take a paper in your right hand, fold it in half, and put it on the floor." (3 points)		______
Read and obey the following:		
"Close your eyes." (1 point)		______
"Write a sentence." (1 point)		______
"Copy this design." (1 point)		______
Total Score	**30**	______

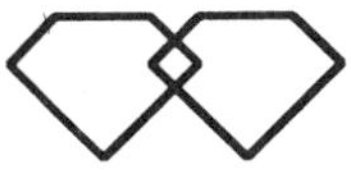

≥26 normal 21–25 non-diagnostic ≤20 moderate–severe dementia

Figure 8-1. The Mini-mental status is a standardized assessment that can be useful when evaluating a patient's mental status and following patients over time. (Adapted with permission from Folstein MF, Folstein SE, McHugh PR. "Mini-mental state." A practical method for grading the cognitive state of patients for the clinician. *J Psychiatr Res* 12:189–98, 1975.)

it from dementia also are listed. These conditions frequently coexist, and over one third of patients with dementia experience depression. Often an empiric trial of antidepressants is appropriate in affected patients to see if this reverses any depression that is contributing to the altered mental status.

Table 8-2. Causes of dementia*

Diagnosis	History	Physical examination
Alzheimer's disease	Prevalence increases with age, slowly progressive, patient often unaware of changes	Mental status changes can be the only abnormality, without other neurologic deficits or pathologic reflexes
Multiinfarct (often multiple, small, white matter lacunar infarcts)	Hypertension; "stuttering" progression, with several episodes of stepwise functional decline	Bilateral pyramidal tract abnormalities (up going toes, hyperreflexia, jaw jerk); "pseudobulbar" signs, such as emotional lability and dysarthria
Depression ("pseudodementia")	History of psychiatric disease, more acute onset, socially withdrawn, anhedonia, sadness, vegetative symptoms (anorexia, weight loss, sleep disturbance)	Other than mental status, no neurologic abnormalities; respond with "don't know," rather than incorrect answers
Vitamin B_{12} deficiency	Gradual onset; gastric or ileal resection; immune-mediated pernicious anemia more prevalent in elderly Scandinavian patients	Paresthesia and posterior column deficits (loss of position and vibratory sense); can have associated megaloblastic anemia
Thiamine deficiency (Wernicke's and Korsakoff's syndrome)	Heavy alcohol use, Caucasian, poor dietary intake	Wernicke's is an acute, reversible syndrome, typified by gaze paresis, confusion, ataxia; Korsakoff's syndrome is irreversible and associated with loss of short-term memory and confabulation
Hepatic encephalopathy	Liver disease can be clinically mild; precipitating event such as GI bleed, dietary protein load, electrolyte imbalance, infection, or new medication	Asterixis; sleep disturbance; apraxia; mild alteration in mental status, progressing to somnolence and coma
Subdural hematoma	Headache, history of head trauma, drowsy	Asymmetry of neurologic findings (lateralizing signs)
Normal-pressure hydrocephalus	6 to 12 month course, history of subarachnoid hemorrhage or meningitis	Triad of memory deficit; gait apraxia (feet appear to "stick to the floor" and inability to coordinate foot movements, such as kick a ball); and incontinence
Brain tumor (rare cause of dementia); dementia also can be a remote effect of malignancies	6 to 12 months of symptoms	Frontal lobe location can result in memory loss, without lateralizing neurologic findings; impaired smell; "primitive" reflexes (snout, root)

*Many other neurologic diseases cause dementia, and these include degenerative diseases (e.g., Parkinson's disease, Huntington's chorea, Tay-Sachs disease, Wilson's disease), endocrine disorders (e.g., hypothyroidism), metabolic problems (e.g., hypercalcemia, hyponatremia), and chronic CNS infections (e.g., syphilis, cryptococcal meningitis).

Delirium

The symptoms of delirium typically develop along a continuum, from slight clouding of consciousness to global cognitive impairment. Delirious patients have a reduced ability to attend to external stimuli (e.g., their attention wanders and questions must be repeated). Thinking is disorganized, and speech is rambling, irrelevant, or incoherent. Additional features include anxiety, insomnia, agitation, and, occasionally, delusions and hallucinations.

Delirium is a frequent disorder and occurs among approximately 10% of hospitalized adults. It is more common in the elderly and those with underlying CNS dysfunction. Delirium can be caused by conditions directly affecting the CNS or by a disorder involving another organ system. The four general categories of causes of delirium and examples of disorders in each are listed in Table 8-3. It can be difficult to distinguish between delirium and dementia, and the conditions often coexist. The typical features of both disorders are listed in Table 8-4.

Table 8-3. Problems causing delirium

Category	Examples
Primary CNS disease	Cerebrovascular infarct, subdural hematoma
Systemic illness affecting brain function	Metabolic disorder (e.g., hyponatremia, hypercalcemia,hypoxia); infection (e.g., urinary tract infection and pneumonia); new or progressive organ dysfunction (as with a myocardial infarction or exacerbation of chronic obstructive pulmonary disease)
Intoxications and medication effects	Benzodiazepine, anticholinergic drugs, amphetamines, phencyclidine, aspirin, NSAIDs
Withdrawal from substances	Alcohol, barbiturates, tricyclic antidepressants, benzodiazepines

Table 8-4. Delirium versus dementia

Characteristic	Delirium	Dementia
Onset	Acute onset; onset often associated with an acute underlying problem	Insidious and slowly progressive
Orientation	Impaired; can mistake surroundings for another place	Impaired late
Memory, attention and mood	Short-term and long-term memory impaired; lack of ability to attend; mood can change rapidly; patient can appear angry, fearful, or hostile	Short-term memory impaired, long-term memory can be retained; ability to attend preserved; mood can be flat
Hallucinations	Can result from altered perceptions	None
Sleep-wake cycle	Always disrupted; severity of symptoms varies during the day and worsens at night ("sun downing")	Can have fragmented sleep

Table 8-5. Assessing patient competence

Item being evaluated	Questions used
Understanding of the situation and illness	Why are you in the hospital? What is the name of your illness? Tell me about your illness (cause, natural history treatment).
Understanding of management plans	What has been recommended for your illness? Tell me about treatment options. Why is one treatment being recommended over the others? What will treatment do?
Understanding of treatment risks	What are the possible "unwanted" effects or complications of treatment?
Understanding of consequences of decisions	What will happen if the illness is not treated?
Personal beliefs and their relationship to decisions	What factors influenced your decision? How would you explain your decision to a family member?

Assessing Competence

Assessing competence begins with mental status testing; this identifies conditions that would affect the competency of decision-making, such as dementia, delirium, and depression with suicidal wishes. However, dementia is not synonymous with "incompetency," in that some patients with dementia can make competent decisions. For patients to be judged competent they must be able to understand the nature of their illness, its proposed management, and the consequences of their actions. A framework for assessing competence is presented in Table 8-5.

Vignette Follow-up

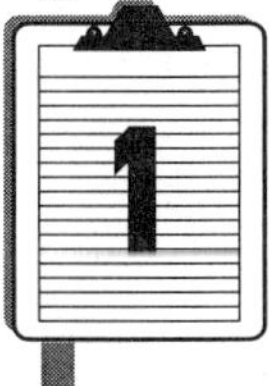

Mr. A's laboratory evaluation does not reveal any metabolic abnormalities. Carotid doppler studies show plaques but no evidence of narrowing. A CT scan demonstrates bilateral old internal capsule and corona radiata infarcts, which are more extensive on the left than right. During follow-up, his blood pressure remains elevated and he is begun on every-other-day hydrochlorothiazide treatment. His findings are most consistent with small-vessel multiinfarct CNS disease, associated with hypertension. Approximately a month after the episode, no deficit can be detected.

Vignette 2

Meningeal signs: physical findings due to inflammation of the meninges, such as a stiff neck, Kernig's and Brudzinski's signs.

MS is a 33-year-old woman seen because of the "worst headache of my life." She has a history of occasional (approximately once every 3 months) headaches, which have primarily been located behind her right eye, occur without warning, last about 24 hours, and are relieved by acetaminophen and rest. Her family history is remarkable for a parent with migraine headaches.

During the past week, several family members have experienced a "runny nose," and the patient has noted rhinorrhea and nasal congestion. She has no fever, earache, or sore throat. In the past 36 hours, a severe, diffuse headache has developed, made worse by movement and associated with nausea and photophobia. She vomited approximately six times this evening and had taken acetaminophen with only minimal relief.

Physical examination reveals an uncomfortable woman, who is shading her eyes. Vital signs: her **blood pressure** is 136/88 mm Hg, **heart rate** is 70 beats/min, and **temperature** is 38.1°C orally. **HEENT:** nontender scalp, no signs of trauma; pupils are equal, round, and reactive to light; fundi are normal, with sharp disks and visible venous pulsations (photophobia is noted during the ophthalmoscopic exam); no sinus tenderness; tympanic membranes and oropharynx are clear; neck shows mild tenderness at the extreme range of flexion and extension, Kernig's and Brudzinski's signs are not present. **Chest:** clear to auscultation. **Breasts:** no masses. **Cardiac:** normal S_1, and S_2. **Abdomen:** normal bowel sounds, soft, no organomegaly or masses. **Extremities:** no edema or cyanosis. **Skin:** without rash, bruising, or petechiae. **Mental status:** alert, oriented to person, place, and date; speech is fluent; remote and recent memory are intact. **Cranial nerves** II through XII are intact. **Reflexes:** 2+ and symmetrical, with plantar flexion (downgoing toes). **Sensation:** intact to light touch. **Cerebellar function:** normal finger-to-nose and heel-to-shin testing.

Vignette Objectives

1. What are causes of chronic recurrent headaches?
2. What life-threatening disorders cause headaches?
3. What history and physical examination features are useful in identifying potential causes of a headache?
4. What neurologic findings indicate increased intracranial pressure?

Headache

Headache is a common complaint. When assessing a patient with a headache, the first consideration is whether a life-threatening problem is present (e.g., subarachnoid hemorrhage [SAH], meningitis, a mass, or another cause of in-

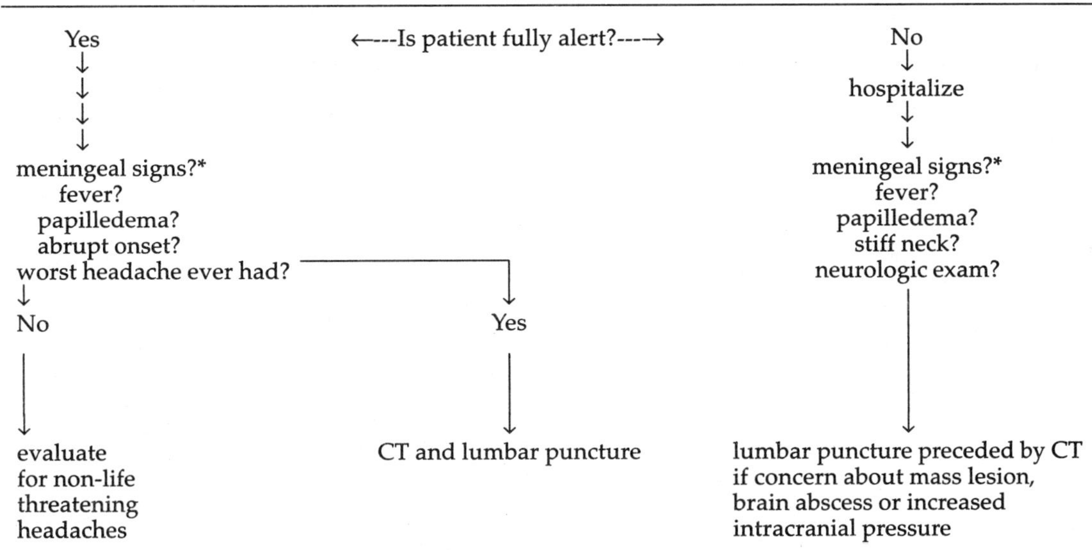

Figure 8-2. The algorithm for headache management demonstrates that patients with altered mental status, fever, meningeal signs, papilledema, or "the worst headache of my life" usually will require urgent evaluation.

creased intracranial pressure). Once these life-threatening causes have been excluded, attention can be focused on causes of non–life-threatening headaches. An algorithm for evaluating a patient with a headache is shown in Figure 8-2.

Causes of headache are listed in Table 8-6. Certain types of headache are associated with unique symptoms and signs. The clinical distinction between muscle contraction, or "tension," headaches and migraine, or "vascular," headaches can be difficult, and symptoms frequently overlap. Vascular headaches are subdivided into three major types, as shown in Table 8-7.

Meningitis

Meningitis is a life-threatening emergency and a concern whenever headache is accompanied by fever. Viral and bacterial meningitis usually develop quickly, over hours to a few days. The major symptoms include fever, myalgia, headache, nausea, vomiting, photophobia, and meningeal irritation (manifested as a stiff neck). Increased intracranial pressure (observed on funduscopic exam as a loss of retinal venous pulsations, progressing to papilledema) and altered mental status also can be findings. Neck stiffness is revealed by the finding of pain with neck flexion and extension. Diffuse neck myalgias are associated with pain in all directions of movements. If the clinician is in doubt about whether meningitis is present, a lumbar puncture must be performed to obtain cerebrospinal fluid (CSF), and evaluate for that possibility.

Table 8-6. Common forms of headache

Forms of headache	Location and character	Onset and duration	Assocations
Muscle contraction ("tension")	Can be over any part of scalp; often begins in occipital area; pressure, aching, bandlike; no nausea or photophobia	Gradual onset; lasts hours to days	Emotional stress; cervical muscle strain
Migraine (20% "classic" with aura, 80% "common" without an aura; rarely, "complicated" with prolonged neurologic deficit)	Any area of scalp; often unilateral; throbbing; nausea, vomiting, photophobia	Gradual or abrupt onset; precipitated by menses, alcohol, red wine, chocolate, onions, citrus fruit, cheese, nuts, MSG, and caffeine withdrawal; lasts hours to days	Positive family history; aura (usually visual field loss or hemidysesthesias) resolves prior to onset of headache; female-to-male ratio 3 : 1
Cluster	Ocular region and temple; unilateral; severe pain	Abrupt onset; can be a cluster of attacks occurring daily; lasts 10 minutes to 2 hours (usually less than 60 minutes)	Ipsilateral nasal congestion and lacrimation, miosis, ptosis, often at night, men > women
Trigeminal neuralgia	One or more division of cranial nerve V, severe pain	Abrupt onset, following trigger of touching area or chewing, lasts minutes	—
Exertional	Diffuse or localized	Precipitated by cough, sexual activity, or exercise; lasts hours to days	Usually onset in mid-50s, men > women, rule out posterior fossa space-occupying lesion
Subarachnoid hemorrhage	Diffuse, occasionally frontal or occipital	Abrupt onset; lasts hours to days	Severe headache ("worst of my life"); nausea, vomiting, lethargy; meningeal signs (nuchal rigidity); localizing signs (partial third nerve paresis)
Meningitis	Diffuse; occasionally frontal or occipital	Onset over hours to a few days, patients become progressively more symptomatic	Fever; nausea, vomiting, lethargy; meningeal signs
Temporal arteritis	Temple or diffuse	Gradual onset, can be constant for days or episodic	Elderly (>50 years old), Caucasian women; tender extracranial vessels; diplopia; jaw claudication; malaise; elevated erythrocyte sedimentation rate*; can be associated with polymyalgia rheumatica

*Because of potential for catastrophic ischemic optic neuritis, assess the erythrocyte sedimentation rate in elderly patients with headache.

Table 8-7. Classification of vascular headaches

Characteristic	Common migraine	Classic migraine	Cluster
Pain	Unilateral or generalized; throbbing or pulsating; aggravated by physical activity	Often unilateral; recurs in same location; throbbing	Orbital, same side each time; severe; boring or sharp
Aura or prodrome	None	Visual field defect (fortification field, flashing lights, zigzag lines), hemisensory symptoms, brainstem symptoms	None
Duration	4 to 72 hours	4 to 72 hours	15 to 120 minutes
Associated findings	No neurologic signs, nausea and vomiting can occur, begins in young adulthood	Prodrome resolves with onset of pain, begins in young adulthood	Conjunctival injection, lacrimation, miosis, ptosis, rhinorrhea; begins in middle age

Brain Abscess and Increased Intracranial Pressure

A complaint of headache raises concern about increased intracranial pressure produced by a mass or other problem (e.g., pseudotumor cerebri or dural sinus thrombosis). The funduscopic and neurologic examination usually can identify patients with these problems. A CSF pressure of greater than 200 mm H_2O abolishes retinal vein pulsations, and a careful neurologic examination often detects signs of a mass. Normal neurologic findings and visible venous pulsations make increased intracranial pressure or a clinically significant mass unlikely.

Fever and headache also can be symptoms of a brain abscess. A lumbar puncture is hazardous in such patients, because the increased intracranial pressure associated with an abscess could cause brain herniation. Unlike patients with meningitis, patients with a brain abscess often have subacute symptoms, with three quarters of them experiencing an illness lasting more than a week. In addition, focal neurologic signs are more common in patients with brain abscess. Because papilledema is unusual in the setting of uncomplicated meningitis, its presence also increases suspicion of a mass. If an abscess or other mass is suspected, brain imaging should be done before performing a lumbar puncture.

Vignette Follow-up

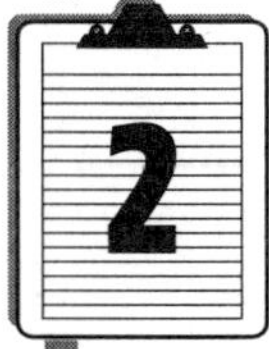

Ms. S's headache and fever are suggestive of meningitis, and a lumbar puncture is performed. CSF examination reveals eight white blood cells/mm^3 (all lymphocytes). She is hospitalized for pain relief and hydration, with a diagnosis of viral meningitis. Her headache abates over the ensuing 36 hours. Her prior recurrent headaches are thought to be common migraines.

Vignette 3

Grand mal seizure: major motor seizure; all extremities show tonic and clonic movements. These seizures result in a postictal (after seizure) state of confusion and, in some cases, focal neurologic deficits.

Petit mal seizure: brief (lasting a few seconds) episode of staring; this type of seizure does not result in a postictal state.

Simple partial seizure: repetitive focal movements; the movements do not involve the entire body (not generalized) and mental status is not affected.

Complex partial seizure: similar to simple partial seizures (focal motor movements), but associated with altered mental status.

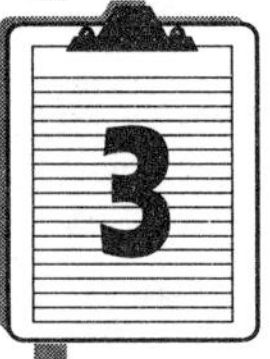

Mr. J is a 38-year-old man who is brought to the emergency room after an episode of loss of consciousness. He has been well and was at dinner with friends. His companions observed him to fall to the floor, and his body began making jerking movements. The abnormal movements lasted approximately 2 minutes, and he did not respond to verbal stimuli for another 10 minutes. Paramedics were called, and Mr. J was brought to the emergency room. People who witnessed the event say that he was behaving normally before dinner. By the time he reaches the hospital (approximately 25 minutes after the episode), he is conversing but feels "a little confused." When questioned in the emergency room, the patient recalls "shaking a little" at the onset. He has a history of a 10-pound (4.5-kg) weight loss, but denies headaches or any other organ-specific complaints.

Six years before this event, he was involved in an automobile accident and sustained a fracture of his left femur and closed-head trauma, with about 30 minutes of posttraumatic loss of consciousness. A CT scan and cervical spine radiographs were normal at that time. He takes no medications. He smokes 1 1/2 packs of cigarettes a day and admits to drinking three beers each evening and a few more on the weekend. He denies any medical problems resulting from drinking. Mr. J is not married and is employed as a bookkeeper.

Physical examination reveals a healthy-appearing man, whose **blood pressure** is 136/78 mm Hg, **heart rate** is 86 beats/min, and **temperature** is 37.1°C orally. **HEENT:** normocephalic, atraumatic; pupils are 3 mm, equal, round, and reactive to light; extraocular movements are full; oropharynx is clear, except for a small laceration on the side of his tongue; tympanic membranes are clear bilaterally; neck is supple; no thyromegaly or adenopathy. **Chest:** clear to auscultation. **Cardiac:** no jugular venous distention (JVD); normal point of maximal impulse (PMI); S_1 and S_2 are normal; no murmur, gallop, or rub. **Abdomen:** soft without organomegaly or masses; stool is occult-blood negative. **Extremities:** no cyanosis, clubbing, or edema. **Mental status:** alert, oriented with fluent speech; remote and recent memory are intact; he is able to abstract and interpret proverbs; serial 7s are intact. **Cranial nerves** II through XII are intact. **Reflexes:** were 2+ in the upper extremities, 2+ in the left lower extremity and 3+ to 4+ in the right lower extremity, with a flexor Babinski's reflex on that side. **Motor:** symmetrical 5/5 strength in the upper extremities; the left lower extremity shows normal strength, but the right lower extremity is noted to be weak on dorsiflexion of the toes and foot. **Sensation:** intact. **Cerebellar:** normal finger-to-nose and heel-to-shin testing.

Vignette Objective

1. Loss of consciousness has many causes. What history and physical examination findings indicate that a seizure has caused a patient's loss of consciousness?

Seizures

Seizures are a consideration in any patient who suffers a transient loss of consciousness. (See also Vignette 6 in Chapter 3 and Table 3-11). A grand mal seizure is typified by transient tonic-clonic motor activity, involving the entire body. It can be generalized from the onset or it can start with focal repetitive movements that progress (or "march") to involve the entire body. The nature of the initial focal movements or postictal neurologic abnormalities, if these occur, can indicate the location of the CNS lesion causing the seizure.

Features that distinguish a seizure from other causes of a loss of consciousness are listed in Table 8-8. A period of postictal confusion, tonic-clonic movements (witnessed by others), and incontinence are features that help distinguish a seizure from these other causes.

Table 8-8. Causes of loss of consciousness

Feature	Seizures	Nonseizure cause (cardiac, vasovagal, hypotension)
Prodrome	Aura can precede (e.g., smell, sensations of coldness, or visual hallucinations)	No aura; history of cardiac symptoms or problems; vagal symptoms (nausea, diaphoresis, salivation) can precede vasovagal syncope
Findings when unconscious	Tonic-clonic movements (can be generalized or focal); incontinence	Usually no repetitive motor movements or incontinence; vasovagal syncope resolves promptly with position change that restores CNS perfusion
Postevent	Confusion; asymmetry of strength and reflexes; localized weakness after the event can indicate the seizure's origin (Todd's paresis); evidence of tongue biting and incontinence	Alert, no neurologic residua (prolonged CNS hypoperfusion can result in seizure activity and neurologic findings)

Many pathologic conditions can cause seizures, and the prevalence of these conditions varies with patient age. Idiopathic epilepsy rarely begins before 3 years of age or after 18 years of age. This disorder and trauma are the most common causes of seizures in adolescents. Head trauma can cause seizures, with the incidence in patients suffering closed-head trauma being much less (at approximately 5%), than the 45% incidence in those with open head injuries. New seizures in young adults (20 to 35 years of age) are more suggestive of a primary CNS malignancy, drug ingestion, or alcohol withdrawal. In patients older than 35 years of age, vascular accidents and metabolic disorders (such as hyponatremia) become additional concerns.

Vignette Follow-up

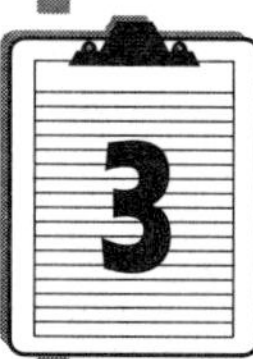

Mr. J had several potential causes for a seizure, including head trauma with CNS scarring, a malignancy (suggested by his smoking history and 10 pound weight loss), and the potential of alcohol withdrawal. Studies for electrolyte and other metabolic abnormalities are normal. The patient is given diphenylhydantoin in the emergency room and undergoes emergency CT scanning. The scan shows a meningioma. He undergoes successful surgery and fully recovers.

Vignette 4

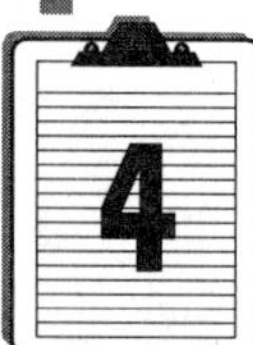

RK is a 58-year-old man who is admitted for the management of depression and a CNS lymphoma. He was well until 6 months ago, when he noted decreased sensation on the left side of his body. At that time he also had problems with depression and impulsive behavior, and he began psychiatric care. The numbness progressed, and he noted loss of coordination in his left arm. A CT scan revealed a uniformly enhancing lesion in the right temporoparietal area, and a craniotomy was done for biopsy, which led to the diagnosis of lymphoma. He began monthly blood-brain barrier (BBB) treatment, consisting of methotrexate, cyclophosphamide, etoposide, and decadron. After his fourth treatment session, he attempted suicide and required hospitalization.

Physical examination reveals a lethargic, apathetic man. His **blood pressure** is 154/76 mm Hg, and his **heart rate** is 78 beats/min. **Mental status** testing shows an increased latency of responses and a sad, expressionless face. He admits to feeling depressed and experiencing insomnia and persistent suicidal ideation. He is oriented and attentive and recalls three of three items at 5 minutes. He denies having hallucinations and delusions. Examination of **cranial nerves** II to XII reveal a left homonymous hemianopia and central left cranial nerve VII deficit (facial weakness that spares the forehead). **Deep ten-**

don reflexes are 1+ on the right and 3+ on the left, with an upgoing toe. Fine **motor** movements in the left arm are slow, and he demonstrated pronator drift of that extremity. No frontal release signs are present. **Sensory** exam reveals left-sided neglect. A CT scan shows reduced tumor size and a hydrocephalus.

Vignette Objectives

1. List the symptoms and signs suggestive of a brain tumor and specify how brain tumor–related headaches differ from chronic tension headaches.
2. What are the remote neurologic effects of a malignancy?

Malignancy and the Nervous System

Malignancy can affect the nervous system, either by direct involvement or by the "remote" effects of a cancer located outside the nervous system. Tumors causing direct effects either have originated in the nervous system or have metastasized there. Such CNS tumors often are associated with seizures and papilledema, and cause lateralizing neurologic abnormalities. Approximately two thirds of patients with CNS malignancies experience headaches. However, only a small percentage of all headaches are due to brain tumors. If neurologic findings are normal, a brain tumor is an unlikely cause of headaches. The mechanisms by which malignancies elsewhere in the body produce neurologic abnormalities usually are not understood. The types of problems that can occur are listed in Table 8-9.

Table 8-9. Remote neurologic effects of malignancies

Neurologic affect	Comments
Metabolic encephalopathy	Malignancies can cause organ failure and electrolyte abnormalities that lead to lethargy, confusion, and behavioral disturbances; examples include uremia, hepatic encephalopathy, respiratory failure with hypoxia and CO_2 narcosis, hypercalcemia, hyponatremia, hypoglycemia, and medication effects.
Cerebellar degeneration	Symptoms are gait unsteadiness, progressing to slurring of speech and involvement of the upper extremities.
Myasthenic (Eaton-Lambert) syndrome	Usually associated with lung tumors. Characteristic feature is initial muscle weakness, but repeated muscle contractions result in increased strength. (Myasthenia gravis results in decreased strength with repeated muscle contraction.)
Dementia	Malignancies can result in a "limbic encephalitis."

Vignette Follow-up

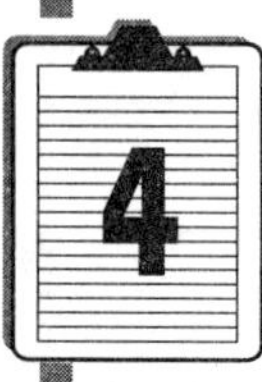

Mr. K continues to undergo treatment for both depression and lymphoma. A ventriculoperitoneal shunt is placed to relieve the hydrocephalus. Physicians do not want to initiate BBB treatments while antidepressants are in his bloodstream, and because most antidepressants have a long half-life, he is placed on ritalin therapy. In the short term, Mr. K shows minimal improvement in his mental state.

Vignette 5

Lacunar infarct: deep white matter, small-vessel infarct.
Stroke and cerebrovascular accident (CVA): generic terms that encompass several types of acute CNS vascular events, resulting in CNS infarction.
Transient ischemic attack (TIA): neurologic deficit due to a transient vessel occlusion, which resolves within 24 hours of onset.

LH is a 66-year-old man hospitalized because of the acute onset of right-sided weakness and inability to speak. He was well until the day of admission, when he called his daughter to tell her that his right upper extremity felt numb and weak. By the time his daughter arrived (approximately an hour later), he was unable to stand or talk. Mr. H has not reported any previous similar episodes, nor has he complained of visual loss, headaches, or head trauma. His daughter calls her brother, and they bring him to the emergency room.

Mr. H has a 20-year history of hypertension, which has been well controlled over the past 3 years. Although he has no history of angina or myocardial ischemia, an old inferior myocardial infarct is shown by his electrocardiogram, evidenced by the presence of Q waves in the inferior leads [II, III, and AVF]. He has been a two-pack-a-day smoker for 40 years. He is a widower and lives near his four children and their families.

Physical examination reveals an overweight man resting supine on a stretcher. Vital signs: **blood pressure** is 188/105 mm Hg in both arms; **heart rate** is regular at 68 beats/min. **HEENT:** normocephalic, atraumatic; pupils 3 mm, equal, round, and reactive to light; fundi have sharp disks, with arterial narrowing, no hemorrhages or exudates; oropharynx is clear; neck is supple; carotids are 2+ without bruits. **Chest:** clear to auscultation. **Cardiac:** S_1 normal, S_2 physiologically split, S_4 present, no murmur. **Abdomen:** soft without organomegaly or masses. **Extremities:** no rash, edema, or evidence of arthritis. **Mental status:** alert but cannot speak; over the next 2 hours, he becomes more lethargic and sleeps when not aroused; he is able to nod his head in response to questions and follow commands. **Cranial nerves:** abnormal findings include a right-sided visual field cut and a right central seventh cranial nerve paresis. **Motor:** right upper and lower extremities are weak at 3–4+/5. **Reflexes:** symmetrical at 2+, but a right-sided extensor plantar response (positive Babinski's reflex) is noted. **Sensation:** response to pinprick seems to be intact bilaterally, but sensation on the right side is extinguished, as shown by double bilateral simultaneous stimulation. **Cerebellar:** not tested.

Vignette Objective

1. Mr. H's inability to talk and his right-sided weakness point to several possible diagnoses. What are these potential causes and explain how the history and physical examination findings differ for each?

Strokes and Cerebrovascular Accidents

There are several different types of CVAs, and these are listed in Table 8-10. TIAs are reversible (resolving within 24 hours) neurologic vascular events that can precede a CVA. Their identification can allow interventions to be instituted to prevent a subsequent permanent deficit. The symptoms of a TIA depend on a vessel's distribution. Events occurring in the carotid artery distribution (anterior circulation) cause amaurosis (transient monocular blindness), aphasia, and hemisensory or motor symptoms. TIAs in the vertebro-basilar artery distribution cause brainstem symptoms, such as transient dysarthria, vertigo, diplopia, and ataxia.

TIAs can be a prodrome of a thrombotic or embolic CVA. A thrombotic stroke typically is present on awakening and the deficit can progress in a stepwise fashion. In contrast, an embolic stroke deficit is maximal at the onset and usually there is a reason for the emboli (e.g., atrial fibrillation or a mural thrombosis stemming from a recent myocardial infarction).

Carotid plaque ulceration and stenosis are associated with CVAs, and carotid bruits can be a sign of stenosis. However, carotid bruits are a nonspecific finding and relatively common among elderly people. They are a marker for vascular disease and associated with an increased risk for cardiac and cerebrovascular events. Their absence, however, does not rule out the presence of significant stenosis.

Because lacunar strokes affect smaller blood vessels and deep white matter tracts, rather than larger cortical vessels, they typically are associated with more circumscribed abnormalities without cortical dysfunction. Four examples of lacunar strokes syndrome are pure motor hemiplegia, pure hemisensory defect, clumsy hand plus dysarthria, and leg paresis plus ataxia.

Approximately half of intracerebral hemorrhages occur among people with hypertension. Other causes include anticoagulation, thrombolytic agents, arteriovenous malformation (AVMs), and neoplasms; 15% of hemorrhages are idiopathic. Intracerebral hemorrhages are abrupt in onset. In addition to neurologic abnormalities resulting from bleeding, the acute increase in the intracranial pressure results in a severe headache, an elevated systolic blood pressure, and depressed consciousness. Approximately one quarter of the cases are associated with a seizure. Hemorrhage is the likely CNS event when, in addition to a neurologic deficit, one or more of the following findings are present: severe headache, vomiting, anticoagulation, or a systolic pressure of more than 220 mm Hg. A CT scan can show whether a CVA is due to a hemorrhage or ischemia from an occluded vessel. However, in the latter case, the CT scan can be normal during the first 12 hours after the event.

Table 8-10. Characteristic features of "strokes"

Characteristics	Embolus	Large-vessel thrombosis	Intracerebral hemorrhage	Lacunae	Subarachnoid hemorrhage
Predisposing conditions	Arrhythmia, recent myocardial infarction, endocarditis	Risks for atherosclerotic vascular disease	50% associated with hypertension; other causes include anticoagulation, thrombolytics, vascular malformations, and neoplasms	Hypertension	Polycystic kidney disease, onset with exertion
Location	Cerebral cortex (depends on vessel's distribution)	Variable (depends on vessel), deficit in distribution of cerebral vessel	Primary location in small arterioles in the basal ganglia, putamen, thalamus, and cerebellum (cortical defects also can occur due to dissection of blood vessel or increased intracranial pressure due to the blood)	Pons, internal capsule	Vessels of the circle of Willis (usually few or no focal signs)
Onset	Sudden, while awake (maximum deficit at onset)	Can be sudden or stepwise progression; onset while asleep; TIAs can be warning	Sudden, while awake (deficit develops over minutes to hours)	Can be sudden onset; while asleep or inactive	Sudden onset, typically while awake and active
Headache	Sometimes; level of consciousness not affected initially; edema maximum after 3 to 4 days, and then can be associated with depressed consciousness	Similar to embolus	Usually; depressed consciousness can develop soon after onset	No	Always (meningeal signs present)

A SAH usually is due to bleeding from an aneurysm in the circle of Willis. SAHs account for 10% of CVAs and result in a severe headache, altered consciousness, and occasionally focal neurologic abnormalities. A CT scan, which is superior to an MRI scan in its ability to detect blood, can identify blood in the subarachnoid region in approximately 90% of patients. Normal CT scan findings should preclude the performance of a lumbar puncture, however, if SAH is suspected strongly. The mortality associated with SAH is high, with half of patients dying within 24 hours.

If an ischemic stroke occurs in a young person, the likelihood of more unusual causes is increased. These include disorders of vessels (arteritis, traumatic arterial dissection), drug use (cocaine), coagulation disorders (circulating anticoagulants, antithrombin III deficiency), sickle cell disease, thrombocytosis, paroxysmal nocturnal hemoglobinuria, complicated migraine, oral contraceptive use, and cardiac disorders that result in the formation of emboli (cardiomyopathy, atrial fibrillation, endocarditis, myxoma, mitral valve prolapse, and other heart valve diseases).

Vignette Follow-up

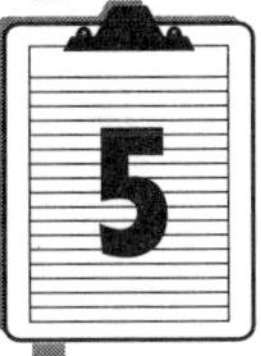

A CT scan is obtained approximately 24 hours after Mr. H's admission and shows a hypodense area in the left hemisphere. Mr. H is in the hospital for 2 months, including 6 weeks in a rehabilitation unit. He is home and living with a caretaker. He is capable of minimal speech and can walk short distances with a cane but does most of his traveling by wheelchair. He has not required subsequent hospitalizations.

Vignette 6

"Dizzy": an imprecise term that can refer to many disorders. Patients may use it to describe perceptions of vertigo, hypotension, and dysequilibrium due to sensory disturbances. Complaints of dizziness need to be clarified to more precisely identify what the patient is experiencing.

Dysarthria: slurred or nonarticulate speech.

Vertigo: instability of balance, experienced as a perception of movement and rotation in space; the symptom can be accompanied by nausea and vomiting.

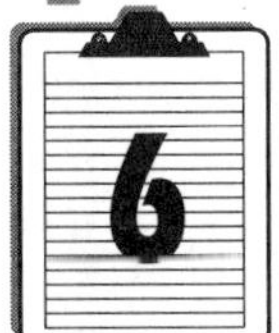

TM is a 79-year-old woman who comes to clinic with the complaint of "dizziness." She had been well until the past 2 days, when mild nausea developed. Today, she woke feeling unwell, with a "swimming" feeling in her head, and vomited several times. She does not complain of fever, double vision, difficulty talking, weakness, headache, tinnitus, or head trauma. Her only medication has been aspirin, and she takes up to four tablets per day for "aches and pains."

Physical examination reveals an anxious woman. Vital signs: **supine blood pressure** is 148/80 mm Hg; **heart rate** is 86 beats/min. When **sitting, her**

blood pressure is 128/90 mm Hg and her **heart rate** is 110 beats/min. **HEENT:** atraumatic, normocephalic; pupils are equal, round, and reactive to light; fundi are normal; oropharynx is clear; left tympanic membrane is clear, right tympanic membrane is obscured by cerumen; neck is supple; carotids are 2+ without bruits; no thyromegaly. **Chest:** clear to auscultation. **Cardiac:** normal S_1, and S_2, no murmur or gallop. **Abdomen:** soft without organomegaly. **Extremities:** no edema, and pulses are present and symmetrical. **Mental status:** alert and oriented to person, place, and time; able to spell "world" forward and backward. She recalls three of three items after 3 minutes. **Cranial nerves:** II to XII are intact, except for sustained lateral nystagmus. During the exam, head movements precipitate nausea, feelings of spinning, and nystagmus. **Motor** exam: tone and strength are 5/5 and symmetrical. Deep tendon **reflexes** are 2+ and toes are downgoing. **Sensation:** intact to vibration and light touch. **Cerebellar:** finger-to-nose and heel-to-shin testing are normal, normal rapid alternating movement. **Gait:** not tested.

Vignette Objectives

1. What symptoms indicate that "dizziness" is vertigo?
2. What are the common causes of vertigo and how would the findings vary with these conditions?

Vertigo

Dizziness can be a complaint in the setting of diverse conditions, including cardiac arrhythmias, hypotension, visual problems, and drug effects, such as those produced by ototoxic drugs and salicylates. A frequent cause of dizziness among the elderly is a combination of sensory deficits (e.g., a peripheral neuropathy plus cervical myelopathy plus visual impairment). Useful questions to ask patients to evaluate vertigo are given in Table 8-11. Most cases of acute labyrinthitis or vestibulitis resolve in a few days. Chronic vertigo, lasting more than 3 weeks, usually is due to a vestibular disorder, psychiatric problem, or a combination of factors.

Vignette Follow-up

Ms. M is dehydrated as the result of her nausea and vomiting, and she is hospitalized overnight to receive hydration therapy. In addition, she is given oral diazepam for the treatment of presumed labyrinthitis and prochlorperazine for the treatment of nausea. Her symptoms persist, and over the next 2 weeks, an MRI and electronystagmogram (ENG) are obtained. Imaging, including that of the posterior fossa, shows normal findings. The ENG shows a persistent right-beating nystagmus in four of six head positions. The diagnosis is viral labyrinthitis, and subsequent benign positional vertigo (her eye movements are characteristic of that syndrome). Her symptoms resolved over several weeks, and she has done well without recurrence during the ensuing 2 years.

Table 8-11. Assessment of patients with vertigo

Question	Findings
Are symptoms related to head position?	• Benign positional vertigo occurs with head turning or position change and lasts seconds to minutes • Most acute vestibular disorders that cause vertigo are exacerbated by position change.
Is there tinnitus or deafness? (Signs of eighth nerve dysfunction)	• Test hearing with audiometry, a high-frequency tuning fork, or ability to identify softly spoken words. • Acute labyrinthitis can affect hearing; vestibular neuronitis has similar vertiginous symptoms, without auditory signs or symptoms. • Meniere's disease usually occurs between 30 and 60 years of age, and the episodes of vertigo are accompanied by tinnitus and hearing loss. • An acoustic neuroma causes tinnitus, decreased hearing, and dysequilibrium.
Is there a history of head trauma?	• Posttraumatic vertigo is common, and symptoms usually subside over several weeks.
Are there symptoms or signs of headache, diplopia, dysarthria, or numbness?	• As an acoustic neuroma grows into the cerebellopontine angle, cranial nerve dysfunction develops (e.g., loss of the corneal reflex, facial weakness). • Vertebro-basilar vascular insufficiency and central causes of vertigo usually are accompanied by brainstem symptoms (diplopia, slurred speech, numbness, trouble swallowing) or signs (cranial nerve dysfunction, motor or sensory loss). • Cerebellar hemorrhage can begin with vertigo, and patients also experience vomiting, inability to walk, and severe headache.

Vignette 7

LM is an 83-year-old man who has moved to the area to be near his daughter and comes in to establish care. He has a history of Parkinson's disease, which was diagnosed approximately 15 years ago on the basis of the findings of tremor and bradykinesia. Mr. M was a professional featherweight boxer for 11 years, and his Parkinson's disease is thought to be a consequence of boxing. He functioned independently, with the help of neighbors, until last year. However, his ability to care for himself has gradually declined, and progressive limitations necessitated his moving near his daughter. His additional medical problems include hypertension and peripheral vascular disease.

Physical examination reveals an alert man, with a resting tremor of the right upper extremity. **Blood pressure** is 150/85 mm Hg, and **heart rate** is 82 beats/min. **Skin:** actinic keratoses over his face and upper chest. **HEENT:** depressed nasal bridge and deviated septum; oropharynx is clear; no thyromegaly; carotids are palpable, without bruits. **Chest:** clear to auscultation. **Cardiac:** no JVD; sustained, nondisplaced PMI; S_1, S_2, and S_4 are present, with no murmur. **Abdomen:** no bruits; no hepatosplenomegaly; because of moderate obesity, his abdominal aorta cannot be assessed. **Rectal:** moderate prostate enlargement, no nodules; occult-blood–negative stool. **Extremities:** no edema; absent pulses in his feet and bilateral femoral bruits; absence of hair over both feet. **Mental status:** alert and oriented; long latency of response; remembers two of three items; no complaints of depression. **Motor:** symmetrical tone with cogwheel rigidity. Proximal and distal strength are normal bilaterally. **Reflexes:** 1+ bilaterally. **Gait:** festinating gait (usually uses a walker); however, he is able to shadowbox and once started, briskly throws punches.

Vignette Objectives

1. What are the typical history and physical examination findings in patients with Parkinson's disease?
2. What are characteristics of different types of tremors?

Movement Disorders

Parkinson's Disease

Parkinson's disease is due to basal ganglion dysfunction, and affects approximately 1% of persons over 65 years of age. Although its manifestations vary, primary findings in most patients consist of tremor, rigidity, bradykinesia, and posture instability. The most common finding is a unilateral resting tremor that is extinguished with voluntary movement. It is the initial finding in two-thirds of patients with Parkinson's disease.

Parkinson's disease is infrequent before 40 years of age, and early onset should prompt a search for other causes, such as Wilson's disease, exposure to toxins (MPTP), and CNS malignancy. Drug-induced Parkinson's disease is the most frequent secondary cause, and the offending medications usually are phenothiazine-like drugs. Once the drugs are discontinued, symptoms generally resolve slowly over several weeks.

Gait

Assessing gait is a means to screen for disorders of coordination, muscle strength and tone, and sensory function. It usually involves watching the patient walk normally and then on the toes and heels to assess strength. The patient's ability to turn also is observed, and the patient walks back using a tandem gait. Disorders associated with characteristic gaits are listed in Table 8-12.

Table 8-12. Gait disturbances*

Disorder	Description of gait
Upper motor neuron, such as a thrombotic CVA of the right middle cerebral artery causing a hemiparesis	Increased extensor tone in lower extremities, upper extremities flexed; hemiplegic gait involves circumduction of the affected leg, and the toe scrapes the floor; manifestations of a mild deficit can be only a loss of associated movement (e.g., no arm swing affected side) when walking
Frontal lobe apraxia, due to multiple lacunar infarcts in periventricular white matter and basal ganglia or to normal-pressure hydrocephalus	Shuffling gait, difficulty picking up feet and mimicking movements (e.g., kicking a ball); reduced balance; associated with urinary incontinence
Cerebellar degeneration, as occurs with familial syndromes or alcohol use	Wide-based, unsteady gait; instability and inability to maintain stance with eyes either open or closed during Romberg's test
Parkinson's disease	Stooped posture; shuffling, short steps and stiff turns; difficulty initiating walking, then, once walking, speeds up (festinating gait); decreased arm swing
Myelopathic gait, often due to chronic spinal cord compression resulting from osteophytes of the cervical spine	Spasticity and hyperreflexia of legs; urinary urgency; walks with stiff legs and reduced toe clearance
Sensory loss	High-stepping and slapping foot strike of both legs (to increase sensory input about foot position); Romberg's test positive when eyes closed; abnormal sensory exam
Muscular weakness	Proximal muscle weakness results in characteristics waddling gait, with weight shifting and leg swinging forward at the hip
Lower motor neuron (e.g., peroneal palsy [foot drop])	High step of affected leg (so that foot does not scrape floor) results in a slapping foot strike
Antalgic gait (gait limited by pain, rather than neurologic disorder)	Joint pain and asymmetrical mechanical abnormalities (e.g., unilateral knee osteoarthritis) can result in reduced joint range of motion; limp; tentative and unsteady gait

*10% to 20% of the elderly with a gait disorder have no cause defined (termed *essential senile gait disorder*).

Tremor

It is important to classify a tremor, because this bears on the prognosis and management. There are four types of tremors, and these are summarized in Table 8-13.

Vignette Follow-up

Mr. M continues taking his carbidopa-levodopa and verapamil (for hypertension). Although Muhammad Ali's illness has drawn attention to the association between boxing and Parkinson's disease, it is a rare disorder.

Table 8-13. Tremors

Type of tremor	Characteristics	Additional findings
Accentuated normal or physiologic tremor	Frequency 6 to 12 Hz	Provoked by anxiety, fright, thyrotoxicosis; responds to beta blocker therapy
Essential tremor	Frequency 6 to 11 Hz; causes movement in flexion and extension; primarily involves extremities, but can involve head and neck	Can be inherited (autosomal dominant), sporadic, or senile; increased by conditions that accentuate a physiologic tremor; reduced with alcohol and beta blockers
Parkinson's disease	Frequency 3 to 7 Hz at rest and 7 to 12 Hz with action; causes movement in supination and pronation; rarely involves head and neck; disappears with sleep and voluntary movement	Other features are bradykinesia, rigidity, and postural instability; also can be accompanied by intention tremor
Cerebellar	Frequency 3 to 5 Hz; elicited by movements (e.g., finger-to-nose testing)	Cerebellar degeneration; associated with multiple sclerosis, Wilson's disease

Vignette 8

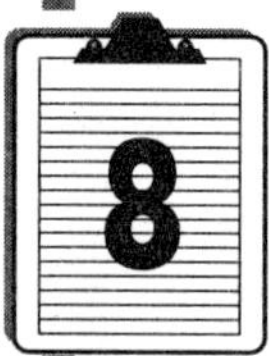

BV is a 44-year-old woman who is followed in the university's multiple sclerosis (MS) clinic. She comes in to get established with a primary care provider. Her primary problem is gradually progressive MS, which had its onset approximately 15 years ago. Her initial symptoms were occipital headaches and tingling in both hands. At that time, she was evaluated with a myelogram, which was normal. However, CSF findings were abnormal and indicative of MS. Her symptoms spontaneously resolved.

Approximately 4 years later, decreased vision developed in her right eye and she experienced profound fatigue and weakness in her left hand. These abnormalities resolved over 3 months. Two years later, while in the process of a divorce, she began to have trouble walking. This problem abated, but she did not regain her ability to walk normally. Over the past 2 years, her gait progressively has deteriorated. She drags her left leg and began using a cane about a year ago. She recently purchased a wheelchair to use at work. She has no bowel or bladder problems. She has noted that heat exacerbates her symptoms. Her family history is notable for early atherosclerotic disease. She does not smoke or drink alcohol. She is married and has three grown children. Ms. V works three-quarter time doing data entry for a local retail store.

Physical examination reveals an overweight woman (**height,** 66 inches [1.6 m]; **weight,** 186 pounds [84 kg]) who is sitting in a wheelchair. **Blood pressure** is 125/80 mm Hg, and **heart rate** is 80 beats/min. **Mental status:** including speech, is normal. **Cranial nerves** II to XII are intact, except for decreased visual acuity in the right eye (20/40). She has a Marcus-Gunn pupil and pallor of the optic disk on the right. Her extraocular movements are full, with no nystagmus, and she has normal pursuit and saccadic movement. **Motor** tone in the upper extremities is normal, but fine motor movement and dexterity are reduced in the left upper extremity. Grip strength in the right hand is 160 pounds and 80 pounds in the left. The left lower extremity is weak (4+) at the hip, knee, and ankle. Deep tendon **reflexes** are 4+ in all extremities, with clonus and flexor plantar responses. **Cerebellar** evaluation reveals a mild intention tremor (left more than right) on finger-to-nose and heel-to-shin testing. **Position sense** is decreased in the left toes. She is able to walk with her cane 25 feet (7.5 m) in 10 seconds.

Vignette Objective

1. What are the history and physical examination findings expected in a patient with MS?

Multiple Sclerosis

Multiple sclerosis (MS) is a disorder characterized by neurologic deficits that are separated both in time and location in the nervous system. For example, the patient in Vignette 8 had discrete episodes of symptoms over several years, and deficits were in different nervous system locations. The illness is more prevalent in the midlatitudes, being rare near the equator. Asians are rarely affected. Because an increased body temperature further hampers neuron transmission, affected patients often relate that their illness transiently worsens after a hot shower or bath.

Overall, about 20% of affected patients have one or a few isolated episodes of deficits and recover completely. Symptoms often arise suddenly and can last from a few minutes to a few weeks. Of those in whom a chronic disability develops, one-third experience a steady decline in function. Others partially recover between exacerbations; however, over time, their functional level gradually decreases. Those showing a steady decline often have findings of a myelopathy, with progressive spasticity of their limbs, and bowel and bladder dysfunction.

Certain neurologic findings are characteristic of MS. It is the most common cause of an intranuclear ophthalmoplegia, which results in an inability to abduct the affected eye. Optic nerve involvement can cause a Marcus-Gunn pupil, which is a pupil that constricts more when light is shown in the contralateral pupil (i.e., the consensual response is greater than the direct). This finding can be present even if acuity is preserved, and it is due to a reduction in the affected eye's afferent input. In addition, fatigue that is unexplained by abnormal laboratory findings or neuromuscular deficits is a frequent manifestation.

The natural history is variable, which makes rendering a prognosis and assessing the effects of treatment difficult. Poor prognostic features are onset at over 40 years of age, male sex, and a high frequency of episodes early in the illness. In general, approximately half of patients are disabled enough to require a cane 5 years after the initial diagnosis.

Vignette Follow-up

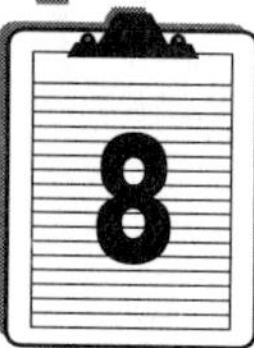

Over the ensuing 2 years, Ms. V receives intermittent solumedrol infusions for the treatment of MS exacerbations but experiences a progressive decline in function. In addition, a spastic neurogenic bladder and recurrent urinary tract infections develop. She was able to ambulate with support until 1 year ago and now is confined to a wheelchair.

Vignette 9

Coma: mental status of a patient who cannot be aroused by external stimuli; also referred to as being unconscious.

Concussion: transient loss of consciousness resulting from a blow to the head.

Postconcussive syndrome: a disorder that can follow head trauma; it includes headache, vertigo (often positional), insomnia, poor concentration, memory impairment, lack of energy, irritability, anxiety, and depression.

Stupor: marked lethargy, so that a patient appears to be sleeping and only transiently can be aroused by sensory stimulation (loud voice, vigorous shaking, or pain).

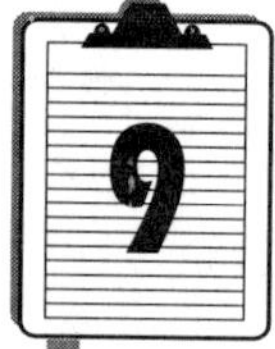

LL is an 86-year-old woman brought to the emergency room after a fall at her nursing home. She was walking to the bathroom and tripped, striking her right chest on the toilet. She denies head trauma and loss of consciousness. Because of chest pain and concern about a fracture, she was brought to the hospital.

Six weeks before this fall, Ms. L tripped in her apartment and fractured her hip. After hip pinning, she was discharged to a nursing home, with plans to return home in a few weeks. She is a widow, and has no children. Up until the time of her hip fracture, she was in good health, with only rare visits to a physician. Two nieces are her closest relatives.

Physical examination shows a frail, slender woman. She is alert, but a mental status and detailed neurologic exam are not performed. Vital signs: **supine blood pressure** is 180/80 mm Hg, with a **heart rate** of 80 beats/min; **sitting blood pressure** is 150/80 mm Hg, with **heart rate** of 80 beats/min. **Chest:** tenderness to palpation along the right sixth rib in the anterior axillary line; clear lung fields to auscultation. A chest radiograph shows marked osteoporosis and a hairline rib fracture. She is returned to the nursing home, where she receives two acetaminophen-plus-codeine tablets for pain. The nurses note that she sleeps well, but in the morning, she cannot be aroused.

Vignette Objectives

1. Outline a systematic approach for assessing a patient with an altered mental status, including coma.
2. What components of the history and physical examination are most important when evaluating a patient with head trauma?

Evaluating a Patient with Coma

Various labels have been used to refer to an altered mental status, such as *lethargy, stupor,* and *coma,* and scales have been developed to define the depth of coma. The Glasgow coma scale is one such scale, and it is presented in Table 8-14. Rather than using the terms *lethargy* and *stupor,* however, it is preferable to describe the patient's level of alertness. For example, "responds to questions appropriately with short answers, but sleeping when not being questioned" is more informative than indicating that the patient is "lethargic."

Evaluation of the comatose patient usually involves obtaining a history from family and friends, a rapid directed physical examination, assessment of specific laboratory results, and, when necessary, CNS imaging. These evaluations often are done simultaneously. A systematic approach to managing a patient with altered mental status is presented in Table 8-15. When Plum and Posner initially formulated this scheme, CT scanning was not readily available and the neurologic findings determined whether the patient required an emergent cerebral angiogram. The examination is focused on symmetry and the level of impairment of motor response, pupils, eye movements, and breathing (as presented in Fig. 8-3). Today, the neurologic examination is relied on less, and after the patient's condition is stabilized, a focused history and physical examination are performed, laboratory tests are obtained, and patients usually undergo head CT scanning to identify structural lesions.

Table 8-14. Glasgow coma scale

Glasgow score	Eye response	Verbal response	Motor response
1	None	None	None
2	Opens to pain	Moans	Decerebrate to pain
3	Opens to loud command	Nonsense	Decorticate to pain
4	Spontaneously opens	Confused	Not purposeful
5	Spontaneously	Converses	Withdraws to pain
6	Spontaneously	Alert	Follows commands

Table 8-15. Steps in approach to patients with altered mental status

ONE:	Measure blood glucose and give thiamine, glucose, and naloxone	Hypoglycemia causes irreversible CNS damage; giving glucose is not detrimental to any patient and it is preferable to not treating hypoglycemia. Glucose is administered as a "cocktail," with thiamine (to reverse Wernicke's encephalopathy and prevent Korsakoff's syndrome) and naloxone (to reverse opiate toxicity).
TWO:	Mental status is altered by 1) cortical disorders, when both hemispheres involved and 2) disorders of the ascending reticular activating formation of upper brainstem and thalamus	Bilateral hemisphere or brainstem dysfunction cause an altered mental status. An event involving only one hemisphere (such as an embolic CVA) does not alter consciousness, unless that edematous hemisphere also affects the other side.
THREE:	Three broad categories of problems cause an altered mental status	1. Seizures (either ongoing or postictal state) 2. Structural lesions 3. Diffuse CNS abnormalities
FOUR:	Four types of diffuse abnormalities can alter the mental status	D = delirium (and all the problems that cause it [see Table 8-3]) D = drugs, toxins (both intoxication and withdrawal) I = infection (such as meningitis and encephalitis) M = metabolic (electrolyte, oxygenation, organ dysfunction [uremia, hepatic encephalopathy])

Head Trauma

Most head injuries are nonpenetrating or "blunt." The term *concussion* implies a violent blow to the head, resulting in a transient loss of neurologic function. The evaluation of a patient with head trauma involves both identifying acute signs of injury and performing sequential assessments to detect cerebral edema or an enlarging mass. The aspects to include are (1) describing the patient's level of consciousness; (2) assessing the patient's ability to carry out mental tasks; (3) recording pupillary size and reaction; (4) examining for asymmetry and abnormalities of the neurologic exam; (5) documenting the patient's heart rate and blood pressure (increasing intracranial pressure causes the "Cushing response," consisting of blood pressure elevation and bradycardia); and (6) evaluating for direct signs of trauma, such as the tympanic membranes for evidence of basilar skull fracture (blood or CSF behind the tympanic membrane) and scalp for localized trauma. All except the last one are repeated for sequential "neuro checks."

Five to ten percent of patients with head trauma resulting from a fall or motor vehicle accident have a major injury to the cervical spine. Any unconscious patient's neck must therefore remain immobilized until a cervical spine injury is excluded on the basis of cervical radiograph findings.

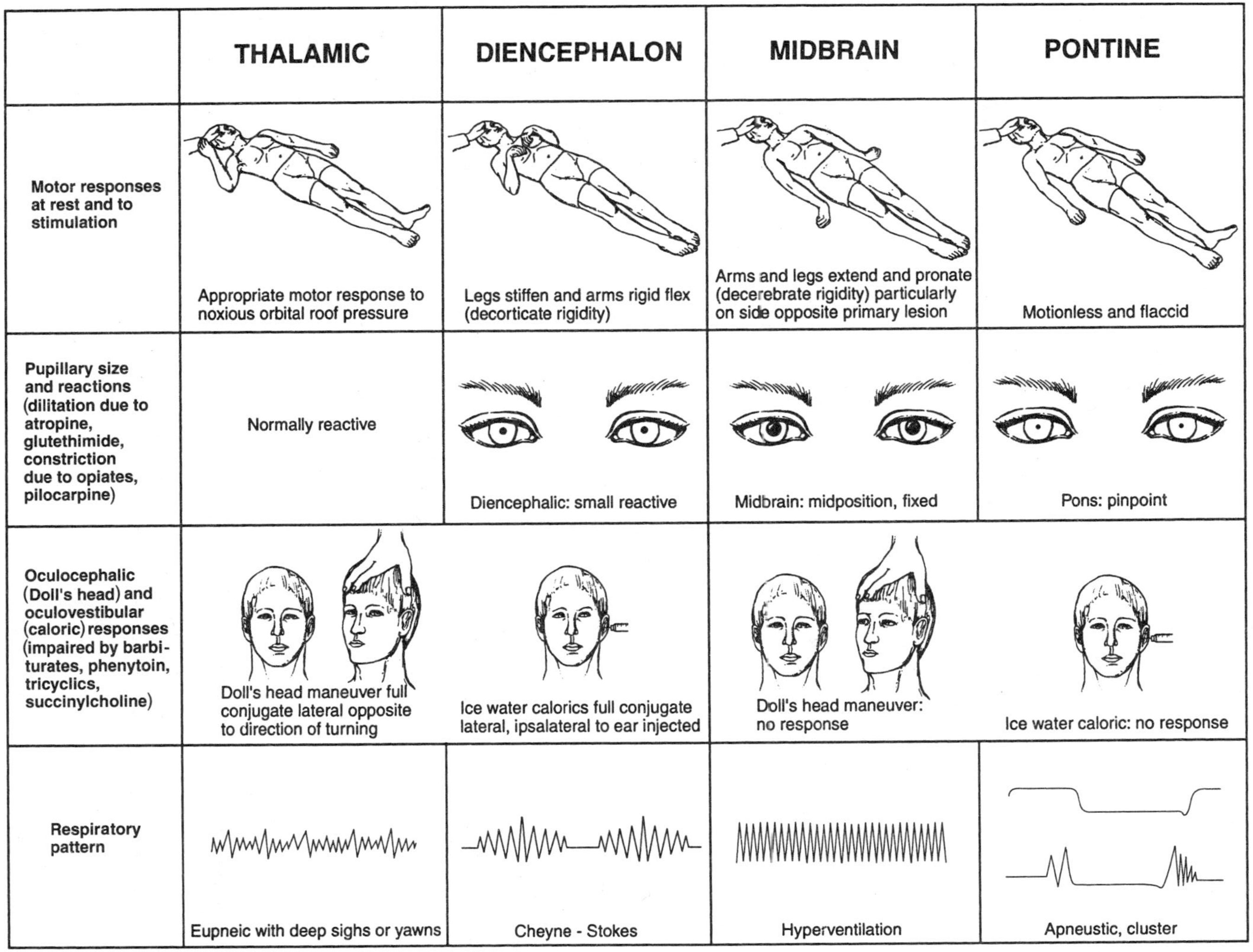

	THALAMIC	DIENCEPHALON	MIDBRAIN	PONTINE
Motor responses at rest and to stimulation	Appropriate motor response to noxious orbital roof pressure	Legs stiffen and arms rigid flex (decorticate rigidity)	Arms and legs extend and pronate (decerebrate rigidity) particularly on side opposite primary lesion	Motionless and flaccid
Pupillary size and reactions (dilitation due to atropine, glutethimide, constriction due to opiates, pilocarpine)	Normally reactive	Diencephalic: small reactive	Midbrain: midposition, fixed	Pons: pinpoint
Oculocephalic (Doll's head) and oculovestibular (caloric) responses (impaired by barbiturates, phenytoin, tricyclics, succinylcholine)	Doll's head maneuver full conjugate lateral opposite to direction of turning	Ice water calorics full conjugate lateral, ipsalateral to ear injected	Doll's head maneuver: no response	Ice water caloric: no response
Respiratory pattern	Eupneic with deep sighs or yawns	Cheyne - Stokes	Hyperventilation	Apneustic, cluster

Figure 8-3. Evaluation of the symmetry and character of motor response, pupillary size and reaction, oculocephalic (doll's eyes) response, and breathing pattern help determine the extent and progression of CNS impairment.

Neurologic Sequelae of Head Trauma

Head injury can result in the development of an acute epidural or subdural hematoma. An epidural hematoma usually is caused by high-pressure arterial bleeding, as with a skull fracture and tearing of the middle meningeal artery, which results in blood accumulating between the skull and dura mater. The patient's condition can deteriorate steadily after the trauma, or the patient can experience a "lucid interval," then manifest a decline in neurologic function.

A subdural hematoma often originates from bridging veins, and the low-pressure venous bleeding results in slower blood accumulation. Unlike injuries causing an epidural hematoma, which usually are apparent immediately, the head trauma causing a subdural hematoma can appear trivial. Symptoms can develop gradually, with the initial effects apparent weeks after the event. The disorder is more common among the elderly, because of the fragility of their vessels and propensity to fall. Head trauma, with or without loss of consciousness, also can cause the postconcussive syndrome. This disorder includes headache, vertigo (often positional), light-headedness, irritability, anxiety, and memory difficulties.

Vignette Follow-up

Ms. L undergoes urgent CT scanning, which shows an epidural blood accumulation and a midline shift. She is brought to the operating room where the blood is evacuated. Her postoperative course is difficult, with rebleeding and the development of pneumonia. She recovers only partial CNS function and is discharged to a nursing home.

Vignettes 10 and 11

Paresis: incomplete loss of strength.
Plegia or **paralysis:** complete loss of strength.
Monoparesis: weakness in a single extremity.

MB is a 48-year-old woman who is referred from the ENT clinic, where she was seen for dysphagia. Ms. B has had a long history of psoriasis and recently has suffered weight loss, weakness, and difficulty swallowing. She has dysphagia for both solids and liquids, and review of systems reveals a history of Raynaud's phenomenon. She has a 60 pack year smoking history, and because a chest radiograph shows an area of atelectasis, her initial evaluation focuses on a search for an intrathoracic malignancy. Her only medication has been topical steroids for the treatment of her psoriasis.

Ms. B is a thin woman who is seated in a wheelchair. Her **blood pressure** is 140/90 mm Hg, and **heart rate** is 86 beats/min. **Skin:** psoriatic lesions are noted over the elbows and knees. **HEENT:** full extraocular movements; fundi are normal; oropharynx shows normal mucosa without ulcers or leukoplakia. Her neck shows no thyromegaly or adenopathy, and her trachea is midline. **Chest:** bibasilar crackles. **Cardiac:** jugular venous pressure is estimated to be 7 cm H_2O; S_1 and S_2 are normal, and no other sounds are heard. **Breast:** no masses or tenderness. **Abdomen:** liver span is 9 cm to percussion; no masses or tenderness; occult-blood negative stool. **Extremities:** there is evidence of an inflammatory arthritis of both wrists, with erythema, warmth, and synovial thickening. **Neurologic** examination reveals proximal muscle wasting and tenderness. She is unable to rise from a chair without using her arms. **Mental status, reflexes, sensation,** and **cerebellar** findings are all normal.

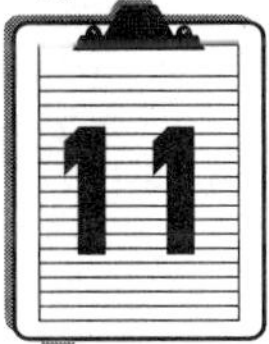

DP is a 38-year-old, healthy man who works as a carpenter and is seen because of weakness and a tingling pain in his right hand. The problem has made it difficult for him to work, and he often needs to switch hands to hammer and use a screwdriver. The symptoms began about 4 months ago. The tingling occasionally wakes him up at night. At work the tingling "turns to pain," and he shakes his hand to try to relieve the discomfort. Most recently, he has noticed that fine motor skills, such as buttoning his shirt, are difficult to perform with his right hand. Mr. P's father had a stroke at 56 years of age (about 5 years ago), and Mr. P is worried his problem means that he is going to have a stroke. The patient smoked for 10 years (approximately one pack-per-day) but quit 2 years ago. He is married and has three healthy children.

Physical examination reveals a healthy-appearing man, who occasionally makes a fist with his right hand. Vital signs: **blood pressure** is 132/88 mm Hg, and **heart rate** is 72 beats/min. **HEENT:** normocephalic; pupils are equal, regular, and reactive to light; extraocular movements are intact; fundi are normal. Neck is supple; no pain with rotation, flexion, or extension; and his symptoms are not exacerbated by cervical movement. **Chest:** clear to auscultation. **Cardiac:** S_1 and S_2 are normal; no murmur or gallop. **Neurologic** examination: cranial nerves II to XII are intact; deep tendon reflexes at the biceps; triceps, brachioradialis, patella, and achilles tendon are 2+ and equal bilaterally. Tinel's sign is positive, and right wrist flexion (Phelan's sign) also increases symptoms. No thenar atrophy or weakness is noted, and two-point discrimination is normal in his right hand.

Vignette Objectives

1. Weakness is a nonspecific symptom. How does the history and physical examination identify whether weakness due to problems with muscles, nerves, or the neuromuscular junction?
2. What are potential causes for a peripheral neuropathy and what findings are suggestive of each diagnosis?

Disorders of Muscles, Motor Neurons, and the Neuromuscular Junction

The complaint of "weakness" is nonspecific and can be due to disease in any organ system. For example, anemia, congestive heart failure, and movement restriction resulting from pain can all result in a feeling of weakness. True muscular or motor weakness is a reduction in strength or ability to sustain muscle function. It can be due to problems with the muscles, nerves, or the neuromuscular junction. Features of muscular weakness are listed in Table 8-16.

Patients with a myopathy usually first notice a loss of strength in the larger proximal muscles. For example, they experience trouble getting out of a chair or brushing their hair. In addition, myopathies result in muscle atrophy, but because it does not require much muscle strength to maintain normal reflexes, the deep tendon reflexes in patients with myopathies usually are preserved, despite the atrophy.

Disorders of the neuromuscular junction are distinguished by a weakness that fluctuates with the muscle's repeated use, and repetitive contractions can result in either a decrement or increase in strength. Myasthenia gravis is such a disorder and is characterized by weakness that increases with activity. The ill-

Table 8-16. Findings associated with different forms of muscular weakness

Disorder	History	Motor findings	Sensory findings	Reflexes
Myopathy (hereditary, inflammatory, drug-induced, infections)	Family history, distribution of involved muscles; symptoms of inflammatory (e.g., muscle pain and tenderness); drugs, toxins	Strength is lost proximally more than distally; can be atrophy; muscle tone normal	No sensory abnormalities	Normal until severe weakness
Peripheral nerves (lower motor neuron)	History of a disorder accompanied by a peripheral neuropathy, most commonly diabetes or alcoholism	Strength lost distally more than proximally; atrophy usually present; tone decreased; fasciculations	Distal stocking and-glove distribution; loss of sensation; some peripheral neuropathies characteristically primarily affect motor function (as occurs with lead poisoning)	Decreased
Upper motor neuron	History of CNS event	Muscle bulk normal; tone increased; spasticity; loss of fine movements	Can be loss of higher sensory functions (e.g., graphesthesia, stereognosis)	Increased; can have pathologic reflexes, such as Babinski's response

ness usually presents among either young people (women more than men) or those in their sixties (men more than women). Most experience generalized skeletal muscle weakness, ptosis, and diplopia. The reflexes and the neurologic findings are normal, except for the weakness.

Additional neuromuscular junction disorders include drug-induced myasthenia (such as that resulting from penicillamine, aminoglycoside, or procainamide use) and the Eaton-Lambert syndrome (presented in Table 8-9). The latter sometimes is called *reverse myasthenia,* because the weakness improves with repetitive contractions.

Upper motor-neuron weakness caused by CNS lesions usually affects groups of muscles that reflect the CNS event. For example, a cortical CVA can cause a hemiparesis, and a lacunar stroke can cause a monoparesis. Upper motor neu-

Table 8-17. Common compression and entrapment neuropathies

Nerve	Syndrome or location of entrapment	Clinical findings
Median	Carpel tunnel	Numbness, tingling, and hand pain; weakness of thumb abduction; thenar eminence atrophy; sensory loss in the nerve's distribution, especially tips of middle and index fingers; Tinel's sign (tapping over transverse carpal ligament at the wrist reproduces symptoms) has limited utility in diagnosis; most useful diagnostic tests are Phalen's maneuver (flexed wrists cause symptoms within 60 seconds) and having patients draw the distribution of their hand numbness
Ulnar	Guyon's canal in palm or ulnar groove at the elbow (cubital tunnel)	Numbness on the medial side of the hand; weakness with finger abduction; atrophy of hypothenar muscles
Radial	"Saturday night palsy"; nerve is compressed in upper arm when arm is draped over the back of a chair for long time	Wrist drop; primarily motor loss in nerve's distribution
Thoracic outlet syndrome	Ulnar sensory, median motor	Hand tingling with arm abduction; weakness in median nerve distribution; winging of scapulae if long thoracic nerve involved
Sciatic	Piriformis muscle	Foot drop; decreased ankle jerk
Peroneal	Fibula head	Foot drop; sensory loss in the web space of first and second toes
Posterior tibial	Tarsal tunnel	Burning heel; weakness of intrinsic foot muscles
Lateral femoral cutaneous (pure sensory nerve)	Meralgia paresthetica	Numbness of lateral thigh
Femoral	Femoral neuropathy	Weakness in knee extension; decreased patellar reflex

ron weakness is associated with increased muscle tone (spasticity), increased reflexes, and extensor plantar responses.

Lower motor-neuron weakness is characterized by muscle fasciculations, atrophy, and decreased tone (flaccidity). The reflexes usually also are depressed. The distribution of lower motor neuron disorders depends on the nerves affected, and peripheral neuropathies are generally "distal" (occurring in a stocking-and-glove distribution) or the result of local damage to a peripheral nerve (as occurs in a radiculopathy, plexopathy, or mononeuropathy). Localized nerve drainage can result from trauma, ischemia, or entrapment. The common entrapment neuropathies are presented in Table 8-17.

Distal weakness is a typical finding in the setting of a diffuse peripheral polyneuropathy. Unlike the proximal weakness occurring in a myopathy, patients with a peripheral neuropathy complain of difficulties with distal muscle function, such as trouble turning a key in the ignition or with grip strength. The weakness is accompanied by distal muscle atrophy, often observable as an atrophy affecting the interosseous muscles of the hand or as flexion deformities of the toes.

Distal peripheral neuropathies usually cause both sensory and motor symptoms. The sensory symptoms can consist of impaired sensation or a burning or lancinating pain occurring in a symmetrical distal distribution. Distal vibratory sense often is decreased, and reflexes usually are depressed. The list of disorders associated with a diffuse peripheral neuropathy is long. The mnemonic DANG THERAPIST is a convenient way to remember potential causes, and the causes of neuropathies and their findings are summarized in Table 8-18 according to this mnemonic.

Table 8-18. Peripheral polyneuropathies: DANG THERAPIST

Type	Description
Diabetic	Long-standing diabetes can result in a diffuse polyneuropathy, or its vascular changes can cause a mononeuropathy (often involves cranial nerve III or VI); in addition, involvement of the lumbosacral plexuses can cause proximal lower extremity pain, weakness, and muscle atrophy ("diabetic amyotrophy")
Alcoholic	Diffuse distal sensorimotor neuropathy
Nutritional	Water-soluble B vitamins, thiamine (beriberi), niacin, B_6; B_{12} deficiency (see Table 6-3, p. 167)
Guillain-Barre	Inflammatory demyelinating neuropathy; primarily motor; respiratory and facial muscles can be affected
Toxic	Vincristine, *cis*-platinum (sensory), isoniazid (B_6 antagonism), penicillamine, gold salts, lead, arsenic, acrylamide hexacarbon solvents (occupational, glue sniffing)
Hereditary	Charcot-Marie-Tooth disease (autosomal dominant inheritance; slowly progressive, predominantly motor; high arches, stork legs due to loss of distal musculature; nerve enlargement)
Recurrent	Relapsing form of inflammatory neuropathy; often responds to immunosuppressive treatment
Amyloidosis	Circulating paraproteins (myeloma); idiopathic and hereditary forms
Porphyria	Motor neuropathy, can progress rapidly
Infections	Diphtheria, leprosy
Systemic	Associated with collagen vascular diseases, uremia, sarcoidosis
Tumor	Pure sensory or sensorimotor neuropathy; can be combined with myopathy

Vignette Follow-up

Ms. B is thought to have mixed connective tissue disease, evidenced by the combination of polymyositis (documented by muscle biopsy findings), Raynaud's phenomenon, esophageal dysmotility, and laboratory results. She is treated with high-dose prednisone and weekly methotrexate injections. Her weakness resolved, and she continues with this treatment 3 years later.

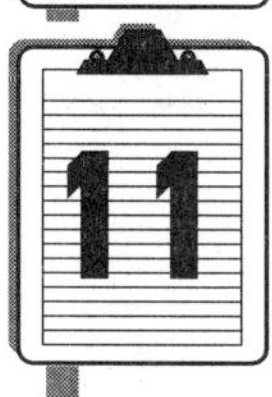

Mr. P has the tentative diagnosis of carpal tunnel syndrome confirmed by nerve conduction studies. Night-time wrist splinting and a corticosteroid injections cause his symptoms and signs to resolve.

Objectives Review

1. What are the criteria for a diagnosis of dementia? What history and physical examination findings indicate potential diagnoses in a patient with dementia?
2. Describe the typical symptoms and signs observed in patients with Alzheimer's disease and multiinfarct dementia.
3. How would the history and physical examination findings differentiate among depression, delirium, and dementia?
4. What are the characteristics of a patient who is competent?
5. What are causes of chronic recurrent headaches?
6. What life-threatening disorders cause headaches?
7. What history and physical examination features are useful in identifying potential causes of a headache?
8. What neurologic findings indicate increased intracranial pressure?
9. Loss of consciousness has many causes. What history and physical examination findings indicate that a seizure has caused a patient's loss of consciousness?
10. List the symptoms and signs suggestive of a brain tumor and specify how brain tumor–related headaches differ from chronic tension headaches.
11. What are the remote neurologic effects of a malignancy?
12. The inability to talk and right-sided weakness point to several possible diagnoses. What are these potential causes and explain how the history and physical examination findings differ for each?
13. What symptoms indicate that "dizziness" is vertigo?
14. What are the common causes of vertigo, and how would the findings vary with these conditions?
15. What are the typical history and physical examination findings in patients with Parkinson's disease?
16. What are characteristics of different types of tremors?

17. List the history and physical examination findings expected in a patient with MS.
18. Outline a systematic approach for assessing a patient with altered mental status, including coma.
19. What components of the history and physical examination are most important when evaluating a patient with head trauma?
20. Weakness is a nonspecific symptom. How does the history and physical examination identify whether weakness due to problems with muscles, nerves, or the neuromuscular junction?
21. What are potential causes for a peripheral neuropathy and what findings are suggestive of each diagnosis?

Suggested Reading

Callahan CM, Hendrie MB, Tierney WM. Documentation and evaluation of cognitive impairments in elderly primary care patients. *Ann Intern Med* 1995;122:422–9.
A quarter of people with dementia are not identified by their care providers as having a dementia; having a dementia is associated with increased hospitalization and mortality.

Carpenter RR, Petersdorf RG. The clinical spectrum of bacterial meningitis. *Am J Med* 1962;33:262–75.

Dawson DM. Entrapment neuropathies of the upper extremities. *N Engl J Med* 1993;329: 2013–8.
Brief clinical summary of the features, diagnosis, and management of carpal tunnel syndrome, ulnar neuropathies, and the thoracic outlet syndrome.

Drachman DB. Myasthenia gravis. *N Engl J Med* 1994;330:1797–1810.
The author presents the clinical features, differential diagnosis, and management of myasthenia gravis; the pathophysiology and immune mechanisms are summarized well.

Ellis GL. Subdural hematoma in the elderly. *Emerg Med Clin North Am* 1990;8:281–93.
Discussion of subdural hematomas, including their pathophysiology, range of presentations, and management; the author emphasizes the problem's unique manifestations among elderly people.

Fisher CM. Lacunar strokes and infarcts: a review. *Neurology* 1982;32:871–6.
Description of the many different deficits seen in patients with lacunar infarcts.

Francis J, Kapoor WN. Delirium in hospitalized elderly. *J Gen Intern Med* 1990;5:65–79.
Review of studies on the prevalence of delirium among hospitalized patients; the authors discuss causes, settings, and management; findings from outcome studies summarized; overall mortality is increased approximately two to four times among delirious patients.

Friedman JH. Progressive parkinsonism in boxers. *South Med J* 1989;82:543–6.
Case report and review; the author also discusses other CNS sequelae of boxing.

Goldstein LB. Clinical assessment of stroke. *JAMA* 1994;271:1114–20.
Part of the Rational Clinical Examination series; points out the limitations in the examination and that examiner's skills improve with training; examination can determine that something is wrong but cannot always localize deficit or identify type of stroke.

Jankovic J, Fahn S. Physiologic and pathologic tremors. *Ann Intern Med* 1980;93:460–5.
Reviews different types of tremors: accentuated physiologic, essential, Parkinson's, and cerebellar.

Kroenke K, Lucas CA, Rosenberg ML, et al. Causes of persistent dizziness. A prospective study of 100 patients in ambulatory care. *Ann Intern Med* 1992;117:898–904.

Half of people whose dizziness persisted for more than 2 weeks were found to have vestibular disorders; the next most frequent diagnosis was a psychiatric problem; approximately half had multiple causes; unrecognized life-threatening conditions were rare.

Kumar KL, Cooney TG. Vascular headache. *J Gen Intern Med* 1988;3:384–95.
The authors summarize information concerning migraine (common, classic, and complicated), and cluster headaches, benign exertional headache, and chronic paroxysmal hemicranial headaches; differential diagnoses as well as abortive and prophylactic managements are presented.

Olsky M, Murray J. Dizziness and fainting in the elderly. *Emerg Med Clin North Am* 1990; 8:295–305.
Review of the causes, evaluation, and management of patients with vertigo and syncope.

Plum F, Posner JB. *The diagnosis of stupor and coma.* Philadelphia: Davis, 1982.
Original edition was written 30 years ago; book remains a classic, with information on the many conditions altering mental status.

Sauvé J-S, Laupacis A, Ostbye T, et al. Does this patient have a clinically important carotid bruit? *JAMA* 1993;270:2843–5.
Analysis of information concerning auscultation of the carotid arteries, the significance of detecting a bruit, and bruits' implications in terms of surgical risk.

Standaert DG, Stern MB. Update on the management of Parkinson's disease. *Med Clin North Am* 1993;77:169–81.
This review focuses on newer forms of management; however, the authors also succinctly outline the differential diagnosis, characteristic features, and their implications for prognosis and management.

Stolinsky DC. Paraneoplastic syndromes (Medical Progress). *West J Med* 1980;132: 189–208.

Sudarsky L. Geriatrics: gait disorders in the elderly. *N Engl J Med* 1990;322:1441–6.
The author describes normal gait physiology and briefly outlines patterns of gait abnormalities seen among the elderly.

Swartz MN, Dodge PR. Bacterial meningitis—a review of selected aspects: general clinical features, special problems and unusual meningeal reactions mimicking bacterial meningitis. *N Engl J Med* 1965;272:725–31.
Classic description of meningitis in the context of the antibiotic era.

Verghese A, Gallemore G. Kernig's and Brudzinski's signs revisited. *Rev Infect Dis* 1987; 9:1187–92.
Reviews the original (Kernig in 1840 and Brudzinski in 1909) descriptions and other signs of meningitis; nuchal rigidity is present in more than 80% of patients with meningitis, being least sensitive among infants.

Weingarten S, Kleinman M, Elperin L, Larson EB. The effectiveness of cerebral imaging in the diagnosis of chronic headache. *Arch Intern Med* 1992;152:2457–62.
This study demonstrated the large variability among practitioners in their use of CT imaging; CT scans were not useful in finding pathology in patients with isolated chronic headaches.

Weinshenker BG. Natural history of multiple sclerosis. *Ann Neurol* 1994;36:S6–S11.
The author describes subsets of patients: chronic progressive, relapsing-remitting, and a few acute isolated attacks; overall, at 5 years, about half of patients are disabled enough to require a cane; MRI findings, immunologic profiles, and response to treatment among the different patient groups are presented.

Yesavage J. Differential diagnosis between depression and dementia. *Am J Med* 1993; 94(S5A):23–8.
Both conditions are common, and they often can coexist; the author reviews causes for dementia and features that distinguish it from depression.

9 Endocrine and Metabolic Problems

Objectives

List history and physical examination findings for the following problems:

- Addison's disease
- Amenorrhea
- Anorexia nervosa
- Bulimia
- Cushing's syndrome
- Diabetes
- Diabetic retinopathy
- Dysfunctional uterine bleeding
- Dyspareunia
- Gynecomastia
- Hirsutism
- Hyperlipidemia
- Hyperparathyroidism
- Hyperthyroidism and hypothyroidism
- Impotence
- Menometrorrhagia
- Osteoporosis
- Pelvic pain
- Pheochromocytoma
- Premenstrual syndrome
- Virilization

Pertinent Points

History

Problems with your glands?
Thyroid problems?
History of an abnormal blood glucose level?
- Family history of diabetes
- During pregnancy
- Polyuria, polydipsia
- Blurred vision

For people with established hyperglycemia:
- Current management: diet, activity, insulin, oral agents, how monitored, level of control, episodes of hypoglycemia (does patient know and recognize symptoms)
- Recent changes in treatment or level of control
- Onset, how diagnosed
- Complications
  - Eyes (last ophthalmologic exam)
  - Feet: ulcerations, callous and vascular, neurologic and infectious problems
  - Neurologic: peripheral neuropathy, autonomic neuropathy (gastrointestinal or genitourinary symptoms), mononeuritis
  - Accelerated atherosclerotic vascular disease (ASVD): angina, myocardial infarction, claudication
  - Hypertension, nephropathy

For patients with diabetic ketoacidosis:
- Adherence to management—medication, diet
- Blood glucose levels
- Urine ketone levels
- Symptoms of infection (upper respiratory tract infection, bronchitis, pneumonia, urinary tract infection, skin)
- Chest pain
- Abdominal pain, nausea, vomiting
- Pregnancy
- New medication

For patients with hyperlipidemia:
- Family history of hyperlipidemia or premature (younger than 50 years of age) ASVD
- Diet (percent calories from fat and unrefined sugars [dietary fat remembered as MEDIC = *m*eat, *e*ggs, *d*airy, *i*n baked goods, *c*ooking method])
- Alcohol use
- History and symptoms of ASVD
- Abdominal pain
- Medications (oral contraceptives, thiazide diuretics, beta-blockers)
- Findings of hypothyroidism

For those with suspected hypothyroidism or hyperthyroidism:
- Prior thyroid disease or goiter
- Cold or heat intolerance
- Changes in skin texture or hair
- Frequency of bowel movements
- Weight change (gain or loss)
- Hoarseness
- Tremor, change in eyes, palpitations, weakness of proximal muscles
- Menses, gynecomastia
- Recent iodine exposure (e.g., intravenous contrast agent)

For women with hirsutism:
- Hair distribution
- Voice change
- Family history of "hairy" women
- Menstrual function
- Temporal balding
- Change in body musculature

For those with primary amenorrhea (absence of onset menses at 16 years of age):
- Weight change, growth curve
- Development of axillary and pubic hair, breast enlargement
- Symptoms of an eating disorder
- Exercise habits
- Symptoms of hypothyroidism

For those with secondary amenorrhea (cessation of menses for 3 to 6 months):
- Sexual activity, possibility of pregnancy
- Prior menstrual pattern
- Menopausal symptoms
- Symptoms of hypothyroidism or galactorrhea
- History of weight loss
- Symptoms of an eating disorder
- Exercise habits
- Prior dilatation and curettage or other uterine surgery
- Medication or other drug use

For men with impotence:
- Onset
- Libido
- Medications or alcohol use
- Claudication or other symptoms of ASVD
- Illness associated with impotence (e.g., diabetes, depression, multiple sclerosis, alcoholism, causes of primary testicular disease)
- Morning erections, erections with masturbation
- Partner's reaction

For males with gynecomastia:
- Medications, drug and alcohol use
- Liver, renal, or thyroid disease
- Chest wall trauma
- For adolescents, sexual development

For women with dyspareunia or vaginismus:
- Libido
- Arousal, orgasm
- Pain on penetration or thrusting
- History of pelvic problems
- Partner's reaction

When assessing osteoporosis risk:
- Family history
- Weight-bearing exercise
- Calcium intake
- Smoking and alcohol use
- Estrogen status
- Medications (e.g., thiazide diuretics, corticosteroids, thyroid hormone)

When evaluating for endocrine causes of hypertension:
- Episodes of headaches, sweating, pallor, palpitations
- Weight change
- Changes in face, skin, new striae (stretch marks), easy bruising, nephrolithiasis

For those with a suspected eating disorder:
- Secretive eating
- Self-induced vomiting, binge eating
- Laxative, diuretic, or "diet pill" use
- Depression, substance abuse
- Level of physical activity
- Weight loss
- Satisfaction with current eating patterns
- Perception of current weight (overweight, too thin) versus desirable weight
- Menses
- Musculoskeletal injuries, stress fractures

For those with unintentional weight loss:
- Documentation of weight loss
- Ability to obtain and pay for food
- Food intake
- Oral problems (such as ill-fitting dentures)
- Anorexia, dysphagia, early satiety
- Fever, night sweats
- Symptoms of malabsorption (frequent, foul-smelling, floating feces that do not flush well)
- Polydypsia, polyuria, polyphagia
- Feeling depressed, vegetative symptoms, anhedonia, sleep disturbance, prior episodes of depression
- Smoking, cough, hemoptysis

Physical Examination

Vital signs
- Blood pressure and heart rate (check for orthostatic changes if suspect pheochromocytoma or diabetic autonomic neuropathy), respiratory rate (hyperventilation occurs with ketosis)

Nutritional state

Body habitus (musculature, fat distribution)
Weight, height (lost with osteoporosis), growth curve
Assessment of secondary sexual characteristics or **Tanner stage**
Skin
Striae, texture, bruising, abnormal pigmentation, lipodystrophy (atrophy of subcutaneous fat at sites of insulin injections), xanthoma, xanthelasma, acne, hair distribution (hirsutism or virilization)
HEENT
Facial appearance, eyebrows, arcus senilis, proptosis, extraocular movements (lid lag), visual acuity, fundi, palpate and auscultate thyroid
Chest
Auscultate breath sounds
Breast
Inspect
Palpate
Cardiac
Jugular venous pressure (JVP)
Palpate point of maximal impulse (PMI)
Auscultate heart sounds
Abdomen
Inspect
Auscultate (renal arteries for bruit)
Percuss liver span
Palpate for liver edge, spleen, masses
Pelvic
Inspect external genitalia
Inspect vaginal and cervical mucosa
Bimanual examination for tenderness, pain with cervical motion, uterus and adnexal enlargement
Genitourinary (male)
Inspect, palpate for masses and testicular size
Extremities
Palpate pulses
Edema
Inspect feet for fungal infection, blisters, calluses
Neurologic
Mental status
Cranial nerves II to XII
Muscle mass, strength
Reflexes
Sensation (light touch, proprioception and vibratory sense)

Vignettes 1 and 2

EP is a 56-year-old woman, who is a new patient being seen for the management of hypertension. She had her blood pressure measured 2 weeks ago at the dentist's office, and it was found to be 150/105 mm Hg. She has checked it twice since at the drug store, and it has been elevated in this range. When measured approximately 9 months before the dental visit, her blood pressure was 130/80 mm Hg. She relates good general health, except some achiness in her knees that she treats with aspirin, as needed. She has no family history of hypertension. Her only medication is conjugated estrogen (0.625 mg a day), which she has taken since a TAH-BSO (total abdominal hysterectomy–bilateral salpingo-oophorectomy) 7 years ago for uterine fibroids.

Physical examination reveals an obese woman, whose **height** is 65 inches [162.5 cm], **weight** is 215 pounds [96 kg], and **blood pressure** is 155/105 mm Hg in both arms. Physical examination findings are remarkable only for generalized obesity (a pear-shaped body habitus with a waist to hip circumference ratio of 0.7) and the absence of the stigmata of sustained hypertension, such as eye-ground changes and a sustained PMI. She has no striae or abdominal bruits. Her initial laboratory findings are notable for a random glucose level of 214 mg/dl; other blood chemistry values (including electrolytes and renal function) are normal.

SH is a 58-year-old woman with the complaint of lower extremity swelling. She was in good general health, except for a history of a goiter treated with exogenous thyroxine. For the past 2 weeks, she has noted bilateral lower extremity swelling, which has been worse at the end of the day. She initially thought it was caused by the hot weather and ignored it. However, it became more prominent, such that she could not wear her shoes. She does not describe symptoms of congestive heart failure, and other than the leg swelling, she is feeling well. She had a hysterectomy at 37 years of age for metrorrhagia and believes only her uterus was removed. She has never taken estrogen replacement therapy.

She was noted to have the goiter 1 year ago. She saw an endocrinologist when she first noticed that her neck was "swollen." Although she was found to be euthyroid, thyroxine treatment (0.1 mg per day) was initiated in an attempt to decrease the goiter. A few months later she began to notice progressive scalp hair loss. However, the endocrinologist did not think it was due to the thyroid supplementation. He had an overnight dexamethasone suppression test performed, which she claims was normal, and referred her to a dermatologist. The dermatologist began her on topical minoxidil, and she has been using it twice a day for about 4 months.

Physical examination reveals a pleasant woman whose **height** is 66 inches (165 cm), and **weight** is 165 pounds (74 kg), which is down 5 pounds from a year ago. Her **blood pressure** is 118/70 mm Hg, and her **heart rate** is 70 beats/min. **HEENT:** clear oropharynx; thyroid gland is palpable and about 50% symmetrically enlarged, without palpable nodules; no cervical adenopathy. **Chest:** clear to auscultation. **Breasts:** no masses. **Cardiac:** no jugular venous distention; normal S_1 and S_2; no murmur or gallop. **Abdomen:** no striae, soft without organomegaly or mass. **Pelvic** and **rectal** exam: normal vaginal vault; adnexa cannot be appreciated; stool is occult-blood negative. **Extremities:** symmetrical and full pulses; 1+ bilateral edema. No calf tenderness or Homan's sign. **Reflexes:** 1+ to 2+ and symmetrical, with normal relaxation.

Vignette Objectives

1. Most patients with hypertension (>95%) have primary "essential hypertension" (i.e., without an identifiable cause). Secondary hypertension is due to an identifiable cause and should be considered whenever hypertension is newly diagnosed or whenever control becomes more difficult in the absence of an identified reason (e.g., noncompliance with therapy, NSAID use, weight gain or alcohol consumption). How would the history and physical examination findings differ for patients with different causes of hypertension?
2. Hypertension and obesity are both common problems that can indicate hypercortisolism. However, most hypertensive, obese patients do not have a cortisol excess. What additional history and physical examination findings can indicate cortisol excess?

Cushing's Syndrome

Although Cushing's disease is rare, the effects of cortisol excess or Cushing's syndrome are not rare, as many patients take corticosteroids for treatment of other conditions (e.g., asthma, collagen vascular disease, and following transplantation). They, too, can show the effects of a cortisol excess. The adrenal gland produces glucocorticoids, aldosterone, and dihydrotestosterone, and their elevation results in specific changes (Table 9-1). Corticosteroid excess can cause thin skin and increased capillary fragility, leading to bruising and ecchymosis. More than half of patients with Cushing's syndrome have wide (greater than 1 cm) violaceous striae. These differ from the less pigmented "stretch marks" seen in weight gain and pregnancy.

The amount of body fat usually is increased and redistributed in patients with Cushing's syndrome, such that they exhibit truncal or central obesity (defined with a waist to hip circumference ratio of greater than 0.8 for women and 0.95 for men). Fat deposits also develop in the supraclavicular areas, over the upper back (buffalo hump), and on the face (moon facies) (Fig. 9-1). If the cortisol excess is due to an elevated ectopic adrencorticotropic hormone (ACTH) level, hyperpigmentation can also be present. Increased adrenal androgen production promotes the development of acne, and hirsutism and oligomenorrhea or amenorrhea can also develop.

Hypercortisolism also affects the skeleton. Children with Cushing's syndrome exhibit early epiphyseal closure and reduced linear growth. Excess cortisol also causes osteoporosis, which can result in back pain as the result of vertebral compression fractures. In addition, approximately two thirds of patients with Cushing's syndrome have reversible psychiatric manifestations, ranging from emotional liability to psychoses.

Table 9-1. Findings in adrenal hormone deficiency and excess abnormalities

Adrenal hormone	Potential findings with hormone deficiency	Potential findings with hormone excess
Glucocorticoid	Anorexia and vomiting, weight loss	Truncal obesity and moon facies; thinning skin, violaceous striae, increased capillary fragility, ecchymosis; emotional lability, psychosis; weakness, muscle wasting
Aldosterone*	Salt-craving, hypotension; impaired water excretion; hyponatremia, hyperkalemia	Hypertension, hypokalemia
Dihydrotestosterone	Lack of axillary hair in women	Acne, folliculitis
ACTH	Manifested as deficiency of glucocorticoids (aldosterone production is preserved)	Hyperpigmentation (especially over the knuckles and scars formed subsequent to ACTH elevation

*Aldosterone levels usually parallel those of glucocorticoids. However, isolated increase (Conn's syndrome) or decrease (as sometimes occurs in patients with long-standing diabetes or interstitial renal disease) also can occur.

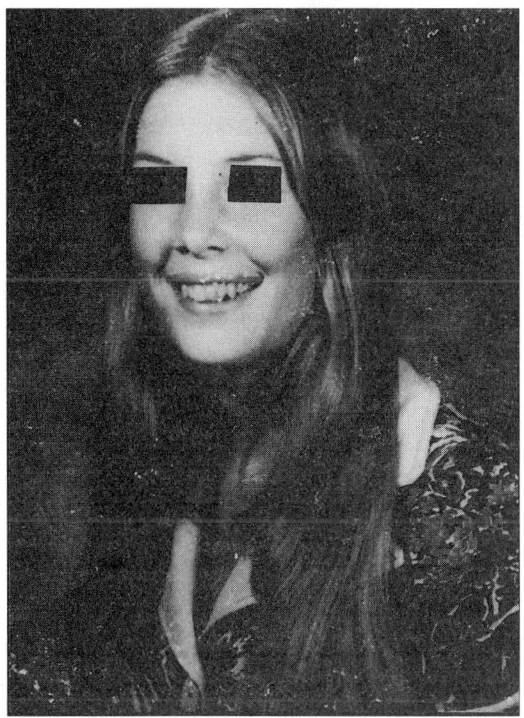

A

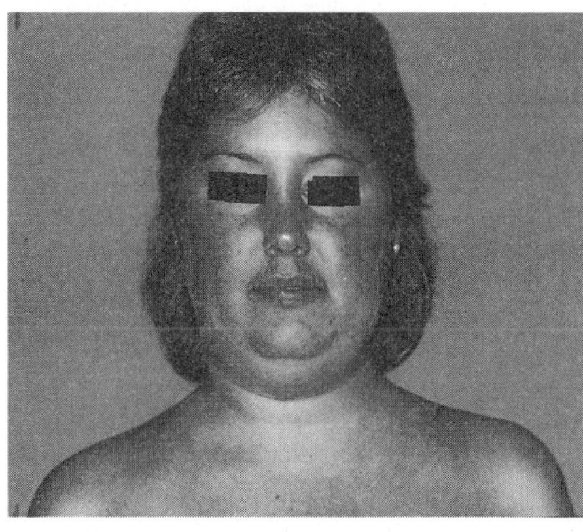

B

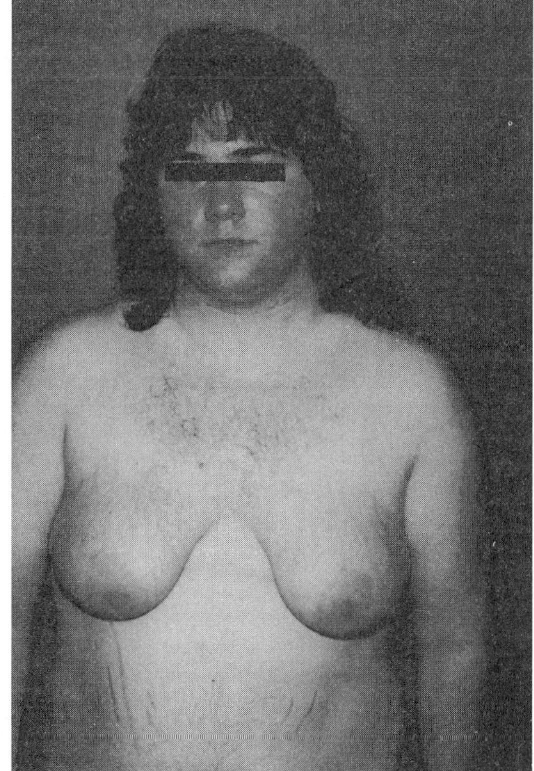

C

Figure 9-1. Cushing's syndrome. Patient's appearance before (A) and after (B) development of Cushing's syndrome. (C) Young woman with stigmata of Cushing's syndrome, including hirsutism, acne, and violaceous striae.

Adrenal Insufficiency

Adrenal insufficiency is a rare disorder, and its symptoms are nonspecific (anorexia, weight loss, orthostatic light-headedness, and generalized fatigue). The typical findings seen in patients with the disorder are listed in Table 9-1. The deficiency usually is due to a primary adrenal gland disorder (Addison's disease), with dysfunction due to immune destruction, infection (especially cytomegalovirus in those with advanced HIV disease), adrenal hemorrhage, or metastatic malignancy. More than 80% of the adrenal glands' function must be lost, however, before adrenal insufficiency occurs. Secondary adrenal insufficiency results from ACTH deficiency.

The hyperpigmentation resulting from an elevated ACTH level in the setting of primary insufficiency is best seen on the gingiva, knuckles, and areola and in scars that have formed after the onset of the elevated ACTH level. Unlike patients with adrenal gland destruction, in patients with ACTH deficiency, adrenal stimulation by the renin-angiotensin system preserves mineralocorticoid production, and hypotension is less problematic. An infrequent but significant finding in patients with adrenal insufficiency is calcification of the auricular cartilage.

The most common cause of adrenal insufficiency is iatrogenic, resulting from withdrawal from long-term exogenous corticosteroid therapy or inadequate replacement during times of "stress." Those on chronic corticosteroid therapy or replacement doses for chronic adrenal insufficiency cannot generate that compensatory increase and an acute "adrenal crisis" can develop at time of stress (e.g., infection, trauma, or surgery). Findings in such patients include hypotension, nausea, vomiting, and certain abdominal laboratory findings (including hyponatremia, hyperkalemia, hypocalcemia, and eosinophilia).

Hypertension

The evaluation of hypertensive patients is discussed in Vignette 2 in Chapter 3. Certain endocrine disorders can cause secondary hypertension, and the diagnostic features of these disorders are listed in Table 9-2.

Hair Loss

The finding of hair loss in women raises the possibility of an endocrine disorder. A hair shaft has three phases: anagen (active growth, 90% of hairs are in this phase), catagen (brief transitional phase), and telogen (3 months of resting before being pushed out by the new hair). Examination of a hair can identify its phase. Causes of hair loss are listed in Table 9-3.

Table 9-2. Secondary causes of hypertension

Condition (prevalence for each is <1% among all those with hypertension)	Symptoms	Signs
Renovascular hypertension (fibromusculary disease and atherosclerotic narrowing)	Arteriosclerotic more common in older patients with risks for and symptoms of ASVD; may have unexplained exacerbations of CHF Fibromuscular arterial disease more common in young women	Lateralizing renal artery bruit (sensitivity of approximately 50% but is more specific if bruit heard in both systole and diastole); other findings of ASVD
Pheochromocytoma	Symptoms often paroxysmal and include headaches, diaphoresis, palpitations, blanching, dizziness, nervousness	Tachycardia, sustained or paroxysmal hypertension, postural drop in blood pressure, weight loss, cafe au lait spots or axillary freckling (neurofibromatosis)
Primary aldosteronism (Conn's syndrome)	Weakness, muscle cramps, polyuria, polydipsia	Hypertension, findings due to hypokalemia
Cushing's syndrome	Weakness, weight gain, backache, history of nephrolithiasis	Moon facies, central obesity, hirsutism, ecchymosis, purple striae, psychological disturbances
Coarctation of the aorta	Asymptomatic hypertension in childhood	Ankle blood pressure lower than that of arm; delayed pulses in lower extremities (compared at radial and femoral artery)
Hyperparathyroidism	Constipation, history of nephrolithiasis or peptic ulcer, usually over 50 years old	—
Hyperthyroidism	Heat intolerance, weight loss, palpitations (see Table 9-11)	Tachycardia, systolic hypertension with widened pulse pressure (see Table 9-11)

Table 9-3. Causes of hair loss

Condition	Etiology and findings
Alopecia areata	Patch(es) of well-circumscribed hair loss; skin normal; regrowth after several months; idiopathic or due to stress; exclude syphilis
Trichotillomania	Behavioral problem of hair pulling
Telogen effluvium	"Stressful" event results in an increase in percentage of telogen hairs and accelerated hair loss; occurs several weeks after the stressful trigger; examples of stressors include childbirth, protein deficiency, surgery, and certain drugs (beta-blockers, lithium, allopurinol)
Androgenic alopecia	"Balding" in male pattern; women can experience this but show diffuse thinning without the "male" pattern; assess for evidence of hirsutism and virilization
Scarring alopecia	Disorders that scar the skin can cause hair loss; examples are lupus erythematosus, herpes zoster, and physical injury

Vignette Follow-ups

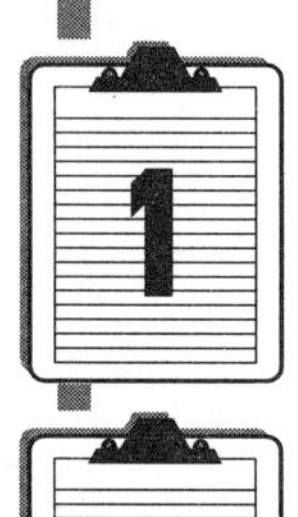

EP begins a walking program and loses approximately 6 pounds (2.7 kg), but her blood pressure remains elevated. She requires treatment with both antihypertensive medications and an oral hypoglycemic agent.

After extensive evaluation, the only nonexcluded cause of Ms. H's lower extremity edema is found to be minoxidil use. She has a normal serum albumin level and no evidence of congestive heart failure, cirrhosis, nephrotic syndrome, pelvic mass, or local venous obstruction. The medication is discontinued, and her edema resolves.

Vignette 3

KS is a 38-year-old man admitted to the hospital with complaints of nausea, feeling "weird," and an elevated blood pressure. The patient has a 6-month history of hypertension, which was detected during a routine physical examination. Treatment with beta-blockers resulted in "fatigue" and was discontinued. He then was treated with a diuretic, which resulted in his blood pressure decreasing into the normal range.

On the day of his admission, Mr. S awoke feeling well. He had tomato juice and later a fudgesicle and root beer. About that time, he began feeling nauseated, light-headed, and unsteady. He reported that he felt "weird," and "noises seemed far away and echoed." He became anxious and fearful that he was going to lose consciousness, and about 9:30 A.M., he called paramedics. He did not experience headache, chest pain, palpitations, or abdominal pain. The paramedics noted that his blood pressure was 210/130 mm Hg, and his heart rate was 110 beats/min. He was brought to the emergency room, where his blood pressure was found to be 190/124 mm Hg, with a heart rate of 88 beats/min.

He does not smoke but admits to drinking about 6 beers a day. He has no history of medical problems from drinking, does not drink in the morning, and has never been told to cut back on his drinking. He takes no medications other than the diuretic, and admits to no other drug use. Review of systems is remarkable for a voluntary loss of approximately 20 pounds (9 kg) over the past 6 months.

Physical examination reveals a healthy, anxious-appearing man. His **blood pressure** is 190/110 mm Hg in both arms, and his **heart rate** is 110 beats/min, without any orthostatic change. **Skin:** normal. **HEENT:** fundi show no arterial narrowing, hemorrhages, or exudates, and disk margins are sharp; the oropharynx is clear; the neck is supple without thyromegaly or adenopathy. **Chest:** clear to auscultation. **Cardiac:** no jugular vein distention; normal PMI; normal S_1, physiologically split S_2; no murmur, gallop, or rub. **Abdomen:** soft without organomegaly, masses, or bruits. **Extremities:** no edema. **Neurologic** exam: alert and oriented to person, place, and times. He can remember three objects after 3 minutes, spell "world" forward and backward, and perform serial 7s without errors. **Cranial nerves** II through XII are intact. Deep tendon **reflexes** are 2+ and symmetrical; **motor tone** and **strength** are normal and symmetrical. **Cerebellar** function is intact. An ECG obtained in the emergency room is normal and unchanged from previous tracings.

Vignette Objective

1. What are the symptoms and signs of a pheochromacytoma?

Pheochromocytoma

More than 90% of patients who have a pheochromocytoma ("pheo") have hypertension. However, a pheochromocytoma is a rare cause of hypertension (less than 1% of hypertensive patients). Approximately 30% of patients with a pheochromocytoma have sustained hypertension, 60% experience paroxysms of elevated blood pressure, and 10% are normotensive.

Orthostatic hypotension can be a clue to the diagnosis of pheochromocytoma. The orthostatic changes are caused by a reduced intravascular volume, resulting from chronic vasoconstriction and reduced baroreceptor sensitivity. A paroxysm or an acute blood pressure elevation is due to a sudden increase in catecholamine release from the tumor. In addition to an increased blood pressure, paroxysms can manifest in the form of headache, excessive sweating, facial pallor, palpitations, and a feeling of apprehension. They can be provoked by exercise or palpation of the tumor, but usually have no identifiable precipitant. Occasionally the diagnosis becomes apparent when a paroxysm is precipitated by anesthesia induction or after the administration of radiopaque dyes.

Approximately 10% of affected people have a family history of endocrine disorders and multiple endocrine neoplasia type IIa or IIb. These autosomal dominant disorders are associated with pheochromocytoma, medullary thyroid carcinomas, and hyperparathyroidism (type IIa) or with the first two and mucosal neuromatosis (type IIb).

Vignette Follow-up

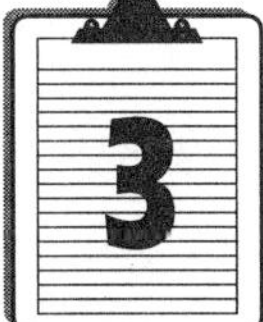

Mr. S's blood pressure is lowered acutely with clonidine and remains normal with treatment using his prior medications. Twenty-four–hour urine collections reveal a vanillylmandelic acid level of 6.3 mg/24 hours (normal, 1.8 to 7.1 mg/24 hours) and metanephrine level of 0.4 mg/24 hours (normal, <1.0 mg/24 hours). With subsequent questioning, he admits that he was drinking excessively the night before admission. That morning, he took 60 mg of pseudoephedrine for nasal stuffiness. His symptoms and elevated blood pressure are attributed to the combined effects of those two events.

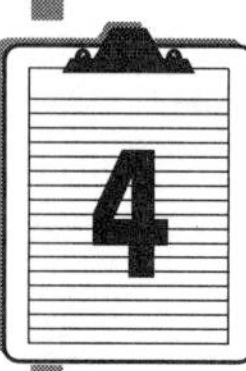

Vignette 4

BJ is a 34-year-old woman who has neurofibromatosis. She is referred for a new finding of an elevated blood pressure. She has felt well and denies headache, palpitations, or episodes of diaphoresis. Physical examination reveals a **weight** of 127 pounds (57 kg) and **height** of 5 feet, 2 inches (1.5 m). Her **blood pressure** is 148/98 mm Hg in both arms, and it does not vary going from supine to standing. Her **physical examination** is remarkable for the finding of freckles in both axilla and the absence of an abdominal bruit or stigmata of sustained hypertension.

Vignette Objectives

1. What are the criteria for a diagnosis of neurofibromatosis?
2. What causes of secondary hypertension are more prevalent among patients with neurofibromatosis?

Neurofibromatosis

Neurofibromatosis 1 (NF-1) is an autosomal dominant disorder, also known as von Recklinghausen's disease. Criteria for the diagnosis are listed in Table 9-4. It affects approximately one in 4000 people. Endocrine disorders that can be associated with it are pheochromocytoma, hypothyroidism, either precocious or delayed sexual development, and hyperparathyroidism. Patients with NF-1 are also at increased risk for two causes of secondary hypertension: (1) renal vascular stenosis (due to renal artery changes or an abdominal aorta coarctation) and (2) pheochromocytoma.

Table 9-4. Criteria for neurofibromatosis-1

1. ≥6 café au lait macules
2. ≥2 neurofibromas
3. Axillary or inguinal freckling
4. Optic glioma
5. Iris hamartoma
6. Osseous lesions
7. First-degree relative affected

Vignette Follow-up

Evaluation of Ms. J for a pheochromocytoma (assessed by measuring the urine metanephrine level) and renal artery stenosis (evaluated with a renal perfusion scan after the administration of an ACE inhibitor) yield normal findings. Ms. J's blood pressure is treated effectively with antihypertensive therapy.

Vignettes 5 and 6

AM is a 55-year-old woman who is concerned about "my bones." Her history reveals that at age 39 she had a TAH-BSO for endometrial cancer, followed by radiation therapy. Because of her malignancy, she has never taken estrogen replacement therapy and is worried about osteoporosis. She relates that she drank milk as a child but does not drink milk as an adult. She eats yogurt, cheese, and ice cream. She recognizes her need for calcium and usually takes about two calcium carbonate tablets a day. She enjoys square dancing on the weekend but is involved in no other exercise program. She recalls that her mother lost height and became "stooped." She does not smoke, drink alcohol, or take medication. She has not experienced any fractures, nor does she complain of back pain.

Physical examination reveals a slender Caucasian woman. Her **height** is 66 inches (165 cm) (which she believes is down from her maximum height of 66 3/4 inches [166.8 cm]), and her **weight** is 112 pounds (50.4 kg). Her **blood pressure** is 118/70 mm Hg, with a **heart rate** of 68 beats/min. Her general physical examination findings are normal.

Laboratory studies show normal serum levels of vitamin D, calcium, phosphate, albumin, and creatinine. Her spinal bone density is found to be 55% of the predicted norm for a 40-year-old woman and 63% of the norm predicted for age-matched controls.

AR is a 20-year-old college junior who is seen at the insistence of her mother because of amenorrhea of 6 months' duration and persistent foot pain. Although in excellent health all her life, she considered herself "mildly obese" until the summer after graduating from high school. That year she worked as a life guard and lost approximately 30 pounds (13.5 kg) by dieting and exercise. When she began college, she lost an additional 10 pounds (4.5 kg). Her weight has been stable for the past 2 years. She reports that she is eating three meals a day, but these consist mainly of fruits and salads. She exercises in her physical education class 3 days a week, and on the other days, she runs 3 to 4 miles.

AR reports that her menses were regular until the past few years, when they became less frequent, occurring two to three times per year. She has been sexually active in the past but not for the past 8 months. Earlier this year, she noted pain and tenderness along the lateral aspect of her left foot. A podiatrist diagnosed a "stress fracture" on the basis of the clinical findings of point tenderness, and radiographic and bone scan results. She switched to stationary cycling for 4 weeks. The symptoms initially resolved but have recurred in the past 2 weeks.

Physical examination reveals a pleasant woman who is in no acute distress. The **percentage of body fat**, as determined with measurement of skin folds, is 14% (normal for women is 19% to 25%). Her general physical examination (including a pelvic examination) findings are normal except for tenderness in the midshaft of her fourth left metatarsal. Her bone density is normal at 117% of the predicted norm for age-matched controls.

Vignette Objective

1. What aspects of the history and physical examination are relevant when assessing the risk of osteoporosis?

Osteoporosis

Osteoporosis is asymptomatic during the process of bone demineralization, and manifestations develop late in its natural history. Findings include fracture after minimal trauma (especially hip or wrist fractures), spinal compression fractures, and skeletal pain. The risk factors, which account for about one third of individual variability, are represented by the mnemonic SKELETON and are listed in Table 9-5 according to this mnemonic. (See also discussion in the section on menopause later in this chapter.)

Decreased estrogen levels, either due to menopause or hypoestrogenic amenorrhea, will accelerate bone loss. Whereas weight-bearing exercise results in preserved or increased bone density, that effect is diminished when decreased estrogen levels are present. Young amenorrheic exercisers are at increased risk for stress fractures and scoliosis. They usually have a bone density lower than normal but not one as reduced as that in hypoestrogenic nonexercisers.

Table 9-5. Risks for osteoporosis: SKELETON

Smoking (increases risk)
Kin (family history of osteoporosis)
Estrogen (estrogen deficiency accelerates bone loss)
Lady (women >men)
Exercise (weight-bearing activities lower risk)
Thyroid (hyperthyroidism decreases bone density)
Origin (increased risk among Caucasians)
Nutrition (low calcium intake increases risk)

Vignette Follow-ups

AM does not want to take any medications for her osteoporosis, other than continued calcium supplements. Her bone density is reassessed every 18 months.

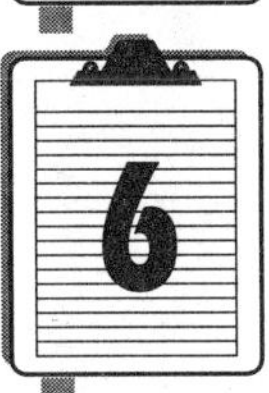

AR is thought to have another or a recurrent stress fracture. Additional history discloses that AR has bulimia (discussed in the next section) and symptoms of depression. She reduces her weight-bearing exercise and enters a counseling program for her psychiatric problems. Over the next 16 months, her weight increases 8 pounds (3.6 kg), her menses resume, and she experiences no further overuse injuries.

Vignettes 7, 8, and 9

TJ is a 15-year-old girl who comes to the clinic because she has not begun menstruation and her breasts are not "developing." She is short (her **height** is 4 feet, 2 inches [1.25 m]), and she and her parents want to know if she is "normal." Physical findings include normal prepubertal **external genitalia** and lack of **breast** development. Her neck is broad, and she has an increased carrying angle at her elbows.

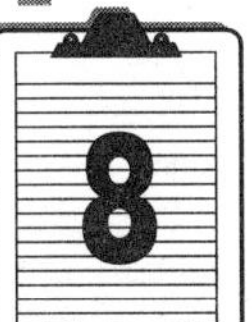

MA is a 16-year-old girl who has just moved to the area. She needs a "sports physical" to participate on her high school's cross country team. Her history reveals that she has not started her menses, although over the past year she has noted breast development. Her mother began menstruating at age 13. The patient has no significant past medical illness and takes no medications. She denies alcohol, cigarette, and other drug use. She is not sexually active. She feels that her weight is appropriate and believes that she eats a balanced diet. She denies bulimic behavior and depressed feelings. She expresses no concern about her sexual development and minimizes the problem. She seems overly cheerful, smiling while saying she dislikes doctor visits. MA has one older brother who is attending college. Her father is a dentist, and her mother owns an antique store. Physical examination reveals an energetic teenager, wearing loose-fitting clothes. Her **height** is 62.5 inches (156 cm), and **weight** is 90 pounds (40.5 kg). **Sexual development** is Tanner stage III to IV.

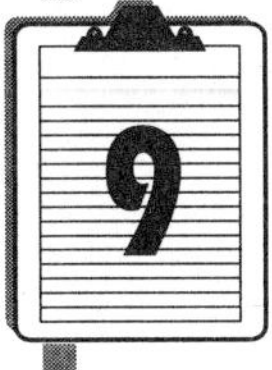

CA is a 19-year-old man complaining of bilateral breast tenderness. He states that his breasts have been enlarged for the past 8 months, but the tenderness has increased over the past 8 weeks. CA lifts weights regularly and wants to become a professional body builder. He reports using anabolic steroids, administered by injection (depot testosterone) and oral stanozolol, among others continuously for over a year. To combat testicular atrophy, he also has used injections of human chorionic gonadotropin (hCG).

Physical examination reveals a muscular man. His **height** is 69 inches (172.5 cm), and his **weight** is 228 pounds (104 kg). His **blood pressure** is 130/86 mm Hg; **heart rate** is 76 beats/min. **Skin:** there is an acneiform eruption over his chest, arms, and back. **HEENT:** no thyromegaly or adenopathy. **Chest:** clear to auscultation. **Breasts:** tender, symmetrical, bilateral breast tissue; tissue diameter is approximately 2.5 cm. **Cardiac:** PMI normal; S_1 and S_2 normal. **Abdomen:** soft, nontender; no organomegaly, mass, or bruit. **Genitourinary:** normal genitalia; testes are descended and of normal size, without mass.

Vignette Objectives

1. What aspects of the examination are most important when assessing a patient with an abnormality of sexual maturation? Describe how sexual maturation is assessed using the Tanner stages.
2. List the features of normal adolescent male gynecomastia and findings indicating pathologic gynecomastia in an adolescent boy.
3. What are the diagnostic criteria and findings for anorexia nervosa and bulimia nervosa?

Sexual Development

Abnormalities of Sexual Development

Sexual maturation proceeds through a sequence of changes, which are assessed using the Tanner stages (Table 9-6). Several conditions cause ambiguous geni-

Table 9-6. Stage of adolescent development*

Tanner stage	Female	Male
1	No pubic hair or breast enlargement	No pubic hair or genital change
2	Beginning growth of pubic hair (axillary hair growth occurs about 2 years later) Breasts bud (Usually 10 to 11 years old)	Beginning growth of pubic hair (axillary hair growth occurs about 2 years later) Scrotal skin coarsens Testes enlarge (Usually 11 to 12 years old)
3	Pubic hair increases and darkens Breast buds enlarge but no separation of areolar contour Growth spurt (Usually 11 to 12 years old)	Pubic hair increases and darkens Penis lengthens Adolescent gynecomastia (Usually 12 to 13 years old)
4	Adult pubic hair distribution Areolae project above breast Menarche (Usually 12 to 13 years old)	Adult pubic hair distribution Scrotal skin darkens Penis enlarges and lengthens Growth spurt (Usually 13 to 14 years old)
5	Pubic hair extends to thighs Areolae recede to share breast contour (Usually 14 to 15 years old)	Pubic hair extends to thighs Adult genitalia (Usually 15 years old)

*All adolescents are assessed for pubic hair, along with either breast (for girls) or genitalia (for boys) development.

talia at birth or abnormalities of sexual maturation. These disorders are listed in Table 9-7. Gonadal dysgenesis (due to an XO karyotype or to XO/XX mosaicism) is the most common cause of primary amenorrhea. Besides amenorrhea, the syndrome includes gonadal abnormalities, short stature (usually less than 58 inches [145 cm]), coarctation of the aorta (10% of patients), a "shield chest" (appearance due to widely spaced nipples), lateral displacement of the forearms (known as cubitus valgus), and renal anomalies (50% of patients). Affected patients need estrogen replacement therapy to promote the development of normal secondary sexual characteristics and menstruation.

Table 9-7. Abnormalities of sexual development

Category	Disorders
Sex chromosome defect	Mixed gonadal dysgenesis (e.g., karyotype 46 XO/XY)
Genetic male with feminization	Lack of testosterone-producing cells Enzymatic abnormality that prevents testosterone synthesis Testosterone receptor defect Inability to metabolize to active dihydrotestosterone
Genetic female with virilization	Exposure to maternal androgens in utero Block in corticosteroid synthesis resulting in excessive androgen production

Gynecomastia

Gynecomastia is enlargement of the male breast and is common among healthy adolescent boys (pubertal gynecomastia). Transient gynecomastia develops in approximately half of boys between the ages of 10 and 16 years, and signs of male sexual development precede its appearance. Pubic hair development, pigmentation of scrotal skin, and testicular enlargement (testes greater than 3 cm in length or 8 ml in volume) typically are present for at least 6 months before the onset of pubertal gynecomastia. The glandular tissue usually is less than 4 cm in diameter and resembles the early stages of female breast development. Pubertal gynecomastia normally resolves within 2 to 3 years. Hypogonadism also can present as gynecomastia near the expected time of puberty. This and other types of pathologic and normal pubertal gynecomastia are compared in Table 9-8.

Among adult men, gynecomastia can be idiopathic, drug related, or associated with aging or an illness (Table 9-9). Anabolic-androgenic steroids are one of the drugs that can cause it. Often users take the equivalent of 10 to 100 times the amount of normal testosterone production. In addition to gynecomastia, males who use these agents can exhibit aggression, acne, and male-pattern balding. Because of the suppressed folicle-stimulating hormone and luteinizing hormone levels, the sperm count decreases and the testes atrophy. Abnormal laboratory findings can include a low HDL-cholesterol level and increased LDL-cholesterol level, along with liver function abnormalities. Male breast enlargement caused by obesity and an accumulation of fat is compressed easily,

Table 9-8. Adolescent gynecomastia

	Normal pubertal gynecomastia	Potential features of pathologic gynecomastia
Onset	10 to 18 years of age	Younger than 10 years of age
Causative drugs	None	Positive history
Chronic illness	None	Liver or renal disease, cystic fibrosis, hyperthyroidism, ulcerative colitis, chest wall injury
Genital disease	None	Orchitis, testes trauma, cryptorchidism, hypospadias
Puberty onset	Before the gynecomastia	Precocious or after development of gynecomastia
Physical examination	Well nourished, testes enlarged, Tanner stage 2 to 4	Malnourished, goiter, small or asymmetrical testes, lack of secondary sexual characteristics (e.g., axillary and pubic hair and changes in testes and scrotum)

Table 9-9. Causes of adult gynecomastia

Condition	Findings
Idiopathic	Prevalence increases at 50 years of age, when may affect 30% of normal men
Drug related	Usually coincides with drug use; drugs include spironolactone, chemotherapy, cimetidine, anabolic steroids, digoxin, anabolic steroids, heroin, marijuana
Breast cancer	Rare; unilateral; mass fixed or ulcerated; suspicious lesions require biopsy
Decreased testosterone level	Chronic renal failure, Klinefelter's syndrome (XXY karyotype), alcoholism
Estrogen excess	Cirrhosis, hyperthyroidism, hCG-producing testicular tumors
Other	Chest wall trauma, hepatoma

nontender and lacks glandular texture. Asymmetric breast enlargement can be part of the spectrum of bilateral gynecomastia, but the finding should prompt careful assessment for breast cancer. Evaluation of a man with gynecomastia includes identification of drugs he is using and any chronic illnesses he may have. Testicular exam (for hypogonadism and hCG-producing testicular tumors) and a search for signs of hyperthyroidism and the stigmata of cirrhosis are important elements of physical assessment in such patients.

Interviewing Adolescents

Adolescents can take an active role in their health care, and it is appropriate to provide a time to talk with them alone during the interview. Parents therefore are routinely asked to leave for part of the interview and physical examination, and most are cooperative when it is explained that, as with any patient, adolescents need a confidential relationship with their physician.

When speaking with an adolescent, the patient should be informed that the conversation is confidential. Except for what is required by law, nothing is repeated unless the teen gives permission or the information revealed would result in harm to the patient or to others (e.g., suicide, incest, and child abuse).

Alcohol, drug, and tobacco use, sexuality, contraception, and sexually transmitted diseases are important aspects of an adolescent's medical history. Because certain aspects of the history (e.g., the sexual history or drug use) can be threatening, questions should be clear and nonjudgmental. Beginning with questions about others (e.g., "Tell me about your friends," "How do your friends feel about having sex?") and progressing to the teen's own behavior ("How do you feel?" "Are you sexually active now?") can facilitate information disclosure. Other important issues to discuss during the interview are school performance, risk-taking behaviors (e.g., using drugs, engaging in unprotected sex, using firearms, not using seat belts, and riding with a drinking driver), the presence or absence of close friends, and behavioral difficulties.

Eating Disorders

Eating disorders are associated with significant morbidity and mortality, but affected people rarely come to attention specifically because of their eating disorder. The patients usually are seen for a consequence of the disorder, such as amenorrhea or an athletic injury. Screening questions to identify anorectic or bulimic persons include: "How do you feel about your current weight?," "Are you satisfied with your eating habits?," "Are you a binge eater?," and "Do you try to control your weight by vomiting, taking laxatives, or diuretics or by overexercising?"

Bulimia

Bulimia nervosa was not appreciated as a distinct and common disorder until the late 1970s. It typically occurs in late adolescence or early adulthood and is found primarily among women. It is characterized by recurrent episodes of binge eating and at least three of the following characteristics: (1) binge consumption of high-caloric food; (2) inconspicuous eating during a binge; and (3) termination of eating episodes by abdominal pain, sleep, social interruption, or self-induced vomiting.

Other behavior patterns in binge eaters include prolonged fasting (approximately 90% of patients), self-induced vomiting (approximately 90%), laxative abuse for weight control (approximately 60%), over-the-counter diet pill use (approximately 50%), and the misuse of diuretics for weight control (approximately 33%). Most patients with bulimia are preoccupied with thoughts of eating and binge-purge cycles interfere with work or social activities in one third of affected patients.

In contrast to the emaciated appearance of patients with anorexia nervosa, there are few outward signs to suggest the diagnosis of bulimia. Such signs can include "puffy cheeks" (related to parotid gland swelling), enamel erosion (resulting from the acidity of vomitus), and finger calluses, due to trauma from self-induced vomiting.

Anorexia Nervosa

Features of anorexia nervosa include (1) an intense fear of becoming obese, which does not diminish as weight loss progresses; (2) a disturbance of body image and "feeling fat," even when emaciated; (3) a weight loss of at least 15% of original body weight (if patient is under 18 years of age, original weight can be projected from growth charts); (4) a refusal to maintain body weight above a minimal normal weight; and (5) among women, an absence of more than three consecutive menses.

The typical person with anorexia nervosa is a young (14 to 17 years old) woman, often from an economically privileged family. Her weight progressively dominates her thoughts, and she secretly may engage in the abusive use of diet pills, caffeine, laxatives, or diuretics to aid weight control. Common subjective complaints include the cessation of menses, cold intolerance, dry skin, hair loss, brittle nails, constipation, chronic abdominal pain, bloating, and insomnia.

Physical findings include cachexia, with loss of both fat and muscle mass, carotenemia (yellow-tinted skin), and lanugo (fine, downy) hair. Anorectic patients can have severe, life-threatening metabolic abnormalities. In some series, the mortality is up to 15% (resulting from sudden death, suicide, and infections), which is the highest death rate associated with any of the psychiatric disorders.

Vignette Follow-ups

TJ was found to have a 45 XO karyotype and gonadal dysgenesis, also known as *Turner's syndrome*. She is started on estrogen therapy.

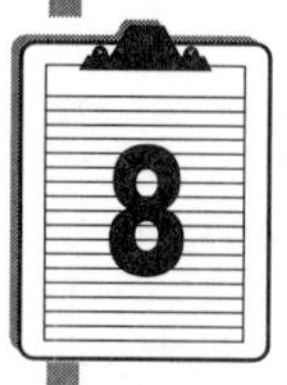

MA is found to be bulimic. She enters counseling, and her eating problems slowly resolve. With weight gain, her menses begin.

CA demonstrates some of the typical findings associated with anabolic-androgenic steroid abuse. CA's thyroid function tests are normal, and he is diagnosed as having anabolic steroid-induced gynecomastia. He has stopped using anabolic steroids for approximately 6 months, but his breast size has not changed. He is considering breast reduction surgery.

Vignettes 10, 11, and 12

SP is a 70-year-old woman who is seen in clinic because of leg swelling, two-pillow orthopnea, and lethargy. She was found to have congestive heart failure 5 years ago, which has responded to digoxin, captopril, and furosemide treatment. During the past 6 months, dyspnea and edema have slowly developed. Her family is concerned about a 30-pound (13.5 kg) weight loss over the past year, which they attribute to "not eating." Her daughter notes that Mrs. P has been disinterested in herself and her surroundings. They have considered her to be forgetful and "a little senile," for the past several years.

Physical examination reveals a lethargic, elderly woman who is incapable of providing relevant historical information about her health. Her affect is flat, and she appears chronically ill. Her **blood pressure** is 130/60 mm Hg; **heart rate** is 140 beats/min (irregularly irregular); **respirations** are 22 breaths/min, and rectal **temperature** is 99.0°F (57.2°C). **General inspection:** dry, wrinkled skin and cool extremities. **HEENT:** blepharoptosis; a multinodular, nontender thyroid gland, estimated to be about 40 gm (nearly twice the normal size) is noted; no thyroid bruit or cervical lymphadenopathy. **Chest:** fine rales bilaterally, which extend from the bases to the midscapular level. **Cardiac:** neck veins are distended at 15 cm of H_2O, with no detectable "a" waves; a diffuse PMI is palpable in the fifth and sixth intercostal spaces, close to the anterior axillary line. S_1 intensity varies, and an S_3 is heard over the apex; a grade 3/6 systolic ejection murmur is present at the base. **Abdomen:** nontender; the liver is palpable 4 cm below the right costal margin and estimated by percussion to be 16 cm in the midclavicular line; no mass; occult-blood negative stool. **Neurologic** exam: in addition to short-term memory deficits, she is unable to raise either her legs or arms more than a few inches above the bed, but her deep tendon **reflexes** appear brisk. Proximal **muscle wasting** is apparent in the upper and lower extremities.

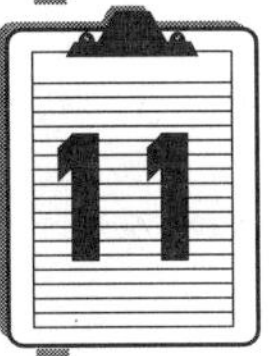

DE is a 42-year-old woman who works as a receptionist and is complaining of "fatigue." She relates that she had "the flu" about a month ago, and symptoms included nausea, malaise, and a low-grade fever. She stayed home only 1 day from work. However, she is not back to her "usual self." She remains fatigued throughout the day and has noticed palpitations. Although her appetite has been good, she has lost about 7 pounds (3 kg). Review of systems is otherwise negative for specific complaints. The patient's general health has been good, and medical history is noncontributory. Family history is positive only for alcoholism.

Physical examination reveals a healthy-appearing woman. Her **blood pressure** is 110/80 mm Hg, with a **heart rate** of 120 beats/min. Her **weight** is 109 pounds (49 kg) (the last weight recorded in her chart was 118 pounds [53 kg] recorded 3 years ago). **Skin:** hands are warm and moist. **HEENT:** no proptosis but lid lag is present; mild, diffuse, nontender thyromegaly, without bruit (over the thyroid). **Chest:** clear to auscultation. **Breasts:** without masses. **Cardiac:** normal PMI; normal S_1, physiologically split S_2; no murmur or gallop. **Abdomen:** soft, without organomegaly or mass. **Pelvic and rectal** exam: cervical and vaginal mucosa is normal, and bimanual exam reveals a nontender, normal uterus and adnexa. Stool is occult-blood negative. **Extremities:** no edema or fingernail abnormalities. **Reflexes** are 2+ and brisk, with a mild resting tremor.

MM is a 28-year-old woman admitted through the emergency room with the diagnosis of "thyrotoxicosis, rule out thyroid storm." Her "thyroid" history began 6 months ago, when she was found to be hyperthyroid and 3 months pregnant. She was treated with propylthiouracil (PTU) to maintain a free-T_4 (thyroxine) level in the normal range. She had no problems during her pregnancy, and approximately 1 month ago, she gave birth to a 7 1/2-pound (3.38 kg) boy, who has done well. Postpartum she was afebrile, had no tachycardia, and remained normotensive. She was discharged on the same dose of PTU. On the morning of admission, she felt weak and had arthralgia in her hips, knees, and ankles. She noted discomfort around her eyes, "as though I've been crying." Additional history includes the fact that the patient's 4-year-old daughter had "the flu," with fever, nausea, and headache. The patient lives with her husband, who is an accountant, and they have three children.

Ms. M's **blood pressure** is 140/70 mm Hg supine and 120/60 mm Hg standing; with her **heart rate** increasing from 115 to 130 beats/min; her oral **temperature** is 39.1°C. **HEENT:** no proptosis or lid lag; fundi are normal; neck is supple without adenopathy; her thyroid gland is 6 × 6 cm and diffusely enlarged; no bruit is audible over the gland. **Chest:** clear to auscultation. **Cardiac:** no jugular venous distention; carotids are 2+ bilaterally, with a transmitted murmur; PMI is located in the fifth intercostal space in the midclavicular line; S_1 and S_2 are normal; a grade 3/6 systolic ejection murmur is noted at the base, with radiation to both carotids. **Pelvic** exam: No erythema or purulent discharge; no tenderness is found on bimanual pelvic examination. **Reflexes** are 3+ and symmetrical, and no clonus or pathologic reflexes are present. **Muscle strength** is symmetrical and normal.

Vignette Objectives

1. What history and physical examination findings are suggestive of hyperthyroidism?
2. What unique features distinguish the hyperthyroidism that occurs among the elderly?
3. What are the findings that indicate thyroid storm?

Thyroid Disease

Hyperthyroidism

Many features of hyperthyroidism mimic aspects of catecholamine excess, such as palpitations, tremulousness, diaphoresis, and anxiety (Table 9-10). An elevated thyroid hormone level causes an increase in the resting metabolic rate and leads to heat intolerance and weight loss, despite a normal appetite. Soft, warm, moist skin and pruritus, hair loss, and onycholysis (separation of the fingernail from the distal nail bed) are characteristic dermatologic findings. If the thyroid is enlarged, the examiner should auscultate the gland. In patients with hyperthyroidism, a systolic bruit (occasionally accompanied by a thrill)

Table 9-10. Clinical manifestations of hyperthyroidism

Type of manifestation	Symptoms	Signs
Skin	Fine hair does not "hold" a permanent wave	Warm, moist skin; fine hair; pretibial myxedema with Graves' disease
Metabolic	Hyperphagia, heat intolerance, diaphoresis	Weight loss
Cardiopulmonary	Palpitations, chest pain, dyspnea on exertion	Tachyarrhythmias, atrial fibrillation, systolic hypertension, systolic flow murmur
Gastrointestinal	Hyperdefecation, nausea, vomiting	—
Genitourinary	Decreased libido, men—impotence, women—oligomenorrhea	Gynecomastia
Neuropsychiatric	Nervousness, agitation, insomnia, depression Weakness	Proximal myopathy Fine distal tremor, brisk reflexes
Other	—	Goiter, proptosis (exophthalmos with Graves' disease), staring gaze and lid lag (present with any type of hyperthyroidism)

can be detectable because of the increased blood flow. Additional physical signs include tachycardia, systolic hypertension and widened pulse pressure, a prominent cardiac apical impulse, staring gaze, and lid lag (delay in descent of the upper eyelid occurring with downward gaze, so that the sclerae transiently are visible above the iris). Several forms of myopathy are associated with hyperthyroidism: (1) a proximal limb girdle myopathy, (2) thyrotoxic periodic paralysis (occurring particularly in Oriental men), and (3) extraocular myopathy (occurring in patients with Graves' disease).

Several disorders can cause hyperthyroidism (Table 9-11), with Graves' disease being the most common. It has unique ophthalmologic and dermatologic findings. Graves' ophthalmopathy is characterized by swelling of the extraocular muscles and an increase in the amount of orbital fat, which leads to proptosis (bulging eyes); this can cause extraocular movements to be restricted and, if severe, can cause the optic nerve to be compressed. Pretibial myxedema is an uncommon feature of Graves' disease. It involves the subcutaneous infiltration of mucopolysaccharide and results in the formation of a painless, sharply circumscribed orange-peel–like induration over the anterior lower leg.

Hyperthyroidism and the Elderly

The symptoms and signs of hyperthyroidism can be absent or atypical in elderly patients, and the diagnosis also is made more difficult by the fact that the onset of hyperthyroidism usually occurs insidiously in this age group. Older patients, with so-called "apathetic" thyrotoxicosis, have minimal sympathomimetic findings. Depression and apathy are the major behavioral manifestations, rather than the anxiety and hyperkinetic state seen among younger af-

Table 9-11. Causes of hyperthyroidism

Condition	Comments
Graves' disease	Most common cause; women >men; diffuse thyroid enlargement; ophthalmopathy and pretibial myxedema are unique manifestations
Thyroiditis	Preceding viral illness causing thyroid inflammation and hormone release; gland can be tender (subacute thyroiditis) or nontender (painless thyroiditis); can occur postpartum
Toxic multinodular goiter	Older patients; large nodular goiter; which is susceptible to hormone release triggered by iodine load (e.g., radiographic contrast agent, amiodarone), causing hyperthyroidism
Toxic adenoma	Nodule >3 cm in diameter
Exogenous thyroid hormone (iatrogenic or factitious)	History of thyroxine use; medical personnel; no gland uptake on thyroid scan
Ectopic production of TSH or thyroid hormone (rare causes)	Hydatidiform mole or choriocarcinoma can produce marked elevation of hCG which crossreacts with the TSH receptor; teratomas can contain functioning thyroid tissue

fected patients. In addition, nearly half of thyrotoxic patients over 60 years of age do not have a detectable goiter.

Thyroid Storm

Thyroid storm is a life-threatening complication of thyrotoxicosis. When it occurs, it usually is precipitated by a "stressor," such as an intercurrent infection, surgery, or labor and delivery. The diagnostic criteria for thyroid storm are (1) a temperature above 100°F (37.7°C), (2) marked tachycardia, disproportionate to the fever, (3) exaggerated manifestations of thyrotoxicosis, and (4) dysfunction of the gastrointestinal, cardiovascular, or central nervous system.

Vignette Follow-ups

Mrs. P is found to have hyperthyroidism (due to a multinodular goiter) and a mild dementia, beside her ischemic cardiomyopathy. Her cardiac function improves with specific therapy for thyrotoxicosis; her affect, muscle strength, and self-care abilities improve, but a dementia persists. No reversible cause of the cognitive dysfunction is identified, and it is ascribed to Alzheimer's disease.

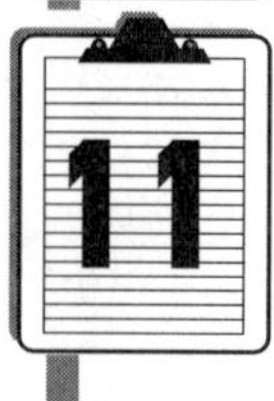

DE is found to be hyperthyroid and to have Graves' disease. She feels better, with less fatigue and palpitations, in response to treatment with beta-blockers. She is treated with radioactive iodine and is being followed with serial thyroid function tests for the development of radiation-induced hypothyroidism or recurrent hyperthyroidism.

On the night of admission, it is thought that Ms. M most likely has a viral infection superimposed on her hyperthyroidism. However, an impending thyroid storm cannot be excluded, and she is therefore treated as if she had this condition. She receives acetaminophen, PTU (200 mg orally every 4 hours), hydrocortisone (100 mg intravenously every 6 hours), and propranolol (20 mg orally every 6 hours). After 36 hours, her free-T4 and thyroid-stimulating hormone (TSH) levels return as normal, and the propranolol, hydrocortisone, and acetaminophen are discontinued. The patient remains afebrile, normotensive, and without tachycardia. All culture results are negative, and her findings are presumed to be due to a viral syndrome.

Vignette 13

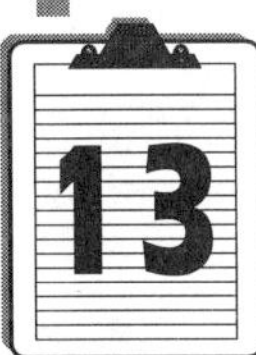

SSZ is a 30-year-old woman who is complaining of headache and fatigue. She reports that she has been healthy, takes no medication, and previously had been an avid exerciser. Two months ago she gave birth to her second child. She states that the pregnancy and birth were uncomplicated and that the baby's health is excellent. SSZ is the public relations director of a large animation studio, and she finds it difficult to breastfeed, nurture her new baby, and work. She felt fine for about 3 weeks after the birth but slowly has become more exhausted. She reported these feelings to her physician, who ordered a complete blood cell count (CBC) and told her that she was "fine" and that it is common for new mothers to feel tired, as the result of the stress of caring for a newborn, sleepless nights, and balancing career and motherhood.

Now more than a month later, she feels worse and comes to the clinic seeking a "second opinion." Physical examination reveals a healthy-appearing woman. Her **blood pressure** is 117/88 mm Hg, with a **heart rate** of 74 beats/min. Her general physical examination findings are normal, including palpation of the **thyroid gland**. The relaxation phase of her **reflexes** is interpreted as normal.

Vignette Objective

1. What history and physical examination findings are suggestive of hypothyroidism?

Hypothyroidism

Hypothyroidism is the flip side of hyperthyroidism (Table 9-12). The historical features are nonspecific and include cold intolerance, coarse hair, dry skin, fatigue, mild weight gain, constipation, myalgias, and arthralgias. Physical examination findings can include facial puffiness, dry skin, thinning hair, bradycardia, galactorrhea, and delayed relaxation of reflexes. Comparing a patient's current appearance with his or her appearance in prior photographs can reveal the changes caused by hypothyroidism (Fig. 9-2). Mild diastolic hyper-

Table 9-12. Clinical manifestations of hypothyroidism

Type of manifestation	Symptoms	Signs
Skin	Prior treatment for hyperthyroidism, complaints of puffy face and eyelids	Thyroidectomy scar, goiter, coarse hair, dry skin Loss of brow and scalp hair, yellow skin (carotenemia)
Metabolic	Cold intolerance	Weight gain
Cardiopulmonary	Dyspnea on exertion	Bradycardia, diastolic hypertension, systolic murmur that decreases with reduced ventricular preload, soft heart tones caused by pericardial effusion
Gastrointestinal	Anorexia, constipation	Ileus
Genitourinary	Decreased libido, menorrhagia, amenorrhea, galactorrhea	Gynecomastia
Musculoskeletal	Arthralgias, myalgia, muscle stiffness and cramps	—
Neuropsychiatric	Fatigue, depression, impaired memory	Psychosis, coma, carpal tunnel syndrome, slowed relaxation phase of reflexes

tension can also be present, and a reversible hypertrophic obstructive cardiomyopathy has been reported to occur. Approximately half of patients experience muscle stiffness and cramps, and over two thirds have elevated creatine kinase levels.

An elevated thyroid-stimulating hormone level is a highly sensitive and specific indicator of hypothyroidism. Assessing thyroid function is a cost-effective procedure in most patients, because the test is inexpensive and effective therapy is readily available.

Myxedema Coma

Impaired CNS function can accompany mild hypothyroidism. It can become more marked as the illness becomes more severe, with development of profound hypothyroidism (myxedema coma) in response to stressful events. Additional findings can include hypothermia, hypoventilation, obtundation (myxedema coma), and pericardial effusion.

Postpartum Hypothyroidism

Postpartum hypothyroidism occurs in approximately 5% of women after pregnancy and appears due to the cessation of gestational "immunosuppression." The postpartum increase in immunologic-mediated thyroid gland inflammation can lead to transient hyperthyroidism. That phase may be followed by hy-

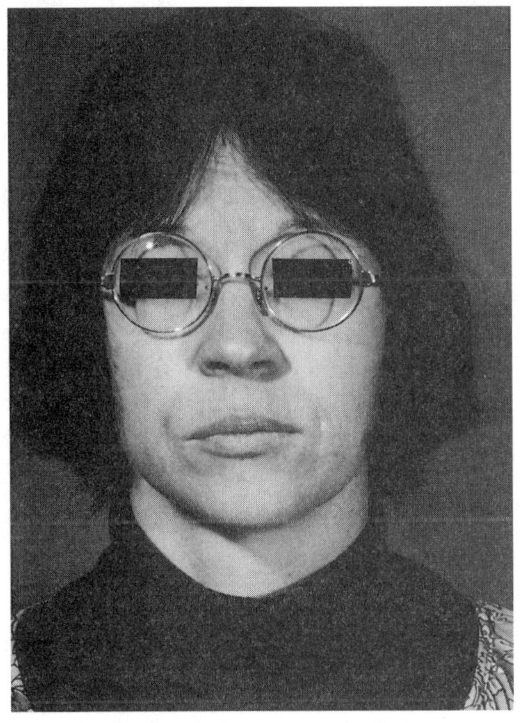

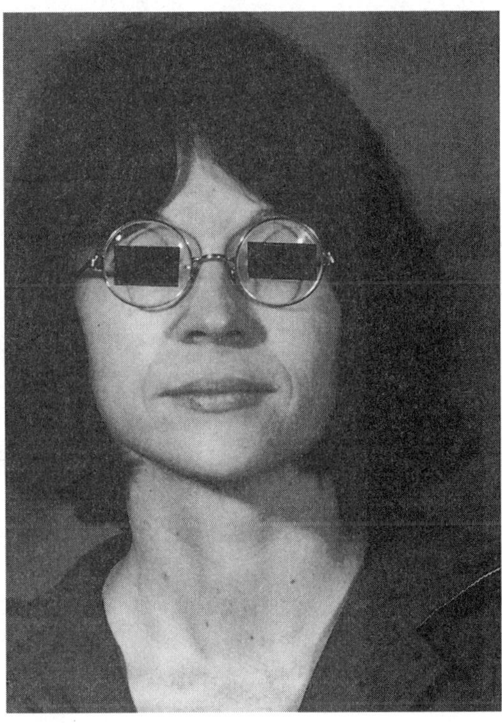

A B

Figure 9-2. A. Woman who complained of fatigue and myalgias but had not noticed a gradual change in her facial features. B. The same patient after thyroid replacement therapy.

pothyroidism, which usually occurs approximately 3 months postpartum, at a time when many new parents are feeling tired and lethargic. Thyroid hormone levels usually return to normal over 6 months.

Vignette Follow-up

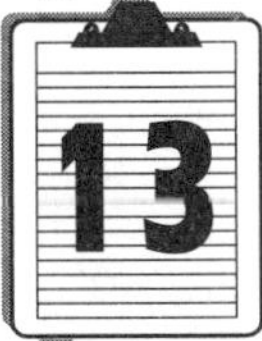

SSZ is found to have an elevated thyroid-stimulating hormone level. She is placed on L-thyroxine therapy, and her symptoms resolve over the next 8 weeks. She remains on thyroid replacement therapy for 8 months, after which it is tapered and discontinued. Five years after treatment, she has had no recurrence of symptoms, and her thyroid hormone level remains normal.

Vignette 14

EW, a 42-year-old man, has been told at a promotional health fair that his cholesterol level is elevated, but he cannot recall the specific value. He relates that his father had "cholesterol problems" and underwent coronary artery bypass surgery at 58 years of age. Mr. W never smoked, and no other modifiable coronary risk factors are present. Because of his work-related travel schedule, he often eats in fast food restaurants, without concern for low-fat choices.

His general physical examination reveals a well-developed, middle-aged man who is comfortable and talkative. His **height** is 70 inches (1.75 m), and his **weight** is 180 pounds (81 kg). His **blood pressure** is 136/84 mm Hg, with a **heart rate** of 78 beats/min. **HEENT:** neck is supple without thyromegaly; no xanthelasma; fundi are without exudate or arterior-venous abnormalities. Lateral earlobe creases are not present. **Chest:** clear to auscultation. **Cardiac:** normal S_1 and S_2, without murmur or gallop. Carotid and femoral pulses are normal, without bruit; radial, dorsalis pedis, and posterior tibial pulses are normal. **Extremities:** no edema or tendon xanthomas. **Skin:** no xanthomas over his elbows or knees or in palmar creases.

Vignette Objective

1. What are the relevant history and physical examination findings in patients with a hyperlipidemia?

Hyperlipidemia

When assessing patients with hyperlipidemias, important historical points include diet, alcohol consumption, drug use, exercise habits, changes in weight, family history, and symptoms due to sequelae of the hyperlipidemia. Physical examination findings suggestive of hyperlipidemia are listed in Table 9-13, and the manifestations are illustrated in Figures 9-3 to 9-9.

Table 9-13. Findings in the hyperlipidemias

Condition	Findings
Familial hypercholesterolemia	Autosomal dominant (heterozygotes 1 in 500); tendon xanthomas; xanthelasma (only 50% of patients with finding have hyperlipidemia); arcus senilis (significant if patient <35 years old); premature atherosclerosis (onset before 50 years old)
Familial hypertriglyceridemia	Autosomal dominant; triglycerides and / or chylomicrons can cause hyperviscosity; lipemia retinalis (milky retinal vessels), eruptive xanthomas, and pancreatitis; link to atherosclerosis unclear
Familial combined hyperlipidemia	Autosomal dominant; premature atherosclerosis
Familial dysbetalipoproteinemia (type III)	Premature atherosclerosis; palmar crease xanthomas
Secondary forms	
Drug induced	Alcohol, oral contraceptives, hydrochlorothiazide, beta-blockers
Hypothyroidism	History and examination findings of hypothyroidism
Nephrotic syndrome	Proteinuria, lower-extremity edema, low serum albumin level

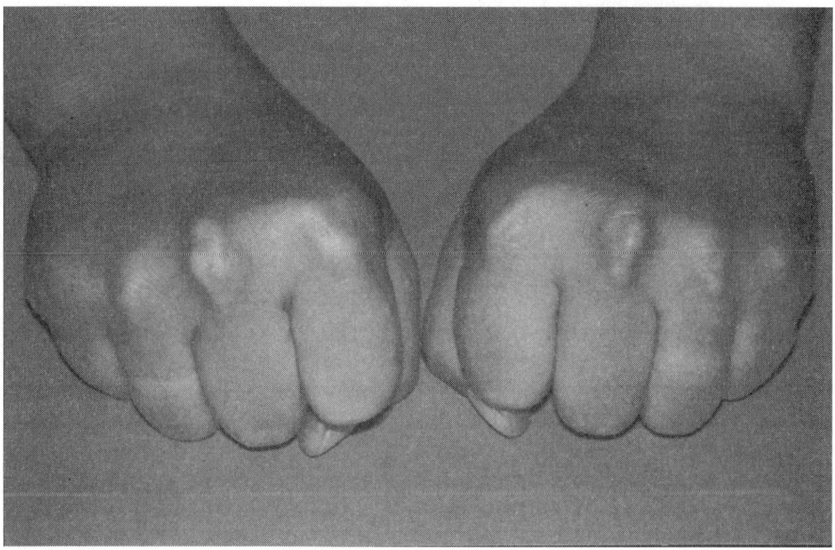

Figure 9-3. Tendon xanthomas in a woman with heterozygous familial hypercholesterolemia.

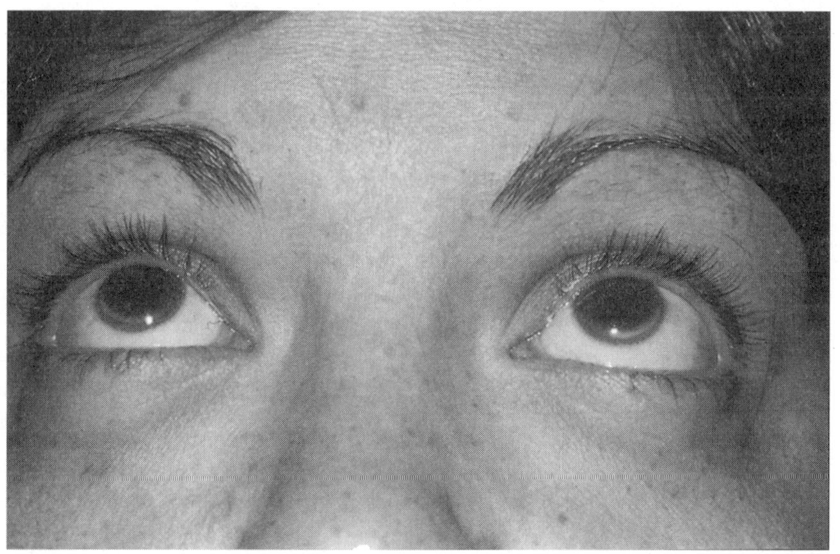

Figure 9-4. Corneal arcus senilis in a 19-year-old woman with severe heterozygous familial hypercholesterolemia.

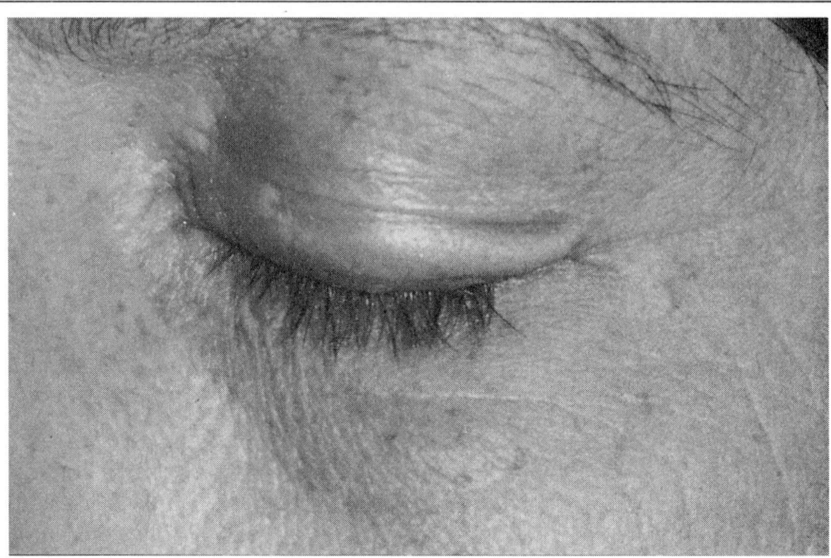

Figure 9-5. Xanthelasma in a woman with heterozygous familial hypercholesterolemia.

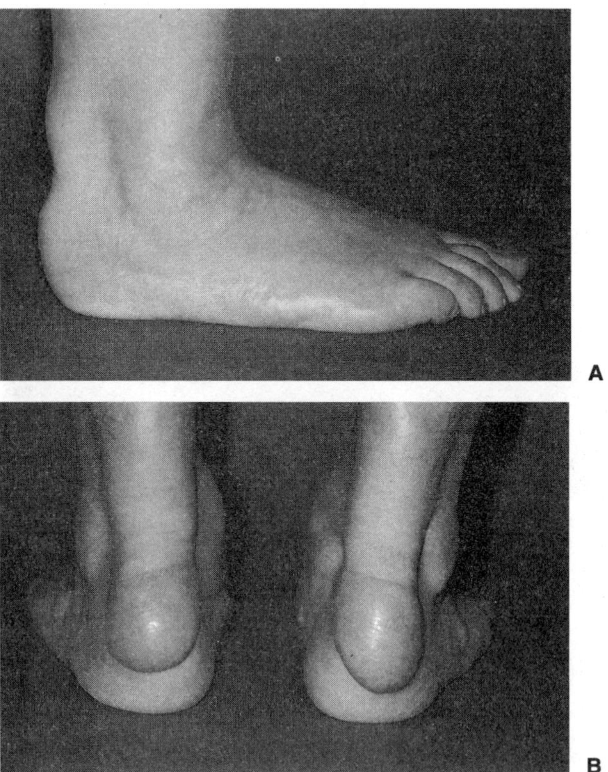

Figure 9-6. Tendon xanthomas in a patient with heterozygous familial hypercholesterolemia.

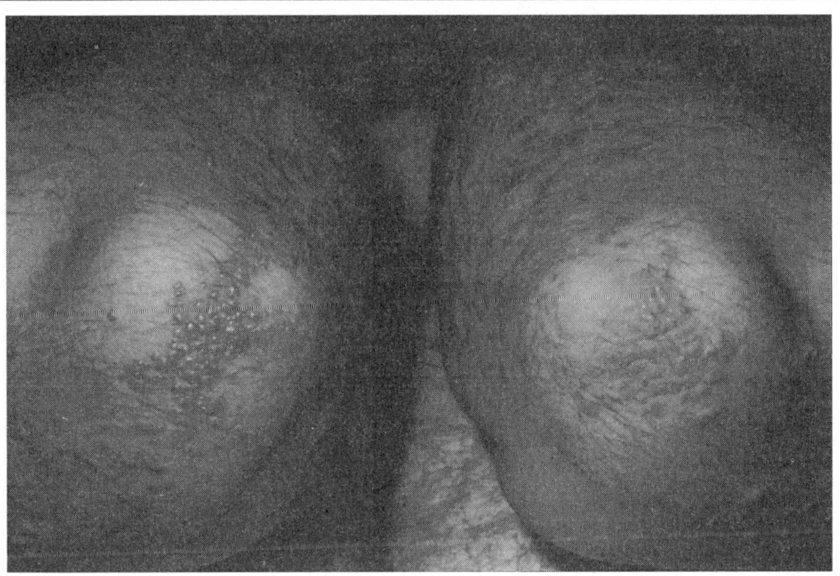

Figure 9-7. Tuberoeruptive xanthoma over the elbows in a patient with type IV hyperlipidemia.

Figure 9-8. Palmar crease xanthomas in a patient with type IV hyperlipidemia.

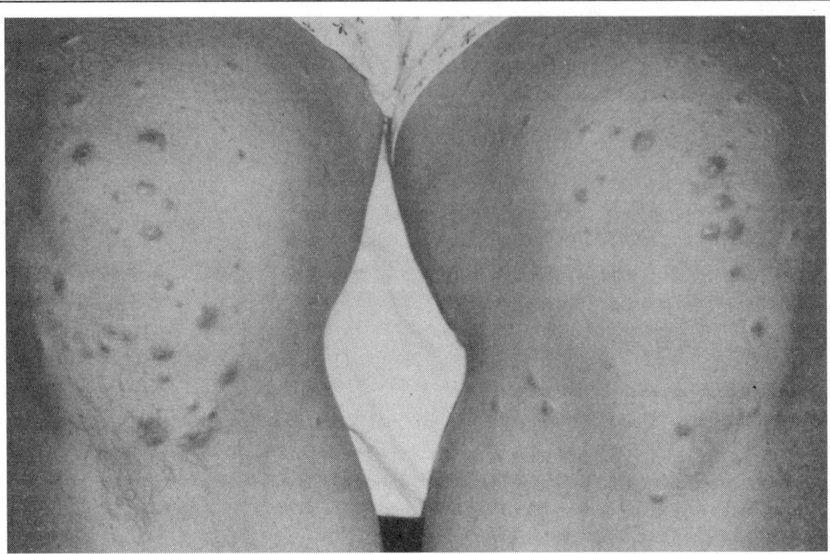

Figure 9-9. Eruptive xanthoma over the knees of a patient with severe type V hyperlipidemia and chylomicronemia.

Vignette Follow-up

EW is placed on a step I low-fat diet (intake of fat less than 30% of total calories) and followed up three weeks later. At his return visit he admits that he was not able to "diet" much, because of a wedding and out-of-town guests. Although he is referred to a dietician, he is "busy" and does not have time to keep the appointment. He is placed on HMG-CoA reductase inhibitor therapy and strongly encouraged to see the dietician and begin a reduced-fat diet.

Vignettes 15 and 16

VA is a 40-year-old man admitted to the hospital with blurred vision of 2 months' duration and pain on the left side of his scrotum for the past day. Physical examination reveals a man in distress because of pain. His **height** is 71 inches (1.78 m), and his **weight** is 207 pounds (93 kg). His **heart rate** is 96 beats/min, with a **blood pressure** of 110/70 mm Hg when supine. When standing, his **heart rate** is 115 beats/min, and **blood pressure** is 110/80 mm Hg. His general physical examination findings are normal, except for a 1.5- to 2-cm swelling on the left lateral aspect of his scrotum. The area is tender, erythematous and draining a purulent discharge.

Laboratory findings are remarkable for a hematocrit of 55%, WBC of 11,300/mm^3 (polymorphonuclear leukocytes, 63%; lymphocytes, 32%); dip stick testing of his urine shows 2+ glycosuria and moderate ketonuria; serum glucose level is 588 mg/dl; serum electrolyte values: sodium, 136 mmol/L; potassium, 4.2

mmol/L, with chloride of 102 mmol/L and bicarbonate of 12 mmol/L. Arterial blood gases: pH, 7.25; $PaCO_2$, 25 mm Hg; and PaO_2, 105 mm Hg. Smear of the scrotal discharge shows gram-positive cocci, with many polymorphonuclear cells.

JD is a 36-year-old man who presents for a preoperative evaluation before vitrectomy. He has had diabetes since 12 years of age, when weight loss and frequent urination developed. He has been taking insulin since that time. Currently he takes 10 units of regular and 25 units of NPH in the morning and 8 units of regular and 12 units of NPH before dinner. With his family's help, he checks his blood sugar level when "he remembers," which is about twice a week. He reports that it usually is in the range of 120 to 140 mg/dl. Regarding the complications of diabetes, he has retinopathy, and during the past 2 years, proteinuria and hypertension have developed. His hypertension has been treated with captopril, with reportedly good control. He denies chest pain, claudication, and symptoms of an autonomic or peripheral neuropathy.

His past medical history, other than the diabetes, is noncontributory. He has no family history of diabetes. He smokes one pack of cigarettes a day and does not drink alcohol. He is married and lives in a small town about 50 minutes from the clinic. He used to work in construction but has been unable to work for over 6 years because of his diabetes and progressive visual loss. Currently he cannot drive a car or read the newspaper. He spends most days home with his children. His wife works as an LPN.

Physical examination reveals a well-nourished man. Supine **blood pressure** is 160/80 mm Hg, with a **heart rate** of 76 beats/min standing; **blood pressure** is 132/80 mm Hg, with a **heart rate** of 86 beats/min. **Skin:** loss of hair over his toes. **HEENT:** fundi show hemorrhages, exudates, and scars from prior laser treatments. The optic disk in the left eye (the one surgery is planned for) is obscured by a recent hemorrhage. Vision is 20/140 in the right eye and finger counting is possible in the left eye. His oropharynx is clear, and his neck is supple without thyromegaly or adenopathy. **Chest:** clear to auscultation. **Cardiac:** no jugular venous distention; sustained, but not displaced, PMI; S_1 is normal, and S_2 is physiologically split; an S_4 is present; no murmur. No dorsal pedal or tibial pulses are palpable, and there are bruits over both femoral arteries. **Abdomen:** soft without organomegaly or mass. Stool is occult-blood negative. **Genitourinary** exam reveals a normal circumcised man. **Extremities:** trace lower extremity edema. **Neurologic:** absent ankle and knee jerks. There is decreased light touch and vibratory sensation in his feet.

Vignette Objectives

1. Diabetes is a common problem. What historical features are important in assessing blood glucose control?
2. Diabetes can result in many potential complications. What historical and physical examination findings would assist in the evaluation for retinopathy, neuropathy (peripheral and autonomic dysfunction), nephropathy, and accelerated atherosclerotic vascular disease?
3. What questions are useful for identifying depression in a patient with a chronic medical illness?

Diabetes

Current Treatment and Control

There are two general types of diabetes mellitus—Types I and II (Table 9-14); this classification reflects the pathogenesis of the disorder, which in turn has implications for management. The signs and symptoms of poorly controlled diabetes occur when the plasma glucose level is above 300 mg/dl; however, an absence of these symptoms does not necessarily indicate that blood glucose control is adequate. The more immediate sequaelae of hyperglycemia are listed in Table 9-15. The osmotic diuresis associated with hyperglycemia causes dehydration, polyuria, and polydypsia. Patients with poorly controlled diabetes also report fatigue and visual blurring, the latter resulting from the osmotic changes in the lens, stemming from the fluctuating glucose levels.

The management of diabetes and the way in which control is monitored must be assessed in all affected patients. Therapy with insulin and oral hypoglycemic agents, diet, and activity all contribute to the success of management. However, although most patients have access to blood glucose monitoring supplies, many perform testing incorrectly. By documenting blood glucose fluctuations levels and monitoring the percentage of glycosylated hemoglobin (hemoglobin A_IC) can assess the adequacy of therapy.

Findings in Long-standing Diabetes

Although the duration and severity of hyperglycemia are correlated with certain complications, there is marked variability among patients. The sequelae of

Table 9-14. Classification of diabetes

	Type I (juvenile)	Type II (adult-onset)
Onset	Before 21 years old (occasionally onset occurs up to 40 years of age)	Older than 30 years old
Family history	Unusual (only 50% concordance between identical twins)	Common (autosomal dominant pattern)
Ketosis	Common	Rare
Obesity	Rare	>80% of patients
Other	—	History of gestational diabetes

Table 9-15. Signs and symptoms of hyperglycemia

Pathogenic feature	Findings
Hyperglycemia causing an osmotic diuresis	Polyuria, polydipsia, dehydration, blurred vision (osmotic changes in lens), fatigue, weight loss
Infection due to impaired WBC function	Vaginitis (especially *Candida*), periodontitis, urinary tract infection, skin infection

Table 9-16. Complications of diabetes

Exam component	Manifestations of the complication
Vital signs	Hypertension, autonomic neuropathy results in loss of heart rate change with the respiratory cycle and orthostatic hypotension (blood pressure drop without coincidental heart rate increase)
Skin	Poor wound healing, lipodystrophy, foot ulceration
HEENT	Diabetic retinopathy (see Table 9-17), cranial nerve palsies (mononeuritis)
Cardiac	Angina, myocardial infarction, diastolic dysfunction
GI	Early satiety; nausea and vomiting due to gastroparesis; constipation or diarrhea due to autonomic neuropathy; fecal incontinence due to reduced sphincter tone
Genitourinary	Proteinuria, azotemia; bladder dysfunction due to autonomic neuropathy; urinary tract infections; pyelonephritis can be associated with papillary necrosis and acute ureteral obstruction; sexual dysfunction
Musculoskeletal	Aseptic necrosis; arthropathy (Charcot joints) due to neuropathy and repeated joint trauma
Neurologic	See Table 9-18

diabetes can affect almost every organ system (Table 9-16). Usually these complications are not found until after patients have had diabetes for at least 5 years. Rarely they are present when type II diabetes first is recognized or they are the initial manifestation of the disorder.

Diabetes accelerates the development of large-vessel atherosclerosis, causing the incidence of peripheral, coronary artery, and cerebrovascular disease to be increased in this patient population. As a consequence, approximately 60% of people with type II diabetes die of atherosclerotic cardiovascular disease and approximately 25% die of cerebrovascular disease.

Diabetes results in several types of cardiac disease. In addition to cardiac ischemia and the sequelae of hypertension, diabetes can affect small vessels and cause diastolic dysfunction. Renal effects start with microalbuminuria and progress to the nephrotic syndrome. Coincident with that progression, hypertension usually develops. Once the creatinine level begins to rise, patients progress to renal failure within a few years. Ophthalmologic findings are listed in Table 9-17. In the United States, diabetic retinopathy is the leading cause of blindness among people younger than 65 years of age. Neurologic sequelae are prominent consequences of diabetes. The diabetic neuropathies can be classified into the categories as shown in Table 9-18. The peripheral neuropathy is predominantly sensory, and symptoms vary from mild paresthesias or numbness to burning or lancinating pain. The discomfort usually resolves as the neuropathy progresses.

Peripheral vascular disease and neuropathy cause the incidence of serious foot infections and amputation to be increased in diabetic patients. This results partially from the fact that the sensory neuropathy often results in foot trauma going unnoticed. In addition, the neuropathy can impair the local vasodilatory response to infections, which along with peripheral vascular disease, predisposes patients to tissue damage and the progression of infection. Diabetic amyotrophy is an infrequent condition. Its manifestations include an asymmetri-

Table 9-17. Classification of diabetic retinopathy

Classification	Findings
Background	Microaneurysms, intraretinal hemorrhages (dot-and-blot hemorrhages), hard exudates, macular edema (sometimes classified as a more advanced stage of retinopathy)
Proliferative	Neovascularization, vitreous hemorrhage, scarring, retinal detachment

Table 9-18. Classification of diabetic neuropathy

Type of neuropathy	Manifestations
Peripheral polyneuropathy (axon demyelination with manifestation in distal extremities)	Gradual onset; symmetrical paresthesias (burning, lancinating pains); hyperesthesia, numbness; decreased vibratory sensation in stocking-and-glove distribution; interosseous muscle wasting; decreased to absent ankle and knee jerks
Peripheral mononeuropathy (nerve infarction due to thrombosis of vasa-nervorum)	Acute onset involving single nerve; intense pain in nerve distribution (e.g., radiculopathy would cause abdominal pain); resolves over several months
Cranial mononeuropathy	Usually affects cranial nerve III (with pupillary sparing), IV VI, and occasionally VII; resolves gradually
Autonomic neuropathies	
Impotence	Gradual onset; retrograde ejaculation
Neurogenic bladder	Residual postvoid urine, chronic infections, hydronephrosis
Orthostatic hypotension	Postural hypotension, loss of normal heart rate variation with respiratory cycle
Gastroparesis	Bloating, nausea, early satiety, vomiting
Enteropathy	Intermittent diarrhea, especially postprandial and nocturnal; fecal incontinence; intermittent constipation
Abnormal diaphoresis	Usually lower body anhidrosis, with upper body hyperhidrosis
Diabetic amyotrophy	Gradual onset; asymmetrical pelvic girdle and proximal thigh muscle wasting and pain; usually resolves in 3 to 6 months

cal proximal muscle weakness, pain, and muscle wasting. It is thought to result from multiple mononeuropathies involving the sacral plexus. As with other diabetic mononeuropathies, it usually resolves over approximately 6 months.

Psychiatric Diagnoses among Patients: Isn't It "Normal" to be Depressed?

Nearly one third of primary care patients suffer from a psychologic disturbance, and perhaps another 20% have significant emotional problems that complicate their physical illnesses. In some, physical complaints are seen as more "legitimate" avenues for the expression of psychiatric problems. Unfortunately, a third to half of psychiatric problems go unrecognized by primary care physicians, and patients often undergo extensive diagnostic studies before a psychiatric disorder is considered.

Identifying depression in the context of a medical illness can be difficult, however, because most serious and chronic illnesses lead to sadness and the illness itself can cause certain problems, such as fatigue, poor ability to sleep, and weight loss, all of which are also common manifestations of depression. However, it is not true that everyone with a serious illness suffers depression. Studies of terminally ill cancer patients have shown that fewer than half demonstrate the signs and symptoms of major depression.

The assessment for depression focuses on four aspects: (1) mood (feeling depressed), (2) vegetative signs and symptoms, such as insomnia and loss of appetite, (3) trouble concentrating, and (4) anhedonia. Questions to evaluate the last symptom include "What do you do for fun?," "What gives you pleasure?," and "When is the last time you had a good time?" Although the first three can be due to a medical illness, anhedonia, or the lack of pleasure from activities, is more specific for depression.

Several instruments have been used to aid in the diagnosis of depression, and these include the Beck Depression Inventory and the Hopkins Symptoms Checklist. In general, their sensitivity and specificity are approximately 75%.

Vignette Follow-ups

VA is admitted and treated with hydration and intravenous insulin. His infection abates with parenteral antibiotics. He is discharged on a regimen of subcutaneous insulin therapy and home blood glucose monitoring.

JD undergoes uncomplicated surgery. Additional questioning about his mood and anhedonia reveals that he meets the criteria for major depression. He has no suicidal ideation. His sleep pattern, mood, and level of function improve with antidepressant therapy.

Vignettes 17 and 18

LV is a 62-year-old Hispanic man seen for follow-up of hypertension. He has had stable coronary artery disease since having an inferior myocardial infarction 3 years ago. His medications include long-acting propranolol (120 mg/day), hydrochlorothiazide (50 mg/day), and aspirin (one a day). On questioning, Mr. V mentions that he has been having some problems with his "nature." On further discussion, it is found that he is experiencing difficulty achieving an erection. He is retired and lives with his wife.

Physical examination reveals a **blood pressure** of 135/80 mm Hg in both arms and a **heart rate** of 62 beats/min. **HEENT:** fundi show arteriolar narrowing. **Chest:** clear to auscultation. **Cardiac:** no jugular venous distention; normal PMI; normal S_1 and S_2, with an apical S_4. **GU:** normal penis and scrotum, testes size and consistency normal. **Extremities:** no edema and normal pulses.

EP is a 40-year-old woman referred for a fourth opinion regarding 3 years of abdominal pain. Despite normal physical examination findings, extensive evaluations, and visits to several physicians, she continues to seek a "diagnosis" for her complaints.

Vignette Objectives

1. What history and physical examination features are important in evaluating a patient with impotence?
2. What questions are useful in evaluating a woman with a history of sexual dysfunction?
3. What questions are used to obtain a history of sexual abuse?

Sexual History

Studies have shown that the sexual history rarely is obtained, despite the fact that patients express the belief that it is appropriate. There are several barriers to obtaining a sexual history; these include concern about patient embarrassment, lack of time, and physicians' personal discomfort and lack of skill in managing these problems. Frequently the sexual history is a component of the gynecologic review of systems. In men, the sexual history often is obtained during the genitourinary history. Suggestions for questions are listed in Table 9-19.

Impotence

Impotence is defined as an inability to consistently achieve or maintain an erection of sufficient rigidity for intercourse. It can be caused by psychogenic, vascular, neurologic, endocrine, or urologic problems. The prevalence of impotence varies with age, as does the relative proportions of various causes. Potential diagnoses and their findings are listed in Table 9-20. Useful information includes

Table 9-19. Sexual history questions

1. Are you currently sexually active? Do or did you have more than one partner? Men, women, or both?
2. Do you have any sexual questions or concerns?
3. How has your illness affected your sexual function?

Table 9-20. Causes of impotence

Diagnosis	Findings
Psychogenic	Depression, preserved morning erections and with masturbation
Neurologic	History of diabetes, spinal cord trauma, multiple sclerosis; following prostate surgery; other signs of a neuropathy, e.g., absent vibratory sensation or orthostatic hypotension
Endocrine (decreased testosterone level, increased prolactin level or hyperthyroidism)	Reduced testicular size; gynecomastia; loss of libido; findings of hyperthyroidism; headache (prolactinoma)
Vascular	Buttock claudication (Leriche's syndrome: buttock claudication, impotence, and absent pulses due to obstruction at the aortic bifurcation), bruits
Drugs and other agents	Alcohol, marijuana, opiates, anabolic steroids, antihypertensives, antidepressants

the onset and circumstances of impotence, possible precipitating events, the status of the patient's libido, and medications he is taking. The physical examination should focus on an inspection of the genitals, the determination of testicular size, and an assessment of vascular and neurologic function.

Psychogenic impotence usually is characterized by the sudden onset of erectile failure and generally occurs in younger (less than 60 years of age) healthy men. These men retain the ability to masturbate and continue to have spontaneous erections when awakening. Organic impotence usually arises in the setting of a chronic illness, such as vascular insufficiency or diabetes mellitus. It is insidious in onset, occurring over months or years. Libido can be intact, and the impotence usually occurs with all partners. Vascular impotence typically causes a gradually decreasing firmness of erection and frequently is associated with peripheral vascular disease. Neurologic impotence occurs in the setting of a progressive neurologic disorder, such as multiple sclerosis or diabetic neuropathy.

In men with endocrine (pituitary or testicular dysfunction) impotence, frequently the testes are small or soft (normal testes are approximately 4.5 cm by 2.5 cm). Libido is decreased, and secondary sexual characteristics are lost. However, the latter can take months to years to occur. Impotence also may be associated with hyperthyroidism, hypothyroidism, and increased prolactin levels.

Sexual Problems Among Women

Women's sexual dysfunction sometimes is categorized in the areas of libido, arousal, orgasm, and penetration. There are a variety of problems within each category. Dyspareunia is the term for genital or pelvic pain that occurs during or immediately after coitus. Vaginismus is the involuntary contraction of the paravaginal muscles and occurs when penetration is imminent. Open-ended questions (e.g., "What have been the problems?," "Tell me more about what has been going on") can be more revealing than specific questions and better define the problem. Questions directed at identifying potential problems can include:

Libido—"Do you desire sexual relationships?"
Arousal—"Do you lubricate during sexual experiences?," "Do you have difficulty becoming or staying aroused?"
Orgasm—"Do you achieve orgasm?"
Penetration—"Do you have pain on penetration or thrusting?," "Does your vaginal opening ever seem to close and prevent intercourse?"

History of Abuse

Abuse includes child abuse, sexual abuse, spouse abuse, and elder abuse. Each is being recognized with increased frequency. Up to 25% of women coming to emergency rooms with trauma have the injuries due to spousal abuse. Childhood sexual abuse is associated with certain problems that appear in adulthood, including undiagnosed physical complaints (especially chronic abdominal and pelvic pain), anxiety disorders, and obesity. A useful question to ask patients to find out about abuse is simply "Have you ever been abused?" The patient defines what constitutes abuse. If the patient asks what you mean by abuse, clarify by asking whether anyone has ever done something to him or her that they should not have done. The questions can either yield a response, or the patient may bring concerns up later, knowing that you are interested in these issues. If you find a history of abuse, the appropriate response is to reassure the patient it was not his or her fault, help the patient find a setting where he or she is safe, and direct a patient to seek ongoing therapy.

Vignette Follow-ups

An additional history is obtained, and Mr. V relates that he is having an extramarital affair and has experienced problems only with his wife.

Ms. P had a history of childhood sexual abuse, an issue that she had not discussed previously. She begins counseling. Her abdominal pain moderately lessens, and she does not seek care from other physicians.

Vignette 19

ST is a 38-year-old woman seeking your advice because she is overweight and has "excessive body hair." She has been in good health all her life. Although she has always been slightly overweight (height, 64 inches [1.6 m], weight, 148 pounds [66 kg]), in the past 3 years, her weight has gradually increased to 192 pounds (86 kg). She is convinced something is wrong and that her metabolism must be "out of balance."

Her menarche occurred at 13 years of age, and sexual development was normal. Her menses always have been irregular, and she has not had a period for 4 months. She has had "excessive" body hair since 15 years of age. She has several hairs on the upper lip and chin, which require shaving, and a few hairs around her nipples and on her abdomen. The amount of hair seems to have increased steadily over the years. Both parents are of Mediterranean origin, and her father and one sister have diabetes mellitus. She takes no medications.

Physical examination reveals an obese woman in no acute distress. Her lying and standing **blood pressure** is 185/100 mm Hg in both arms, and her **heart rate** is 82 beats/min. Her **weight** is 192 pounds (86.4 kg), and **height** is 64 inches (1.6 m). There is no "moon facies," buffalo hump, central obesity, or violaceous striae. She has no stigmata of hypothyroidism, and the body hair is as described in the history. There are no signs of virilization. **Pelvic** examination reveals normal-sized ovaries and uterus. The **reflexes** are brisk, with a normal relaxation phase.

Vignette Objectives

1. What history and physical examination findings pertain to secondary amenorrhea?
2. List potential causes of hirsutism and the findings that relate to these diagnoses.

Menstrual Disorders

Menarche typically occurs between 9 and 16 years of age, and delayed menarche, or primary amenorrhea, is a consideration after age 16. Secondary amenorrhea is defined as the absence of menses for at least 3 months after the establishment of normal menstrual function. The differential diagnosis for primary and secondary amenorrhea differ; the former includes gonadal dysgenesis, genetic disorders, and certain hypogonadotropic states. Secondary amenorrhea can result from disorders of the hypothalamus, pituitary, ovary, and uterus. The most common cause of secondary amenorrhea is pregnancy, and women with secondary amenorrhea should be considered pregnant until proved otherwise.

Various strategies are possible in organizing any differential diagnosis; they can be organized anatomically (what structure could it be?), according to specific

Table 9-21. Causes of abnormal uterine bleeding

Age group	Most common causes	Uncommon causes
Young adults (15 to 35 years old)	Pregnancy (spontaneous abortion, ectopic pregnancy), enovulation, endometritis	Trophoblastic disease, endometriosis
Middle years (35 to 45 years old)	Intrauterine device, pregnancy (spontaneous abortion, ectopic pregnancy), endometritis, large myoma, submucous myoma or endometrial polyp	Adenomyosis, endometrial cancer
Perimenopausal and postmenopausal	Endometrial cancer	Ovarian cancer

processes (what kinds of problems are there? [e.g., vascular, inflammatory, infectious, metabolic]), or perhaps according to a mnemonic. For example, causes of secondary amenorrhea can be remembered using the mnemonic MENOPAUSE (*m*edication, *e*xpectancy [i.e., pregnancy], *n*utritional, *o*varian, *h*ypothyroid, *p*ituitary, *a*drenal, *u*terine, *s*ystemic illness, and *e*motional).

Premenopausal women can have abnormal uterine bleeding, with abnormalities in the amount (menorrhagia) or regularity (menometrorrhagia). Causes of dysfunctional uterine bleeding can be grouped into three broad categories (Table 9-21): (1) anovulation, (2) uterine structural defects, and (3) bleeding disorders (primarily platelet dysfunction). Anovulation can cause amenorrhea or irregular bleeding, as the result of the endometrial hyperplasia. Uterine lesions are a common cause of menorrhagia and include fibroids, endometrial polyps, cancer, and inflammatory or infectious disorders. In addition, a complication of pregnancy, such as miscarriage or an ectopic pregnancy, should be considered for a woman of child-bearing age. Abnormal bleeding after menopause is called *postmenopausal bleeding,* and necessitates an evaluation to exclude an endometrial malignancy.

Dysmenorrhea is lower abdominal cramping resulting from the effect of local prostaglandins on uterine contraction. NSAIDs are effective in inhibiting prostaglandin production and alleviating dysmenorrhea. Dysmenorrhea can be normal or associated with a pathologic condition (e.g., endometriosis or a uterine fibroid). New-onset dysmenorrhea or a worsening of symptoms previously controlled with NSAIDs point toward the presence of uterine disease.

The premenstrual syndrome (PMS) is a constellation of symptoms that occurs in the luteal phase (7 to 10 days before menstruation), which then disappear with the onset of vaginal bleeding. There are no physical signs or laboratory markers of PMS. Symptoms include abdominal bloating, breast tenderness and swelling, pelvic pain, headache, ankle swelling, and changes in bowel habits. Psychological symptoms include irritability, aggressiveness, depression, anxiety, and changes in libido. Charting symptoms for 2 to 3 months can establish the menstrual association and guide therapy.

Hirsutism

Adult hair can be vellus (thin, soft, lightly pigmented) or terminal (thick, coarse, darkly pigmented). Terminal hair growth is androgen dependent and found on the face (beard area), chest, and male escutcheon. The growth of terminal hair outside of a woman's axillary and pubic regions is called *hirsutism.*

Many hirsute women have either familial hirsutism or anovulation. The latter can be due to polycystic ovary syndrome or to another anovulatory problem (e.g., hypothyroidism or an elevated prolactin level). Familial (or idiopathic) hirsutism is not associated with altered hormone levels and may be due to an increase in the responsiveness of hair follicles to normal female androgen levels. Drug-induced hirsutism usually is not associated with other findings of androgen excess (unless the drug is an androgen), and most nonandrogen agents result in generalized hair growth (termed *hypertrichosis*). Drugs in this category include phenytoin, minoxidil, and cyclosporin.

Elevated androgen levels cause virilization, in addition to hirsutism. The physical examination should therefore include a search for signs of virilization and Cushing's syndrome. Often virilization comes on abruptly, followed by rapid progression. It is distinguished by a decrease in the breast size; lowering of the voice; male-pattern hair loss; hair growth on the chest, beard area, shoulders, and upper abdomen; change in the body habitus with increased muscularity and loss of the female fat distribution, and clitoral enlargement. The probability of an ovarian or adrenal abnormality is high in patients with the signs and symptoms of virilization.

Vignette Follow-up

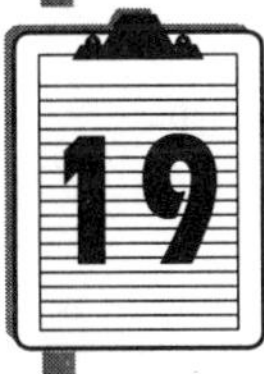

After evaluation, ST is thought to have hirsutism associated with anovulation. She is not pregnant, and after withdrawal bleeding induced by oral medroxyprogesterone therapy, her menses resume a normal pattern. Treatment options are discussed, and Ms. T elects to continue depilatory use.

Vignettes 20 and 21

FP is a 32-year-old woman who came to the emergency room complaining of abdominal pain of 8 hours' duration. She was well until that morning, when diffuse lower abdominal pain suddenly developed while she was watching television. The pain is suprapubic, constant, rated at 7 out of 10, and was alleviated somewhat with a heating pad. She ate and did not experience nausea or vomiting. She is g3, p3003 (three pregnancies [g], with outcomes of full-term deliveries [3], premature births [0], abortions [0], and living children [3]). (The meaning of the four digits can be remembered using the mnemonic,

Florida Power and Light.) She had a normal menses 18 days ago. She is sexually active with her husband and uses a diaphragm for contraception.

Physical examination reveals a woman curled up on the gurney. Her supine **blood pressure** is 110/80 mm Hg; her **heart rate** is 92 beats/min. Her **standing blood pressure** is 100/80 mm Hg and **heart rate** is 110 beats/min. Her **temperature** is 37.9°C. Abnormal findings are confined to those revealed by the **abdominal** examination. Bowel sound are present, but appear to be decreased (one sound per 60 seconds); she has diffuse moderate tenderness, most marked in the left lower quadrant; no rebound tenderness is demonstrable, although she winces when the gurney is moved; the liver span is 8 cm to percussion; **pelvic** exam reveals no cervical motion tenderness, but does show a tender left lower quadrant mass, which seems to be in the adnexal area; **rectal** examination confirms the findings on bimanual examination; stool is occult-blood negative.

MK is a 17-year-old woman who had been in good general health until the past 3 weeks, when anorexia, nausea, and vomiting developed. She intermittently has vomited bilious material. She has no history of gastrointestinal disease. Her medical history is significant for depression, which occurred 3 years ago and responded to antidepressants. Before her depressive illness, she had been using cocaine. However, she has not engaged in subsequent drug use. She currently takes no medications and rarely drinks alcohol. She is a part-time student and also works as a file clerk. Three months ago she moved in with a boyfriend.

Physical examination reveals a healthy-appearing woman. Her **blood pressure** is 100/76 mm Hg, and **heart rate** is 92 beats/min. **HEENT:** no adenopathy, normal thyroid. **Chest:** clear to auscultation. **Breasts:** without masses or galactorrhea. **Cardiac:** normal S_1 and S_2; a 2/6 systolic murmur is noted at the left upper sternal border when she is supine. **Abdomen:** soft without organomegaly or mass. **Pelvic** exam: normal vagina and cervix; she is slightly overweight (**weight**, 158 pounds [71 kg], **height**, 5 feet, 4 inches [1.6 m]), which makes it difficult to feel the limits of her uterus, but her pelvis is freely movable and nontender. No organ enlargement or mass is appreciated. Stool is occult-blood negative. **Neurologic** exam: reflexes are 2+ and symmetrical.

Vignette Objectives

1. List the features of the possible diagnoses unique to women presenting with acute abdominal pain.
2. List the findings associated with early pregnancy.

Abdominal Pain

Identifying the cause of abdominal pain often is difficult. Usually, a disorder's physical examination findings are neither sensitive nor specific. For example, cervical motion tenderness is a sensitive indicator of pelvic inflammatory dis-

Table 9-22. Gynecologic causes of acute pelvic pain

Condition	History	Physical examination
Ectopic pregnancy	Amenorrhea followed by vaginal bleeding; rupture usually occurs at about 2 months of gestation	8-week uterine enlargement; ±adenxal mass; can cause hemorrhage shock
Cyst rupture		
Corpus luteal cyst (Mittelschmertz)	Midcycle, acute onset pain	—
Endometriosis cyst	Prior history of pelvic pain	
Torsion of an adexna	—	Tender adnexa
PID	Risks for PID include prior sexually transmitted disease, IUD use, and multiple sexual partners	Elevated temperature; tender uterus and adnexa; tender adenxal mass; pain with cervical motion
Pelvic abscess	Usually associated with PID; occasionally postoperative or GI related; insidious onset of fever and pain; if abscess ruptures, peritonitis and sepsis can occur	Pelvic mass, low-grade temperature elevation

PID = pelvic inflammatory disease.

ease (PID), but it also is present in half of patients with ectopic pregnancies and a quarter of those with appendicitis. This difficulty is illustrated by the fact that only two thirds of women believed to have PID have the diagnosis confirmed at laparoscopy. Gynecologic causes of acute pelvic pain are listed in Table 9-22.

Diagnosing Pregnancy

Historical information (e.g., sexual activity, contraceptive practices, and the last menses) cannot reliably exclude pregnancy. Symptoms common in pregnancy (e.g., nausea, breast tenderness, and fatigue) are nonspecific. The prevalence of unsuspected pregnancy is not known. However, in one study, 2 of 110 women of child-bearing age hospitalized for nonobstetric reasons and stating there was no chance they were pregnant, were found to be pregnant. Because the history and physical examination are neither sensitive nor specific, laboratory tests are appropriate, especially when evaluating a woman with amenorrhea, pelvic pain or suspected pregnancy, or when ordering radiographic studies in women of child-bearing age.

Tests for pregnancy use monoclonal antibodies to detect the intact molecule or beta-subunit of human chorionic gonadotropin (hCG). Both urine and serum tests are over 90% sensitive at the time of the first missed menses. Home tests also use monoclonal antibodies and have a specificity of more than 95% but are less sensitive. In addition, there is a user error rate of up to 10%.

Pregnancy can be confirmed by other findings. Ultrasound studies can detect a gestational sac at 5 to 6 weeks and a fetal heartbeat at 7 to 8 weeks. Fetal heart tones can be heard by Doppler at 10 to 12 weeks and by fetoscope at 16 to 20 weeks. Quickening (or feeling the fetus move) occurs at 16 to 20 weeks.

Vignette Follow-ups

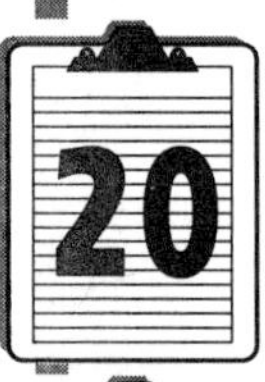

FP is admitted for observation and serial examinations. Her serum hCG level is not elevated, and she undergoes urgent ultrasound scanning, which shows a large adnexal mass, most consistent with an ovarian tumor. A benign ovarian tumor is confirmed at laparotomy. Her acute presentation is thought to be due to bleeding into the tumor.

MK is found to be pregnant.

Vignette 22

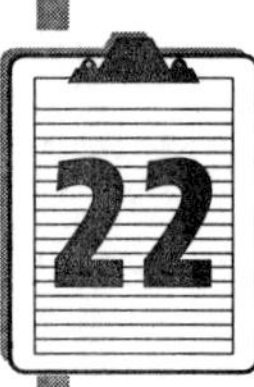

LS is in the clinic because she is wondering whether she should take hormones. She is 48-years-old and stopped having periods about 1 year ago. Although her symptoms have been minimal, she has been reading about postmenopausal hormones and wants to discuss their use. Her general health is good. By her report, pelvic examination, cervical cytology, and mammogram findings were normal 8 months ago. She has no family history of heart disease. Both parents died in their late 80s. She remembers that her mother became "stooped" as she aged.

Vignette Objective

1. List the symptoms of menopause and the risks and benefits of postmenopausal estrogen therapy.

Menopause

The mean age of women at menopause is 50-years-old. Perimenopausal progressive ovarian failure and menopause can result in hot flashes, vaginal dryness, irritability, lability of mood, and insomnia. However, the manifestations vary greatly among women. Some experience problems for 10 years before the complete cessation of menses, while others have minimal symptoms.

The classic menopausal symptom is a hot flash, during which women suddenly feel warm and their skin becomes flushed as skin vessels vasodilate. Estrogen deficiency produces vaginal dryness, failure of sexual lubrication, and pain with intercourse (dyspareunia). Emotional lability, depression, and loss of energy are more difficult to study and are not as clearly related to estrogen deficiency. However, placebo-controlled crossover trials have shown that irritability, anxiety, depression, and headaches respond favorably to estrogen replacement therapy (ERT).

Gall bladder disease is two-fold more common among women using ERT. The risk of endometrial cancer is increased approximately eight times in those who take ERT. However, this risk is preventable if estrogens are administered in combination with progestins. Despite having published findings from over 25 studies, the relationship of ERT and breast cancer is still uncertain, and concerns remain that ERT increases breast cancer risk, especially with more than 10 years of therapy.

The role of estrogen in the prevention of osteoporosis is well established. The risk of osteoporosis is increased with early menopause, Caucasian race, smoking, calcium deficiency, and family history (see Table 9-5). ERT leads to an approximately 60% reduction in the risk of hip and wrist fractures. ERT also leads to an approximately 50% reduction in the risk of cardiovascular disease. The risk reduction is comparable to the additional risk conferred by untreated hypertension (50%) or a sedentary lifestyle (40%).

A major factor in the ERT-mediated reduction in the risk of cardiac disease is its ability to cause an increase in the HDL-cholesterol level and a decrease in the LDL-cholesterol level. However, this effect does not account for all of its ability to reduce the risk of cardiovascular disease, and it also influences vascular tone and has other undefined beneficial effects. When the risks and benefits of ERT are considered, the potential cardiovascular benefits markedly outweigh the risks. One calculation (based on a hypothetical group of 100,000 postmenopausal women) showed that ERT would result in 500 less deaths associated with fractures and 5000 less deaths from cardiovascular disease. Even factoring in an estimated 200 more deaths from breast cancer, ERT would decrease the overall mortality about 40%. However, these data are hypothetical and the actual risks and benefits of ERT will not be known until the results of randomized trials are available.

Vignette Follow-up

Ms. S is given additional educational material on ERT. She schedules another visit and wants to talk more with friends before deciding about ERT.

Objectives Review

1. Most patients with hypertension (more than 95%) have primary "essential hypertension" (i.e., without an identifiable cause). Causes of secondary hypertension should be considered whenever hypertension is newly diagnosed or whenever control becomes more difficult in the absence of an identified cause (e.g., noncompliance with therapy, NSAID use, weight gain, and alcohol consumption). How would the history and physical examination findings differ for patients with different causes of hypertension?
2. Hypertension and obesity are both common problems that can indicate hypercortisolism. However, most hypertensive, obese patients do not have a cortisol excess. What additional history and physical examination findings can indicate cortisol excess?
3. What are the symptoms and signs of a pheochromocytoma?
4. What are the criteria for a diagnosis of neurofibromatosis?
5. What causes of secondary hypertension are more prevalent among patients with neurofibromatosis?
6. What aspects of the history and physical examination are relevant when assessing the risk of osteoporosis?
7. What aspects of the examination are most important when assessing a patient with an abnormality of sexual maturation? Describe how sexual maturation is assessed using the Tanner stages.
8. List the features of normal adolescent male gynecomastia and findings indicating pathologic gynecomastia in an adolescent boy.
9. What are the diagnostic criteria and findings for anorexia nervosa and bulimia nervosa?
10. List important aspects of interviewing an adolescent.
11. What history and physical examination findings are suggestive of hyperthyroidism?
12. What unique features distinguish the hyperthyroidism that occurs among the elderly?
13. What are the findings that indicate thyroid storm?
14. What history and physical examination findings are suggestive of hypothyroidism?
15. What are the relevant history and physical examination findings in patients with a hyperlipidemia?
16. Diabetes is a common problem. What historical features are important in assessing blood glucose control?
17. Diabetes can result in many potential complications. What historical and physical examination findings would assist in the evaluation for retinopathy, neuropathy (peripheral and autonomic), nephropathy, and accelerated atherosclerotic vascular disease?
18. What questions are useful for identifying depression in a patient with a chronic medical illness?

19. What history and physical examination features are important in evaluating a patient with impotence?
20. What questions are useful in evaluating a woman with a history of sexual dysfunction?
21. What questions are used to obtain a history of sexual abuse?
22. What history and physical examination findings pertain to secondary amenorrhea?
23. List potential causes of hirsutism and the findings that relate to these diagnoses.
24. List the features of the possible diagnoses unique to women presenting with acute abdominal pain.
25. List findings associated with early pregnancy.
26. List the symptoms of menopause and the risks and benefits of postmenopausal estrogen therapy.

Suggested Reading

Aron DC, Tyrrel JB, Wilson CB. Pituitary tumors. Current concepts in diagnosis and management. *West Med* 1995;162:340–52.
Two endocrinologists and a neurosurgeon present a thorough review of the clinical manifestations and management of pituitary tumors.

Brander A, Viikinkoski P, Tuuhea J, et al. Clinical versus ultrasound examination of the thyroid gland in common clinical practice. *J Clin Ultrasound* 1992;20:37–42.
Thyroid palpation is an imperfect art; two-thirds of what were felt as solitary nodules were found to be multiple when assessed with ultrasound; there was moderate agreement among observers about gland size.

Braunstein GD. Gynecomastia. *N Engl J Med* 1993;328:490–6.
Gynecomastia is common in men over 50 years of age, and it is idiopathic in approximately one quarter; the author reviews diagnostic considerations and the pathophysiology of conditions associated with gynecomastia.

Burch HB, Wartofsky L. Life-threatening thyrotoxicosis. *Endocrinol Metab Clin North Am* 1993;22:263–77.
Hyperthyroidism plus a "predisposing event" (e.g., surgery or an acute infection) usually lead to thyroid storm; the authors discuss the diagnosis, management, and prevention of this metabolic emergency.

Davis PJ, Davis FB. Hyperthyroidism in patients over the age of 60 years. *Medicine* 1974;53:163–79.
Eighty-five elderly patients (over age 60 years) with hyperthyroidism are described and compared with younger hyperthyroid patients.

Freund KM, Graham SM, Lesky LG, Moskowitz MA. Detection of bulimia in a primary care setting. *J Gen Intern Med* 1993;8:236–42.
These authors found that bulimic patients answered "no" when asked if they were satisfied with their eating pattern and "yes" when asked if they ever ate in secret; these screening questions may be useful in identifying this disorder.

Gifford RW Jr, Manger WM, Bravo EL. Pheochromocytoma. *Endocrinol Metab Clin North Am* 1994;23:387–405.
The authors present this rare disorder's manifestations, evaluation, and management.

Grady D. Rubin SM, Petitti DB, Fox CS, Black D, Ettinger B, Ernster VL, Cummings SR. Hormone therapy to prevent disease and prolong life in postmenopausal women. *Ann Intern Med* 1992;117:1016–37; 1038–41.
Extensive review related to the ACP's Guidelines for Counseling Women about Hormone Therapy, which is in the same issue.

Hamilton CR Jr, Maloof F. Unusual types of hyperthyroidism. *Medicine* 1973;52:195–215.
Graves' disease, multinodular goiter, and toxic nodules are the usual causes of hyperthyroidism; this review describes unusual causes of hyperthyroidism.

Klein I, Levey GS. Unusual manifestations of hypothyroidism. *Arch Intern Med* 1984;144: 123–8.
The authors discuss anemia, myopathy, cardiomyopathy, and rheumatologic manifestations, all of which are associated with hypothyroidism.

Kletter GB, Kelch RP. Disorders of puberty in boys. *Endocrinol Metab Clin North Am* 1993; 22:455–75.
Normal adolescent development and precocious and delayed puberty are reviewed, with information about evaluation and therapy.

Mazzaferri EL. Management of a solitary thyroid nodule. *N Engl J Med* 1993;328:553–9.
The author presents a brief review and outlines management strategies.

Nathan DM. Long-term complications of diabetes mellitus. *N Engl J Med* 1993;328: 1676–84.
The author reviews the many "opathies" due to diabetes, including consequences affecting the eyes, kidneys, vasculature, and nervous system.

Quan M. Diagnosis of acute pelvic pain. *J Fam Pract* 1992;35:422–32.
The author presents causes of acute pelvic pain, including abdominal pain during pregnancy; the utility of the history, physical examination, and laboratory studies is discussed.

Reed BD, Eyler A. Vaginal infections: diagnosis and management. *Am Fam Physician* 1993;47:1805–16.
Vaginitis can be due to Candida, trichomonas, and an altered vaginal ecology (vaginosis); up to one third of women have no specific cause established; this is a practical review of management.

Ricardi VM. von Recklinghausen. Neurofibromatosis. N Engl J Med 1981;305:1617–26. Brief review.

Rosenfield RL, Barnes RB. Menstrual disorders in adolescence. *Endocrinol Metab Clin North Am* 1993;22:491–505.
Genetic disorders need to be considered in adolescents with amenorrhea, and bone age needs to be assessed; the authors describe these disorders and relate them to normal pubertal development.

Van Eljkeren MA, Christiaens GCML, Sixma JJ, Haspels AA. Menorrhagia: a review. *Obstet Gynecol Surv* 1989;44:421–8.
Most bleeding is "essential"; other causes include fibroids, a coagulation disorder, an endocrine problem, or structural disorders; the authors briefly present information on management.

Werbel SS, Ober KP. Acute adrenal insufficiency. *Endocrinol Metab Clin North Am* 1993;22:303–23.
This is a rare disorder; the authors review potential causes, clinical manifestations, results of diagnostic studies, and management.

Yanovski JA, Cutler GB Jr. Glucocorticoid action and the clinical features of Cushing's syndrome. *Endocrinol Metab Clin North Am* 1994;23:487–505.

Glucocorticoids affect all body systems; the authors relate the many manifestations of elevated glucocorticoid levels to the hormones' actions.

10 Rheumatologic and Dermatologic Problems

Objectives

List history and physical examination findings for the following problems:

- Anaphylaxis
- Angioedema
- Ankylosing spondylitis
- Arthritis and arthralgia
- Back pain
- Bursitis
- Carbuncle
- Cellulitis
- Chronic fatigue syndrome
- Degenerative joint disease
- Dysplastic nevi
- Erysipelas
- Fibromyalgia
- Furuncle
- Gout
- Impetigo
- Inflammatory arthritis
- Osteoarthritis
- Palpable purpura
- Podagra
- Polymyalgia rheumatica
- Pseudogout
- Raynaud's phenomenon
- Spondyloarthritis
- Systemic lupus erythematosis
- Temporal arteritis
- Tophi
- Toxic shock syndrome
- Urticaria
- Vasculitis

Pertinent Points

History

Any allergic reactions?
For those with allergic reactions:
- What caused reaction(s) (drugs, insect stings/bites, foods)?
- Symptoms and signs (trouble breathing, hypotension, rash, hives)
- Treatment
- Prior desensitization

Any problems with your muscles? (weakness, pain, spasm) (also see Chapter 8)
Any problems with your joints?
- Arthralgia versus arthritis

For those with pain in one joint (monarticular arthritis):
- Onset, progression, description of pain
- Which movements cause pain?
- Morning stiffness (if present, duration), swelling, redness, pain, warmth
- Prior joint problems
- Fever, rash, cardiac, pulmonary, or gastrointestinal symptoms
- Joint trauma
- Sexual activity, exposure to sexually transmitted disease (STD), genitourinary (GU) symptoms, illness in sexual contacts
- IV drug use
- Tick bites, rash

For those with pain in two or three joints (oligoarticular) or multiple joints (polyarticular arthritis):
- Onset, progression, description of pain
- Migratory versus additive joint involvement
- Morning stiffness (if present, duration), swelling, redness, pain, warmth
- Prior joint problems
- Fever, weight loss, photosensitivity, rash, cardiac, pulmonary, or gastrointestinal symptoms
- Raynaud's phenomenon (episodic sequence of pallor, pain, coolness, cyanosis, and erythema of the distal extremities)
- History of heart murmur, recent dental work
- Rash, tick exposure
- Oral ulcers
- Recent or current "viral syndrome"
- Sexual activity, exposure to STDs, GU symptoms, illness in sexual contacts
- Medications
- IV drug use
- Family history of ankylosing spondylitis

When assessing patients with back pain:
- Onset, trauma
- Occupation, level of physical activity
- Prior problems
- Location, radiation, severity, position effects
- Weakness, numbness
- Bowel or bladder change
- Alleviating factors
- Weight loss, prior malignancy
- Fever, IV drug use
- Corticosteroid use
- Risks for osteoporosis
- Litigation, seeking compensation

Any problems with your skin? Rash?
Any moles that concern you? Sores that have not healed?
For those with skin infection:
- Onset, progression
- Trauma
- Eczema
- IV drug use
- Chronic medical condition(s) (e.g., diabetes, immunosuppression)

For those with a concerning skin lesion:
- Onset
- Change in appearance
- Personal or family history of skin cancer
- Sun exposure

For those with acne:
- Onset, distribution
- Family history
- Exposure to chemicals or cosmetics
- Drug use
- Current treatment

Physical Examination

Vital signs
- Blood pressure (both arms if patient is hypertensive or considering large-vessel vasculitis), heart rate, temperature, respiratory rate

Skin
- Malar rash of systemic lupus erythematosus (SLE), psoriasis, purpura, dermatitis of Reiter's syndrome, Lyme disease (erythema chronicum migrans), rheumatic fever (erythema marginatum)
- Describe any abnormalities

HEENT
- Scalp or temporal artery tenderness
- Alopecia
- Ocular inflammation
- Fundi
- Oral mucosa

Chest
- Chest expansion
- Percussion and auscultation

Cardiac
- Jugular venous pressure (JVP)
- Point of maximal impulse (PMI)
- S_1, S_2, murmur, S_3, S_4, and rub

Abdomen
- Appearance, bowel sounds, tenderness
- Hepatic span, splenomegaly, mass(es)
- Stool for occult-blood

Back
- Inspect
- Range of motion (ROM)
- Paraspinal muscle spasm
- Percuss for tenderness of spine

GU (male)
- Urethral discharge, skin ulcer or rash

Pelvic (female)
- Genital ulceration
- Cervicitis, pain with cervical motion
- Palpate uterus and adnexa

Extremities
- Assess joints for appearance, alignment, symmetry; joint tenderness and synovial thickening, effusion, warmth or erythema; active and passive range of motion (also see Table 10-2) to determine if pain from joint, periarticular structures or referred pain
- Digital skin edema, thickening, or ulceration; nail pitting
- Subcutaneous nodules or tophi
- Trigger points

Neurologic
- Cranial nerves II to XII
- Muscle tenderness, atrophy, or weakness
- Sensation and reflexes

Vignette 1

Angioedema: edema due to mechanisms similar to those that cause urticaria, but involves the deeper dermis and subcutaneous or visceral structures, such as lips, larynx, and gastrointestinal tract.

Urticaria: medical term for hives; it usually lasts less than 24 hours, from time of onset to resolution.

Wheal: pruritic, circumscribed area of edema in the upper dermis; can have central pallor; a collection of several wheals is called *hives*.

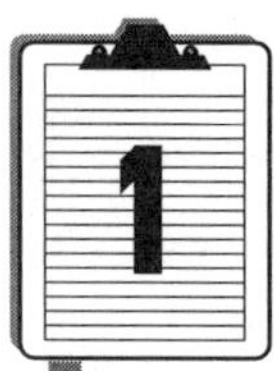

While you are at a graduation dinner for an 18-year-old cousin, a commotion starts at the far end of the table. One of the guests, whom you do not know, begins complaining of an "allergic reaction." The woman says that she is allergic to shellfish and accidentally has eaten a salad containing shrimp. In minutes her palms begin itching. Her voice is normal, but she complains of difficulty breathing. Paramedics are called. After arriving, they note hives on her skin. Her **heart rate** is 110 beats/min; her **blood pressure** is 100/60 mm Hg. Her **respiratory rate** is 28 breaths/min and slightly labored, and her **chest** is clear to auscultation.

Vignette Objectives

1. List the symptoms and signs of anaphylaxis.
2. What are the definitions of and physical examination findings characteristic of urticaria and angioedema?

Anaphylaxis

Anaphylaxis is an immediate, severe reaction to an allergen, resulting from its triggering the release of IgE-associated mediators. Common causes include penicillin, peanuts, fish, and insect venom. Allergic reactions can be localized (e.g., allergic rhinitis) or generalized. The generalized systemic effects result in a spectrum of abnormalities, including urticaria, wheezing, laryngeal edema, and, occasionally, hypotension (Table 10-1).

Hives are transient pruritic, well-marginated edematous dermal plaques. Angioedema is similar to urticaria but involves the deeper subcutaneous and visceral structures. In the early stages of anaphylaxis, people may complain of thirst, light-headedness, shortness of breath, skin flushing, and pruritis (often intense itching of the palms). Laryngeal edema and wheezing develop several minutes later. The life-threatening manifestations of anaphylaxis are airway obstruction and hypotension.

Most patients with mild to moderate symptoms and signs of anaphylaxis respond to epinephrine given subcutaneously. Intravenous administration is essential in patients with more severe symptoms (i.e., anaphylactic shock), because, in shock, the skin is not perfused well and a subcutaneous injection may

Table 10-1. Manifestations of anaphylaxis

Exam component	Findings
General	Sense of foreboding or impending doom
Skin	Flushing, pruritus, urticaria, angioedema
Eyes	Lacrimation, pruritus
Upper and lower respiratory tract	Sneezing, nasal congestion; hoarseness or stridor due to laryngeal edema; wheezing resulting from bronchospasm
Cardiovascular	Hypotension, tachycardia
GI	Nausea, vomiting, abdominal pain, diarrhea
Neurologic	Headache, syncope

not be absorbed. If intravenous access is not available, epinephrine can be delivered endotracheally. Patients with hypotension or laryngeal edema usually are admitted to a hospital for observation. Most patients without these findings can be observed for a few hours and released on a regimen of oral corticosteroids and antihistamines.

Insect bites or stings also can result in a large local reaction, which can be confused with an anaphylactoid reaction. However, local reactions do not lead to a generalized response and, unlike true allergic reactions, are not indications for venom immunotherapy. In addition to an allergen reaction, certain substances (e.g., radiocontrast dyes and narcotics) can degranulate mast cells and result in or anaphylactoid reactions.

Anaphylaxis causes acute urticaria, but urticaria also can be a chronic problem (lasting more than six weeks) or result from a vasculitis. The cause of chronic urticaria (unlike acute reactions) cannot be determined in approximately 90% of patients. Urticarial vasculitis can resemble chronic utricaria. However, the former is associated with autoimmune diseases, its wheals usually last longer than 24 hours, and it is associated with other features of the associated autoimmune illnesses (e.g., SLE or Sjögren's syndrome).

Vignette Follow-up

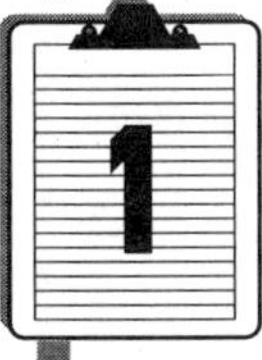

The paramedics begin an intravenous infusion of normal saline, and the emergency room physician orders them to administer epinephrine subcutaneously. When the patient arrives at the emergency room, she is feeling better. She is given diphenhydramine and methylprednisolone intravenously and admitted to the hospital for observation. She recovers uneventfully and is discharged the following morning.

Vignettes 2, 3, 4, and 5

Arthralgia: joint pain without evidence of altered joint anatomy or signs of inflammation.

Arthritis: joint pain, joint inflammation and/or altered joint anatomy; when caused by joint inflammation, it can be manifested by joint effusion, warmth, tenderness, and erythema.

Baker's cyst: herniation of the knee joint synovium into the popliteal fossa; associated with osteoarthritis of the knee.

Bouchard's node: Proximal interphalangeal (PIP) joint enlargement; usually due to osteoarthritis.

Heberden's node: Distal interphalangeal (DIP) joint enlargement; usually due to osteoarthritis.

Podagra: gout involving the first metatarsophalangeal joint; the word's root is the Greek word for 'foot' (the same root used for the word *podiatrist*).

DH is a 78-year-old man with "swelling in his left hand," which began 3 nights ago. At that time, he had pain along the medial aspect of his left wrist, which progressed to involve the entire wrist and was associated with pain and swelling in his hand. He has no history of rheumatologic disorders or trauma. Approximately 4 months ago, however, he did have similar symptoms, which were less severe and resolved over a week. He did not seek care for that episode.

Review of systems reveals that, over the past 6 months, he has been having chest pain, brought on by exertion or intense emotion. The pain is an "ache," which he describes with a clenched fist over his sternum. His chest pains are infrequent, and he had been pain free for the previous 10 days. Medical history is otherwise noncontributory. He is retired and lives with his fourth wife, to whom he has been married for 3 years.

Physical examination reveals a well-nourished man, with a **height** of 70 inches (1.75 cm) and a **weight** of 178 pounds (79 kg). His **blood pressure** is 180/90 mm Hg in both arms, and his **heart rate** is 68 beats/min. **HEENT:** funduscopic exam shows arteriovenous crossing changes, but no hemorrhages or exudates. Disk margins are sharp. His pharynx is clear. Carotids pulses are 2+, with a soft bruit on the left. **Chest:** clear to auscultation. **Cardiac:** no jugular venous distention (JVD); a sustained but nondisplaced PMI; S_1 and S_2 are normal, and an S_4 gallop is heard. **Abdomen:** no organomegaly or masses; liver span is 9 cm to percussion. **Genitourinary** exam: normal male genitalia; no penile discharge or lesions. Prostate is enlarged but without nodules, and stool is occult-blood negative. **Extremities:** no cyanosis or clubbing. Examination of his **left wrist** reveals swelling and warmth, with decreased active and passive ROM. Movement in any direction produces pain. There is no evidence of arthritis involving other joints.

Laboratory findings include the following: uric acid, 5.3 mg/dl; calcium, 9.2 mg/dl; total protein, 8.1 gm/dl; albumin, 3.6 gm/dl; hemoglobin, 11.8 gm/dl; hematocrit, 34.3%, white blood cell count (WBC) 10,300/mm^3 (62 polymorphonuclear leukocytes (PMNs), 8 bands, 20 lymphocytes, 10 monocytes), and an erythrocyte sedimentation rate (ESR) of 105 mm/hr.

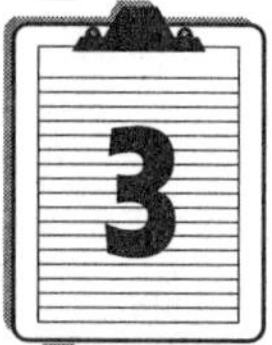

KJ is a 52-year-old man who began experiencing right knee pain approximately 3 months ago. He describes himself as a jogger, running 3 to 4 miles each morning. When his knee began to hurt, he took ibuprofen, but when symptoms persisted, he switched from jogging to stationary cycling. However, the pain has continued and for that reason, he made this clinic appointment. He has no history of knee trauma or prior joint problems.

Physical examination reveals a well-appearing man, whose examination findings are normal, except for a small effusion in his **right knee**. The knee is not warm or erythematous, and the joint line is not tender. Both knees show similar varus and valgus stability. The patella are hypomobile, with the left showing patellar maltracking and moderate crepitance. The Lachman test for anterior cruciate ligament stability demonstrates similar findings in both knees, with less than 1 cm of displacement and a solid end point. The popliteal fossa is normal, without evidence of any synovial herniation (Baker's cyst). **Other joints and lower extremity** alignment are normal.

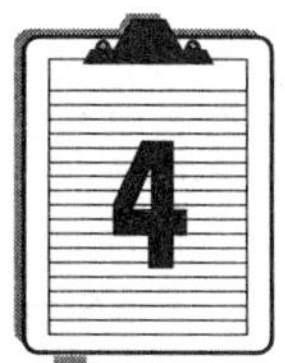

IH is a 76-year-old woman whose chronic problems are severe osteoarthritis of her knees and reduced vision (she is legally blind as the result of macular degeneration and glaucoma). Her husband has brought her to the clinic because her right knee has suddenly become much more painful. Ms. H's only medication is six aspirin tablets per day and "bee pollen."

Physical examination reveals an uncomfortable-appearing woman, sitting in a wheelchair. Her **blood pressure** is 142/76 mm Hg, her **heart rate** is 96 beats/min, and her oral **temperature** is 101.2°F (38.5°C). **HEENT:** testing of visual acuity reveals there is no light perception in the right eye and hand motion can be seen at 2 feet (60 cm) in the left eye. Her neck is supple, without adenopathy. Carotids are 2+, equal, and without bruits. **Chest:** clear to auscultation. **Cardiac:** no JVD; S_1 and S_2 are normal; grade 2/6, early-peaking systolic ejection murmur at the base (noted previously). **Breasts:** no masses. **Abdomen:** normal bowel sounds; no organomegaly or mass. **Extremities:** no edema or clubbing. The **right knee** is exquisitely painful to movement in any plane. There is a tense joint effusion, warmth, and erythema. Her **other joints** show only the changes characteristic of osteoarthritis, which are similar to prior exam findings.

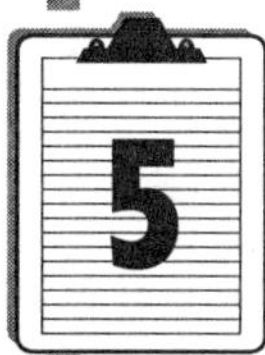

FP is a 62-year-old woman who has returned from a trip to Europe complaining of 24 hours of severe pain in her right foot. She had similar pain while on the trip, but it was much less severe. Now she cannot wear a shoe, and she is "embarrassed" to be wearing a slipper in the clinic. Her medical history is significant for asthma, for which she uses an albuterol inhaler, and hypertension, treated with long-acting diltiazem and hydrochlorothiazide. She took several aspirin when the pain became worse, without relief.

Physical examination reveals a **blood pressure** of 138/85 mm Hg, with a **heart rate** of 72 beats/min. Her general examination findings are normal, and **pertinent negative findings** include no stigmata of sustained hypertension, clear lungs, and no subcutaneous nodules or tophi. The **affected foot** is found to have an erythematous, swollen, warm, and tender metatarsophalangeal joint of the great toe.

Vignette Objectives

1. Describe a general approach to defining which structures are causing joint complaints.
2. What is the differential diagnosis for acute monarticular arthritis, and what history and physical examination findings would relate to these conditions?
3. How do the history and physical examination assist in determining the organism responsible for septic arthritis?

Joint Examination

A patient complaining of "joint pain" usually has one of four problems (Table 10-2). Assessing a joint includes noting: (1) joint deformity and stability, (2) swelling and abnormalities of the articular bones and joint capsule (resulting from synovitis or effusion), (3) tenderness in the joint line (indicative of synovitis) or other periarticular structures, (4) pain or limitations with passive and active ROM, and (5) signs of inflammation (pain, heat, redness, and swelling). Arthritis can be inflammatory or noninflammatory (Table 10-3). The number and distribution of joints involved determines whether the arthritis is monarticular (one joint), oligoarticular (two or three joints), or polyarticular (four or more joints). Causes of monarticular arthritis are listed in Table 10-4.

Table 10-2. Causes of joint pain

Joint pain origin	History	Physical examination
Arthritis	Pain with joint movement in any direction	Joint tenderness; heat and erythema over joint; joint effusion; limitation of movement with active and passive motion in all directions
Periarticular (e.g., tendinitis and bursitis)	Pain in or near the joint, pain with movements using the involved structures	Localized tenderness and swelling of the involved structure; no joint effusion, although fluid can accumulate in bursae; usually normal passive range of motion and decreased active range of motion with movement of the involved structure
Nonarticular (e.g., fibromyalgia and polymyalgia rheumatica)	Pain unrelated to joint movement, atypical pain pattern	Normal joint findings, tenderness of other structures
Referred or neurogenic pain (e.g., shoulder pain due to irritation of the left diaphragm)	Pain follows a dermatome or peripheral nerve distribution	Normal joint findings, cutaneous hyperesthesia in nerve distribution

Table 10-3. Inflammatory and noninflammatory arthritis

Types of arthritis	History	Physical examination
Inflammatory (e.g., rheumatoid arthritis, SLE, and joint infections)	Complaints of red, hot, swollen joints; often rapid onset; episodic flares and remissions; symptoms at rest; prolonged (>1 hour) morning stiffness; can have systemic symptoms and other organ involvement	Erythematous, warm, tender joint; synovial tenderness (usually along joint line) and thickening; effusion; if chronic can have deformity and destruction of joint and periarticular supporting structures
Noninflammatory (e.g., due to osteoarthritis, trauma, and avascular necrosis)	Onset of osteoarthritis usually after 40 years of age; often chronic, with slow progression; <30 minutes of morning stiffness; worse with use, better with rest; often affects weight-bearing joints; can be history of joint trauma	Joint can be tender, but less than in an inflammatory arthritis; joint may be enlarged or deformed due to bony proliferation or noninflammatory effusion; limited range of motion; crepitus or grating

Table 10-4. Causes of monarticular arthritis

Cause	History	Physical examination
SEPTIC		
Gonococcal	Sexually active; prodrome of myalgias, fever, arthralgias, dermatitis; affects women >men	Knee most common site, followed by ankle and wrist; 50% have tenosynovitis; possible skin findings
Nongonococcal	Prior joint damage or prosthesis, IV drug abuse	Monarticular arthritis, stigmata of IV drug abuse or underlying arthritis
CRYSTAL INDUCED		
Gout	Acute onset; exquisite pain; affects distal joints of extremities; affects men >women; precipitated by alcohol, aspirin, trauma; onset at night (distal joints cooler)	Inflammatory monarthritis, tophi, first metatarsophalangeal joint most frequently involved
Pseudogout or CPPD disease (calcium pyrophosphate dihydrate)	Subacute onset; large-joint involvement; can be associated with osteoarthritis, hypothyroidism, hemochromatosis, hyperparathyroidism; men and women equally affected; usually >60 years old	Inflammatory monarthritis, findings of degenerative arthritis (noninflammatory)
LYME DISEASE	History of tick bite, history of typical rash; men and women equally affected; any age	Monarticular or large-joint oligoarticular arthritis, can have CNS and cardiac findings
OSTEOARTHRITIS	Gradual onset of joint pain; prior joint trauma, onset >45 years of age; <30 minutes of morning stiffness; no systemic manifestation	Noninflammatory arthritis, crepitus, knee deformities, Heberden's nodes
TRAUMA	Joint injury, history of joint locking or giving way	Crepitus; tender over one aspect of joint; if acute, can access stability, but with development of effusion and muscle spasm exam is less reliable

Monarticular Arthritis

Septic Arthritis

Joint infection (septic arthritis) leads to rapid joint destruction, and urgent diagnosis and treatment are imperative. Any purulent joint fluid should be considered infected until proved otherwise. Among adults, septic arthritis primarily is due to gonococcal infections, which have disseminated from an asymptomatic infection of the cervix, urethra, rectum, or pharynx.

Before localizing in one or occasionally two joints, the disseminated infection sometimes causes "systemic" findings; this occurs in approximately two thirds of patients. Such findings can include myalgias, migratory arthralgias, fever, dermatitis, and tenosynovitis. The characteristic skin lesions are scattered small papules (less frequently bullae or pustules) on the extremities.

Nongonococcal septic arthritis also is acquired hematogenously, and *Staphylococcus aureus* is responsible for most of the nongonococcal infections. Among adults, these infections primarily occur in debilitated individuals, IV drug abusers, people with altered defense mechanisms, and patients with a damaged or prosthetic joint. In addition, gram-negative organisms (e.g., *Escherichia coli, Pseudomonas aeruginosa*) can be pathogens, especially among IV drug abusers.

Crystal-induced Arthritis

Crystal-induced arthritis usually is due to gout or pseudogout. Gout is an episodic, monarticular (and occasionally oligoarticular or polyarticular) arthritis. Gout results in acute (onset to peak symptoms is less than 24 hours) and exquisite joint pain, effusion, heat, and erythema.

Gout typically occurs in men older than 45 years of age (while women usually do not manifest gout until after menopause). The joint pain develops abruptly, and it can follow trauma (including prolonged walking), surgery, or no discernible precipitating event. The first metatarsophalangeal joint is involved most commonly (podagra). Arthritis resulting from gout usually involves the distal joints, as these are cooler and the uric acid in joint fluid is therefore less likely to remain in solution. If the condition goes untreated, the findings take 1 to 2 weeks to resolve.

Gout has manifestations other than arthritis. Approximately one third of patients have tophi, which are soft-tissue deposits of sodium urate. These are found in bursae (especially the olecranon and prepatellar bursae) and ear cartilage. Uric acid renal stones also eventually develop in about 10% to 20% of patients with gout.

Pseudogout is caused by calcium pyrophosphate dihydrate (CPPD) crystals. Unlike gout, the large joints are involved preferentially in CPPD disease. More than half of the episodes involve the knee. In addition, the shoulder, hip, wrist, elbow, and metacarpophalangeal (MCP) joints can be affected. Although usually less severe than gout, pseudogout can be more protracted, lasting weeks. However, it also can be identical to gout in terms of its intensity and duration. Pseudogout often is associated with osteoarthritis and cartilage calcification, and it can occur in the setting of several metabolic disorders, including hemochromatosis, hypothyroidism, and hyperparathyroidism.

Lyme Disease

Lyme disease first was recognized as a specific illness in 1976. It is caused by the tick-borne spirochete *Borrelia burgdorferi*. Its initial and most distinctive feature is a rash (erythema chronicum migrans), which is observed in 75% of patients. The rash begins as a red papule at the site of the tick bite. It then develops into an annular lesion with central clearing. During this initial phase, systemic symptoms (e.g., fever and chills) often are present.

Weeks to months after the initial infection, symptoms and signs involving other organ systems appear. A relapsing destructive monarticular or oligoarticular arthritis of the knees, shoulders, elbows, ankles, or wrists develops in half of the untreated patients. The duration of the arthritis is variable, lasting from days to weeks, and recurrences are common. Approximately 10% of patients have neurologic problems, (e.g., aseptic meningitis or cranial neuropathies) or cardiac involvement (e.g., conduction blocks or myocarditis).

Osteoarthritis

Osteoarthritis, or degenerative joint disease, is the most prevalent form of arthropathy. The incidence of this "wear-and-tear" joint destruction increases with age, and over half of those over 40-years-old are affected. This noninflammatory arthritis results in joint pain or aching, which slowly progresses. Unlike the prolonged stiffness of an inflammatory arthritis, the joint stiffness occurring after rest ("gelling") rarely lasts more than 30 minutes. The joint swelling is minimal, and effusions are infrequent (except in the knee). Deformities result from marginal bony overgrowth (osteophytes) and loss of articular cartilage. Osteophytes are exemplified by the enlarged DIP joints (Heberden's nodes) typically seen in the hands of patients with osteoarthritis.

Vignette Follow-ups

Mr. H is found to have pseudogout, established on the basis of finding CPPD crystals in wrist synovial fluid. The ESR gradually returns to normal, and a search for other causes of an elevated ESR, including evaluation of a bone marrow specimen (also done to search for the cause of his anemia and assess for myeloma), yields negative findings. He declines further treatment for his chest pain until he presents about 6 months later with worsening pain (crescendo angina). At that time, Mr. H undergoes cardiac catheterization, followed by successful four-vessel bypass.

An MRI of KJ's right knee shows severe degenerative disease of the patellofemoral joint, with lateral subluxation of the patella. There is no meniscal involvement.

Ms. H's knee synovial fluid is found to have many WBCs, and she is admitted for the treatment of presumed septic arthritis. Subsequently, S. aureus is grown from the synovial fluid; blood cultures are sterile. She is treated with parenteral

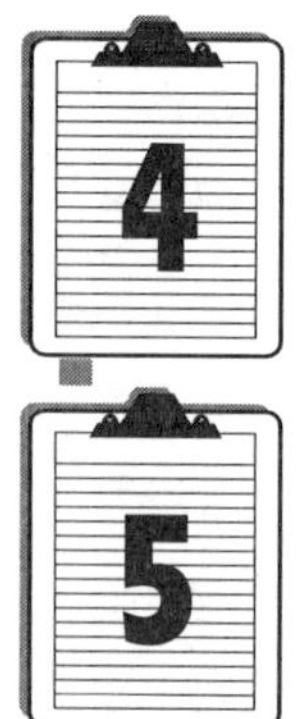

antibiotics and repeated arthrocentesis. Her hospital course is complicated by recurrent atrial arrhythmias, but she eventually does well and returns home.

FP declines arthrocentesis and is presumed to have gout. The thiazide diuretic appears to have increased her uric acid level, which is 10.5 mg/dl. Aspirin also affects uric acid levels. In low doses, it competitively reduces the renal clearance of uric acid; at high doses, it promotes clearance. Ms. P is treated with indomethacin, and her diuretic therapy is discontinued. Two years after this episode, Ms. P's uric acid level remains normal, and she has not experienced a recurrence.

Vignette 6

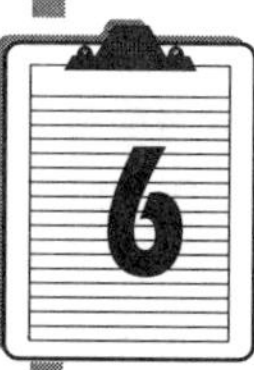

BD is a 47-year-old dentist who is concerned about his shoulder. He is just back from a 2-week vacation at a health spa, where he "worked out" daily, rather than his usual once a week. He reports a dull ache in his right shoulder, which is increased with abduction and elevation of his arm. He has had no prior shoulder complaints or joint problems, and he otherwise feels well.

Physical examination abnormalities are confined to the shoulder. His **neck** is nontender, and neck ROM is normal. On inspection, his **shoulders** appear symmetrical; there is diffuse tenderness over his right shoulder joint, without tenderness of the biceps tendons. Passive shoulder ROM is mildly uncomfortable, and active ROM induces pain with abduction from approximately 45 to 100 degrees. **Sensation** and **strength** in his right upper extremity are normal.

Vignette Objectives

1. Explain how the history and physical examination findings help diagnose the cause of shoulder pain.
2. Describe the physical examination maneuvers used to examine the knee.

Shoulder and Knee Complaints

Shoulder pain is a common problem. The articulations of the humoral head are analogous to a golf ball abutting a horizontal golf tee. The joint itself provides minimal stability, but there are complex periarticular structures that do stabilize the joint and allow motion. Conditions causing shoulder pain and their associated findings are listed in Table 10-5. The assessment for joint ROM involves forward flexion and extension, abduction and adduction, upper arm movement parallel to the floor across the chest, and rotation (elbows flexed at 90 degrees, and forearms moved parallel to the floor).

Acute and chronic knee pain also are common complaints. The physical examination is most useful when evaluating an acute knee injury, before the development of muscle spasm and joint effusion. Several maneuvers have been described as methods to identify the cause of knee pain and localize the structure causing an internal derangement of the knee (Table 10-5A). However, their reported accuracy varies widely, and over half of knee injuries result in more than one abnormality, which are more difficult to identify correctly.

Table 10-5. Shoulder pain

Condition	Etiology and findings
Referred pain from cervical spine disease and nerve root compression or brachial plexus; referred pain in this distribution due to diaphragmatic irritation or cardiac ischemia	Cervical nerve root involvement can cause dysesthesia and weakness during shoulder abduction and external rotation, and neck movement increased symptoms; shoulder is nontender, and passive ROM is not painful
Acute arthritis (e.g., due to joint infection)	Severe pain in all planes of passive and active motion; joint warm, tender, and swollen
Bicipital tendinitis (inflammation of long head of the biceps)	Anterior shoulder pain, tenderness in bicipital groove, pain with resisted shoulder flexion
Subacromion bursitis, supraspinatous tendinitis, or impingement syndrome (because these structures are contiguous, they can be associated with similar findings and sometimes are called the *painful arc syndrome*)	Most common causes of shoulder pain; dull ache, worse at night, and increased with shoulder motion; can be history of recent overuse; tender over greater tuberosity of humerus; pain occurs during abduction from 60 to 120 degrees, but shoulder strength preserved
Rotator cuff injury (partial or complete tear of the supraspinatous tendon)	Younger patients usually have a history of shoulder trauma; in patients 60 to 70-years-old chronic inflammation can cause degeneration of cuff muscles without trauma; weakness and pain noted during abduction at 90 degrees, demonstrated by strength testing or lowering the arm from the overhead position; unlikely if abduction strength is equal for the involved and noninvolved shoulder
Adhesive capsulitis (frozen shoulder) (can be idiopathic or occur among those with a predisposing condition, such as age, diabetes, and after trauma or immobilization)	Dull, aching shoulder; progressively restricted active and passive shoulder range of motion
Shoulder-hand syndrome (reflex sympathetic dystrophy)	Diffuse, constant shoulder pain; hand is edematous and diaphoretic (due to changes in autonomic regulation)

Table 10-5A. Knee pain*

Condition	History	Physical examination
Retropatellar irritation "chondromalacia"	Pain when walking, especially when descending stairs; stiffness in knees after sitting	Abnormal patella alignment and tracking; patellar crepitation when moved medially and laterally; clicking or crepitation behind patella when knee flexed and extended
Patellar tendinitis	Repeated jumping movements; pain inferior to patella	Patella tendon tenderness
Osteoarthritis	Remote history knee injury Knee aches	Genu valgum or varus; crepitation at joint line with knee flexion and extension; small joint effusion
Meniscal tear	Knee locks or catches Sudden knee pain with certain movements; may develop without injury in elderly individuals	Exam may be normal; tenderness at joint line; McMurry or Apley tests
Anterior cruciate	Knee "popped" when injured Knee swelling within 12 hours of an injury	Anterior drawer sign (90° flexion) Lachman test (10° flexion)
Medial ligament	Injury by lateral force on the knee Pain along inner aspect knee	Tender along medial joint line and ligament insertion on tibial plateau; valgus stress produces pain and ± joint laxity
Lateral ligament	Less frequent, as less vulnerable to medial force injury Pain outer aspect knee	Tender along lateral joint; varus stress produces pain and ± joint laxity

*Extraarticular causes of knee pain include prepatellar bursitis (housemaid's knee), anserine bursitis (medial aspect knee between medial collateral ligament and conjoined tendon) and infrapatellar bursitis.

Vignette Follow-up

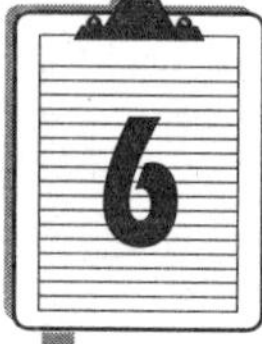

Dr. D's shoulder pain abates with rest, ROM exercises, and NSAID treatment. He reinitiates his exercise program, with gradual increases in intensity, and does not experience recurrent symptoms from presumed subacromion bursitis.

Vignette 7

LS is a 68-year-old man with a 3-week history of left "hip" pain. He is bothered most when he is lying on his left side in bed, and this often wakes him. He had tried taking acetaminophen, aspirin, and ibuprofen, without relief. He is worried that he has arthritis of the hip and needs a hip replacement, like the surgery his wife had about 4 years ago. He denies any other musculoskeletal problems. His medications include verapamil for hypertension and small doses of amitriptyline at bedtime for insomnia.

Mr. S's **blood pressure** is 128/78 mm Hg, with a **heart rate** of 79 beats/min. His **temperature** is normal. **HEENT:** normocephalic, no facial rash, and clear oropharynx. His funduscopic examination reveals mild arteriovenous crossing changes. The remainder of the physical examination findings are normal, except for the **left lower extremity.** The proximal lateral thigh is painful to palpation, directly over the trochanteric bursa. He remarks that this pain is identical to the "hip pain" he experiences at night. There is no abnormality in ROM of the left hip (flexion [neutral to 120 degrees with knee flexion], extension [neutral to 30 degrees], abduction, external and internal rotation with the leg extended [neutral to 45 degrees], and internal and external rotation while the hip and knee are flexed). A left hip radiograph reveals mild degenerative changes of the hip joint.

Vignette Objective

1. Explain how the history and physical examination can establish the cause of hip pain.

Hip Pain

The hip joint is innervated by the femoral, obturator, and sciatic nerves, and hip joint pain can be referred to the groin and the anterior and posterior aspects of the joint. Bursitis of the iliopectineal, ischiogluteal, or trochanteric bursa also can cause "hip" pain. However, the pain of bursitis usually shows point tender-

Vignette Follow-up

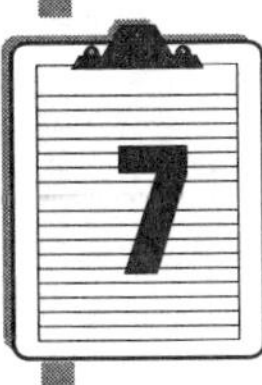

LS receives 2 ml of 1% lidocaine at the site of pain in the area of his left trochanteric bursa. This relieves his pain. Another injection of lidocaine and a glucocorticoid is administered. Four months after treatment, LS remains asymptomatic.

ness, occurring in association with the symptoms. An injection of lidocaine into the bursa can transiently eliminate symptoms and is a diagnostic test. The common causes of hip pain are given in Table 10-6.

Table 10-6. Hip pain

Condition	History	Physical examination
Osteoarthritis	Chronic groin pain that can radiate to the buttock, worsens with exercise and weight bearing	Pain and decreased hip range of motion
Trochanteric bursitis	Lateral thigh pain; worsens when lying on that side, with direct pressure, and during thigh movement	Point tenderness over trochanteric bursa, local lidocaine injection relieves pain
Avascular necrosis of femoral head	Groin pain at rest and with joint movement, underlying predisposing condition (e.g., diabetes, alcoholism, or glucocorticoid use)	Pain with hip motion; infrequently, motion does not cause pain
Femoral neck fracture	History of osteoporosis or trauma	Shortened affected leg, foot held in external rotation, severe pain with hip motion
Osteitis pubis	Groin pain after pregnancy or exertion (especially after sprinting)	Pain with hip abduction, tenderness at symphysis pubis
Referred pain (L-3–L-4 nerve root irritation radiates to anterior thigh	Musculoskeletal back pain; abates when supine	Passive hip motion not painful; findings of an L-3–L-4 radiculopathy

Vignette 8

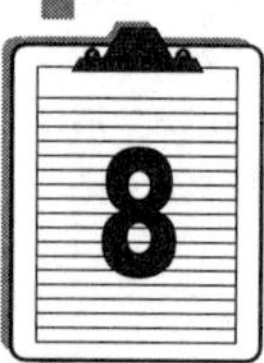

DS is a 42-year-old man who calls the physician's office complaining of back pain. Mr. S is in good general health and has no active medical problems. He relates that he was reaching into the backseat of his car to get a package and felt a sharp pain in his low back and left buttock. He took aspirin and rested, but the pain has persisted and made it difficult for him to walk and drive. The discomfort is relieved somewhat by the aspirin; he has also tried a heating pad, without much relief. He reports no lower extremity dysesthesias or weakness. He asks whether he needs an x-ray.

Vignette Objectives

1. What features of musculoskeletal low back pain indicate the need for radiographs at the initial evaluation?
2. What are characteristics of nerve root irritation at the L-3, L-4, and S-1 levels?
3. What problems other than musculoskeletal ones cause low back pain?

Low Back Pain

Initial Evaluation

Most people have at least one episode of low back pain during their lifetime. More than 80% of these episodes are due to musculoskeletal factors involving the ligaments, paraspinal muscles, disks, facets, or nerve roots. Most episodes of back pain are self-limited. Overall, 60% of patients experience improvement after 1 week and 90% of cases resolve after 2 months.

When assessing patients with low back pain, the challenge is to identify the minority who require a more extensive evaluation. Any of the features listed in Table 10-7 should prompt the early performance of radiologic studies. Limiting these procedures to patients with these findings reduces the inconvenience to the patient as well as the risk and expense of additional diagnostic studies.

Besides malignant, infectious, and musculoskeletal back problems, lumbar pain also can be referred from an intraabdominal process. For example, inflammation of retroperitoneal structures, such as occurs in the settings of pancreatitis, pyelonephritis, and retroperitoneal bleeding, can cause back pain. When this occurs, back tenderness and muscle spasm are absent and the abdominal examination often yields abnormal findings. An aortic dissection is a life-threatening emergency that can also cause back pain. (See Chapter 7, p. 205, for assessment of the abdominal aorta.)

Table 10-7. Indications for radiologic investigation of low back pain

History or physical examination findings	Reason for investigation
Age >50 years or unexplained weight loss	Greater likelihood of malignancy
History of recent trauma, osteoporosis	Assess for fracture
Abnormal neurologic findings;* sensory findings alone are not an indication for radiographs	Objective signs of weakness or reflex asymmetry increase the likelihood of bone or joint abnormalities
History of malignancy	Greater likelihood of bony metastasis and cord compression
Corticosteroid use	Greater potential for osteoporosis and infections
Intravenous drug use, temperature >100°F (37.8°C) (fever has low sensitivity for spinal infection), site of ongoing infection (e.g., indwelling urinary catheter)	Greater potential for epidural abscess and osteomyelitis
Symptoms not reduced over 4 weeks	Greater likelihood of nonmusculoskeletal cause
Seeking compensation	Radiographic documentation often needed for evaluation of injury
Reduced range of motion (Schober's test)	Although test not specific, can indicate ankylosing spondylitis, which usually occurs among young men (<40 years old), with symptoms lasting several months

*Radiographic studies are not specific; up to 30% of normal people (without back pain) will show evidence of disc herniation on CT or MRI studies.

Nerve-Root Syndromes

Mechanical low back pain can result in nerve-root irritation, causing symptoms of a radiculopathy. *Sciatica* is the term for the sharp, burning, or aching pain that characteristically radiates from the area of the sciatic notch down the posterior or lateral leg. It can be due to a radiculopathy or local irritation of the sciatic nerve. The most common site for lumbar disk disease is at L-5–S-1, with S-1 nerve root impingement (Table 10-8). An expeditious way to assess for neurologic deficits is to test the patellar (L-4 nerve root) and ankle (S-1 nerve root) reflexes and to ask the patient to walk on the toes (S-1 nerve root) and heels (L-5 nerve root).

Spinal Stenosis

Spinal stenosis results from spinal canal narrowing, usually stemming from a combination of disk protrusion and the formation of osteophytes. The symptoms are insidious in onset and progress slowly. Along with pain, patients can experience weakness and numbness of both buttocks or thighs. It is given the label *pseudoclaudication* because, like peripheral vascular disease, it causes leg pain when walking. It is relieved within a few minutes by rest, especially if accompanied by flexion of the lumbar spine, or by sitting. If relief occurs when the patient is seated, this tends to differentiate it from nerve root impingement syndromes. Sitting causes pain to be increased in the latter condition, as a result of the attendant increase in the disk pressure.

Cauda Equina Compression

Cauda equina compression is a rare complication of a midline disk herniation or tumor. The disorder can cause incontinence, difficulty walking, and bilateral saddle anesthesia (affecting the perineal area, buttocks, and upper posterior thighs). Ninety percent of those affected also have urinary retention, which is a highly sensitive sign for this disorder. The finding of a normal postvoid residual is strong evidence against the diagnosis of cauda equina compression.

Table 10-8. Lumbar radicular syndromes

Disk level	L-3–L-4	L-4–L-5	L-5–S-1
Nerve root involved	L-4	L-5	S-1
Pain distribution (all may affect low back and buttocks)	Posterolateral leg	Lateral leg and thigh	Posterior leg
Motor defect	Quadriceps (knee extension)	Foot dorsiflexion	Foot plantar flexion
Sensory deficit	Knee and distal anterior thigh	Lateral calf and between first and second toes	Lateral foot and posterolateral calf
Reflex depressed	Patellar	None	Achilles tendon

Vignette Follow-up

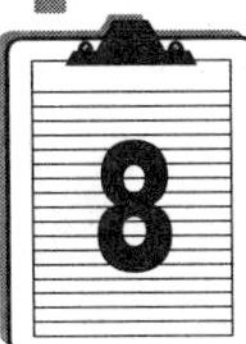

DS has no historical features to suggest problems other than musculoskeletal strain. He is advised to apply ice packs to the lower back, take an NSAID, and anticipate improvement over several days. He is shown general conditioning exercises and specific back exercises to perform once his acute problem has resolved.

Vignettes 9 and 10

TA is a 16-year-old woman being seen for "acne." She has tried several over-the-counter medications, without much benefit. Her general health is good, and she reports no other medical problems. She appears healthy, and her **general physical examination** findings are normal. Examination of her **skin** reveals pustules over her cheeks and chin. In addition, several large (greater than 6 mm in diameter) nevi are noted during examination of the remainder of her skin. She mentions that two of her cousins had "skin cancers."

LB is a 40-year-old woman who is concerned about persistent "athlete's foot." She has tried powders, without much help. She exercises regularly, and she is concerned that her toenails will become involved. She also has a small mole on the middle toe of her left foot. Although it has been present for years, it looks larger than she remembers. She has no family history of skin cancer. Physical examination of the **foot** reveals mild hyperkeratosis and scaling of the sole. The nails are normal, without thickening. A darkly pigmented, 0.8-cm raised lesion with irregular borders is seen on the plantar surface of her middle toe.

Vignette Objectives

1. List terms used to describe skin lesions on the basis of their morphology, location, and configuration.
2. List the features of a pigmented lesion that prompt concern.

Describing Skin Findings

It is important to be able to describe skin findings accurately. The description should include the lesions' distribution and morphology (Table 10 9). Skin lesions can be *generalized,* or they can be *localized* in particular areas, including the acral (distal extremities), facial, truncal, perioral, and periorbital areas, as well as the flexor or extensor surfaces of joints or extremities. Further, lesions

Table 10-9. Describing skin findings

Lesion	Findings
Atrophy	Depressed area produced by thinning of the epidermis, dermis, or panniculus
Bulla	Vesicle >5 mm in diameter
Excoriation	Linear erosion or ulcer caused by scratching
Lichenification	Epidermal hypertrophy with thickening of the skin and accentuated skin markings
Macule	Flat (nonpalpable), circumscribed, ≤1 cm in diameter area with altered coloration; if >1 cm in diameter, it is a macular patch; caused by melanin or vascular changes (e.g., a cafe au lait spot, freckle, vitiligo, petechia, and ecchymosis [purpura])
Nodule	Raised solid lesion >5 mm in diameter; unlike plaque; it can involve deeper structures
Papule	Elevated lesion <5 mm in diameter; caused by vascular or melanocytic proliferation, dermal infiltration, or deposition of a solid substance (e.g., a nevus [mole], cherry angioma, eruptive xanthomas, and vasculitis [palpable purpura])
Plaque	Flat-topped, elevated lesion that is >5 mm in diameter (e.g., psoriasis, mycosis fungoides, and lichen planus)
Pustule	Papule containing a purulent exudate
Ulcer	Loss of deeper layers of skin (epidermis and dermis); if only the epidermis is involved, the lesion is an erosion and heals without scarring
Vesicle	A fluid-filled lesion; <5 mm in diameter; can be beneath the stratum corneum, intraepidermal, or subepidermal (e.g., herpes zoster and herpes simplex)
Wheal (hives)	Erythematous, slightly raised lesion, resulting from vasodilation and edema

can assume a *linear* (arranged in a line), *annular* (forming incomplete circles), or *herpetiform* (grouped vesicles) configuration.

Dysplastic Nevi

Giant congenital and dysplastic nevi are associated with an increased risk of melanoma. Dysplastic nevi usually are larger (5 to 10 mm in diameter) than common nevi. Patients can have one or more than a hundred of these lesions. In general, new nevi are rare after 30 years of age, but dysplastic nevi can continue to appear after this time. The color of the lesion is characteristically variegated (shades of brown, tan, and pink), and lesions generally are macular or have a central papule with a light macular periphery ("fried-egg" appearance). The surface can have a cobble-stone appearance, and the borders often are indistinct. Patients who have dysplastic nevi or a family history of melanoma should have regular total skin examinations to ensure early detection of melanoma.

Skin Malignancies

Pigmented skin lesions are listed in Table 10-10. Melanomas begin in the dermis (or retina) and often their coloring is varied with areas appearing black, red, white, or blue. They appear asymmetrical and have irregular borders. This malignancy is distinguished by its ability to metastasize throughout the

Table 10-10. Pigmented skin lesions

Lesion	Appearance
Blue nevus	Blue-gray, slightly raised papule; usually single and diameter <1 cm
Compound nevus	Well demarcated, round to oval; skin color to dark brown; papillomatous to smooth dome shaped
Hemangioma	Purple nodule, can partially blanch on compression
Junctional nevus	Sharp bordered, flat to slightly raised, finely stippled
Lentigo	Macular, sharp bordered; medium to dark brown; solar variant occurs on the dorsa of hands and face
Pigmented dermatofibroma	Firm, lateral pressure causes dimpling of the skin
Seborrheic keratosis	Waxy; looks "stuck onto the skin"; flesh color to dark brown; more common among elderly and those with certain illnesses, such as HIV disease and Parkinson's disease

body, and metastatic lesions can appear years after resection of the original lesion.

Basal cell carcinomas typically have the appearance of a nonhealing ulcer and often arise in an area of sun-damaged skin. The lesions can have a pearly appearance, with rolled edges and a central depression or ulceration ("rodent ulcer"). They are rare among African-American and Asian people. Squamous cell carcinomas can look like basal cell carcinomas but more often are flat plaques, which can ulcerate.

Acne Vulgaris

Acne is categorized as comedomal (blackheads and whiteheads), papulopustular (less than 15 pustules, occurring in conjunction with comedomes), and conglobata (nodules and cystic changes, which can heal with severe scarring). The onset of acne typically occurs in adolescence, because, during puberty, sebum production increases. This is associated with pilosebaceous plugging, rupture, and inflammation from skin bacteria. The incidence peaks at 18 years of age, and more than 85% of teens are affected. The development of acne is influenced by several factors, such as genetics and exposure to certain chemicals, cosmetics, and drugs (glucocorticoids, progesterone, iodides, and phenytoin).

Vignette Follow-ups

TA's acne abates with changes in hygiene; she changes from using oil-based to using water-based cosmetics and washes her face with a mild soap twice a day, avoiding "scrubbing" her face. None of her skin lesions require biopsy, and she is taught skin self-surveillance and informed of the need for follow-up. She has done well in the 4 years since her original visit.

LB does not have a fungal infection. Dermatophytes infections (fungal skin infections) involve the stratum corneum; an example is "ringworm," which characteristically has erythematous borders with a pale center. Tinea pedis (ath-

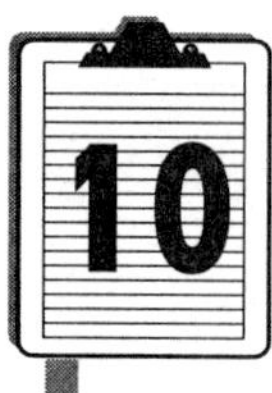

lete's foot) usually involves the toe webs. Her hyperkeratosis is due to dry skin (xeroderma). However, she is found to have a melanoma of her toe. She is treated with isolated lower extremity chemotherapy and surgical removal of her toe. She is undergoing periodic monitoring.

Vignettes 11 and 12

Carbuncle: furuncles connected by subcutaneous tracts.

Erysipelas: superficial skin infection characterized by tenderness, edema, and sharply demarcated, advancing erythematous borders.

Exanthem: skin rash; when it also involves mucous membranes, it is called an *enanthem.*

Furuncle: "boil"; superficial skin abscess, usually beginning in a hair follicle.

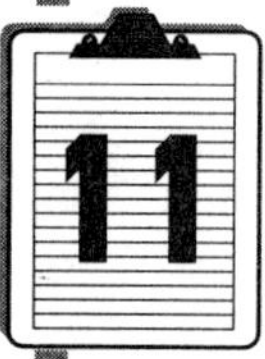

TE is a 24-year-old man complaining of a "sore left arm," fever, and chills. The patient relates that he is an IV drug user and that, several days earlier, he attempted to "shoot" what he thinks was a combination of heroin and cocaine into a vein in his antecubital fossa. He missed the vein and infiltrated his skin with the solution. By the next day, his arm had become sore, warm, and swollen. Past medical history is remarkable for an HIV test that was negative 6 weeks previously.

Physical examination reveals his **blood pressure** is 135/80 mm Hg, his **heart rate** is 88 beats/min, and his oral **temperature** is 100.6°F (38.1°C). **HEENT:** no scleral icterus, normal oropharyngeal mucosa. **Chest:** clear to auscultation. **Cardiac:** no JVD; nondisplaced PMI; normal S_1 and S_1; no murmur. **Abdomen:** nontender; liver reveals 10-cm span to percussion; no splenomegaly or mass. **Genitourinary** exam: normal circumcised male. **Extremities:** hyperpigmented skin over superficial arm veins ("tracks"). Mr. E has a fluctuant erythematous area on the lateral side of his left arm, extending from the deltoid muscle to the elbow. Cutaneous sensation is intact. No crepitance is appreciated; distal neurovascular function (strength, reflexes, sensation) is preserved.

KR is a 51-year-old man whose ongoing problems include hypertension and hypercholesterolemia, treated with diltiazem and niacin. Over the past few days, a "runny nose" has developed, and he experienced facial pain and fever the previous evening. He called a local emergency room and was told that his symptoms were likely due to a sinus infection and that he should see his physician in the morning. Later that evening, his face began to turn red and swell, his fever rose to 102°F (38.8°C), and he experienced chills. He has not had cough, sore throat, sputum production, stiff neck, or gastrointestinal symptoms.

When seen the next day, the physical examination reveals a distressed man with an erythematous face who is complaining of burning facial pain. His **blood pressure** is 140/86 mm Hg, with a **heart rate** of 92 beats/min and an oral

temperature of 38.5°C. **Inspection** reveals a masklike distribution of erythema, with sharp borders. The involved skin is tender and edematous, and no localized lesions are present. **Eyes:** conjunctiva clear; pupils are equal, round, and reactive to light, and fundoscopic exam findings are normal. **Ear** exam shows clear external canals, with normal tympanic membranes. **Mouth:** no circumoral pallor and no "raspberry" or "strawberry" tongue. There is a posterior pharyngeal exudate. His **neck** is supple, and there is no cervical adenopathy orthyroid enlargement. His **skin** does not show any other rash, petechiae, vesicles, or papules. **Neurologic** findings are normal. Specifically, his **mental status** is normal and **cranial nerves** II through XII are intact. The remainder of his physical examination findings are normal.

Vignette Objective

1. What are the symptoms and signs of different types of skin infections?

Skin Infections

The skin may be "infected" with its own saprophytic flora, which consists of gram-negative coryneform bacteria, coagulase-negative staphylococci, and other gram-positive cocci. Skin infection, or pyoderma, can assume several forms. Figure 10-1 provides an algorithm to differentiate among skin infections.

Impetigo

Impetigo is a highly contagious bacterial infection of the superficial dermis, which primarily affects children. Lesions often begin on the face and spread to other areas of the body through autoinoculation of the infection. It is caused by group A beta-hemolytic streptococci, *S. aureus,* or both. Streptococcal infections can be vesicular initially, rapidly progressing to yellow-crusted lesions. If the infection is caused by *S. aureus,* the vesicular lesions can evolve to form large bullae. Streptococcal infections can lead to poststreptococcal glomerulonephritis, which underscores the need for treatment. Occasionally, impetigo in an apparently healthy adult can be an initial manifestation of HIV disease.

Cellulitis

Cellulitis is a generic term and refers to a pyoderma involving structures beneath the superficial dermis. Symptoms and signs of cellulitis are pain, redness, swelling, and warmth. Less frequently, lymphangitis, local lymphadenitis, and fluctuance are present. Erysipelas is a unique skin infection that is usually caused by *Streptococcus pyogenes;* it is characterized by a shiny, swollen bright erythema with sharply demarcated margins.

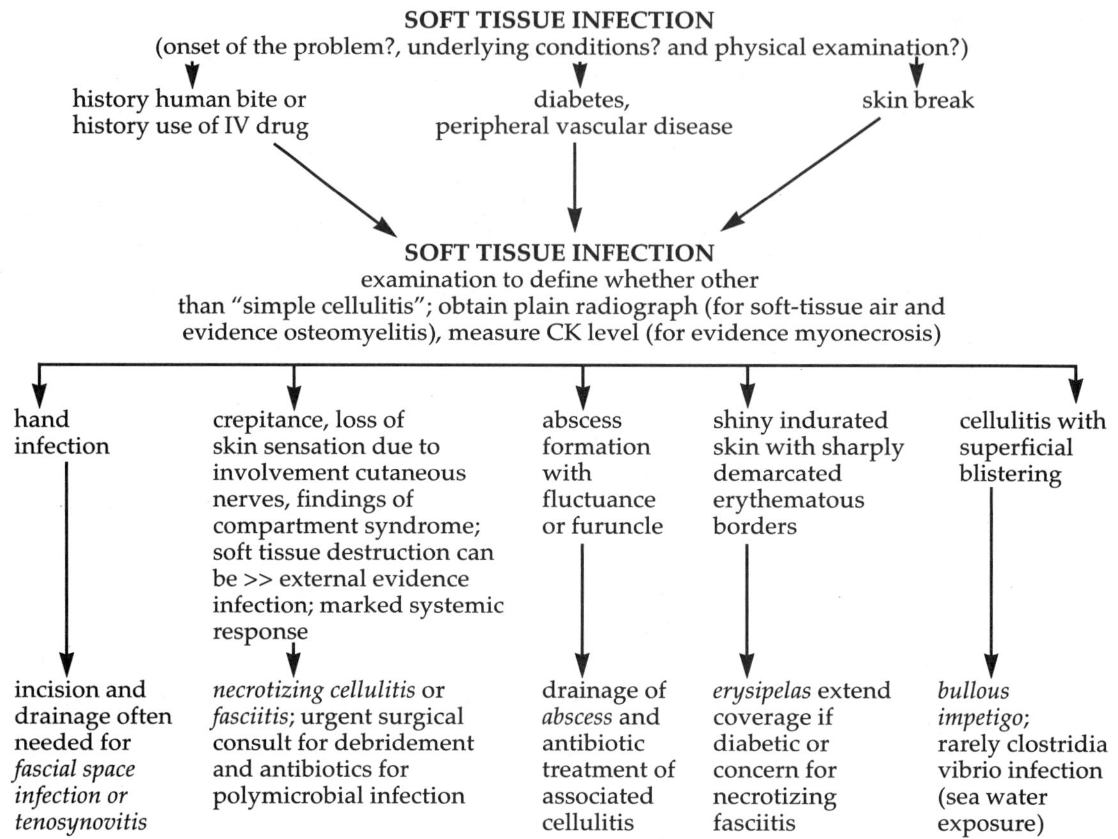

Fig. 10-1. Soft-tissue infections can be differentiated on the basis of patient characteristics and the way in which infecting organisms were introduced. Management is determined by the site of infection, whether an abscess is present, and whether deeper structures are involved.

Abscess

A skin abscess is a subcutaneous collection of pus that often begins with a small skin break or superficial skin infection caused by *Staphylococcus* organisms. The infection results in the formation of a furuncle, or "boil," with a surrounding cellulitis. A cluster of furuncles that are connected subcutaneously are referred to as *carbuncles.* Other organisms besides staphylococci can cause abscesses, and infection with certain organisms is more likely in different settings (Table 10-11). Although antibiotic therapy can control the cellulitis associated with an abscess, the primary treatment of a skin abscess is drainage.

Abscesses in intravenous drug abusers have multiple causes; they can result from (1) use of a needle or drug that is contaminated with bacteria, (2) the inoculation of skin organisms during drug use, and (3) tissue necrosis caused by the drug itself, which leads to the formation of a sterile (without an infectious pathogen) abscess. The last is more likely in those using sympathomimetic

Table 10-11. Organisms causing cellulitis

Condition	Organism(s)	Patient group and predisposing conditions
Impetigo, cellulitis, furuncle (usually staphylococci), erysipelas (usually streptococci)	*S. aureus*, streptococci; can be due to gram-negative bacteria, especially among IV drug abusers	Healthy adults can suffer skin infections; cellulitis and abscesses are common among IV drug abusers
Animal bite infection	*Pasteurella multocida* (gram-negative rod), *S. aureus, Eikenella corrodens, Bacteroides sp., Bartonella henselae* (organism causing cat scratch fever); rabies is a major concern from bites of raccoons, skunks, or bats	Infection risk is increased in puncture wounds due to the difficulty in cleaning these injuries (80% of cat bites become infected versus 15% of dog bites)
Foot infection	*Pseudomonas, Klebsiella, Enterobacter,* anaerobic bacteria	Especially result from puncture wounds; gram-negative organisms can be normal flora of toe webs; if ischemia (e.g., diabetes or peripheral vascular disease), polymicrobial infections, including anaerobic organisms, also can occur
External otitis	*Pseudomonas* (resulting from the organism's colonization of the warm, moist ear canal)	Immunocompromised people (e.g., patients with poorly controlled diabetes mellitus) can suffer rapidly advancing external ear cellulitis (malignant otitis externa)
Erysipeloid	*Erysipelothrix rhusiopathiae* (gram-positive rod)	Handlers of fish, shellfish, or poultry
Furuncles in hot tub users	*Pseudomonas aeruginosa*	Hot tub users with painful and pruritic folliculitis
Tularemia	*Francisella tularensis*	Contact with squirrels, rabbits, and certain ticks; development of ulcer and tender regional lymphadenopathy (ulceroglandular tularemia)
Gas gangrene	*Clostridium perfringens*	Often associated trauma; pain and signs of sepsis out of proportion to the evidence of a local infection; antibiotics and debridement imperative
Necrotizing fasciitis (also known as *Fournier's gangrene* and *Meleney's synergistic gangrene*)	Polymicrobial infection involving streptococci, *S. aureus*, enterococci, and anaerobes	Associated with diabetes and wound infections; rapidly advancing infection; involves structures other than skin and can cause myonecrosis and compartment compression; diagnosis established by demonstrating deep structure involvement; surgical debridement and antibiotics required

agents (e.g., cocaine and amphetamines), which can produce vasoconstriction and tissue necrosis at the injection site.

Necrotizing Soft-Tissue Infections

Necrotizing soft-tissue infections are caused by mixed anaerobic and aerobic organisms and classically appear as an area of tenderness, with blisters, dermal gangrene, edema, and crepitus. Unlike most cellulitis, necrotizing infections can cause a loss of skin sensation as the result of ischemia of cutaneous nerves. The associated myoneurosis and edema can result in compartment syndromes, with an accompanying loss of neuromuscular function. A radiograph of the involved area may demonstrate the presence of soft-tissue gas, and muscle necrosis can result in an elevation of the serum creatine kinase level.

Clostridial infections can cause anaerobic myonecrosis, or gas gangrene. These life-threatening infections usually arise after significant trauma, such as a puncture wound or open fracture. Affected patients experience the sudden onset of severe pain, with mild local swelling and a thin nonpurulent exudate. The amount of local inflammation can appear disproportionately low, given the patient's severe pain and the presence of systemic findings of sepsis. As with necrotizing fasciitis, these infected areas must be promptly debrided and the patients must be given antibiotic treatment.

Toxic Shock Syndrome

Toxic shock syndrome results in a diffuse red rash that is produced by a streptococcal toxin. Most cases are associated with infections due to tampon use, nasal packing, or skin abscesses. Patients with this disorder often have a prodrome of fevers, chills, nausea, headache, and myalgias, after which a rash develops that looks like a sunburn and that can involve the palms and soles. The associated generalized vasodilatation and increased capillary permeability can cause marked hypotension. Abnormal laboratory results can include hyponatremia, hypocalcemia, and thrombocytopenia.

Other diagnoses to consider in a patient with fever, rash, and hypotension are meningococcal infection, Rocky Mountain spotted fever, leptospirosis, and the Stevens-Johnson syndrome (Table 10-12). A diffuse erythematous rash is also produced by the erythrotoxin of the group A beta-hemolytic streptococci causing scarlet fever. However, the rash of scarlet fever typically spares the palms and soles, is preceded by pharyngitis, causes a "strawberry tongue" (white coating with erythematous papillae), and is not associated with hypotension or electrolyte disorders.

Other toxin-mediated skin lesions, such as toxic epidermal necrolysis (TEN), are caused by a toxin produced by *S. aureus.* This disorder (also called the *scalded skin syndrome*) most often affects infants and young children, although it can occur in adults. The erythematous rash begins around the mouth and spreads over the extremities and trunk. Bullae can form, and the skin can become denuded and appear "scalded." One sign of scalded skin syndrome is

Table 10-12. Fever, diffuse rash, and hypotension

Disorder	Findings
Toxic shock syndrome	Staphylococcal toxin; usually due to infection of tampon, nasal packing, or wound; fever, headache, myalgias; erythema extends to palms and soles
Rocky Mountain spotted fever	Rickettsial infection (*Rickettsia rickettsii*) acquired from tick bite; fever, headache, myalgias; macular rash involves wrists and ankles
Leptospirosis	Exposure to contaminated water; dogs are urban reservoir of infection; can be mild "viral" illness or high fever, myalgias, meningeal symptoms, nonexudative conjunctivitis, and rash (maculopapular to purpuric) of the trunk
Stevens-Johnson syndrome	Severe blistering form of erythema multiforme; results from drug reactions and certain infections; annular target-like lesions that begin on distal extremities and can involve palms, soles, and mucous membranes; can have renal manifestations
Meningococcemia	Infection (sepsis or meningitis) with *Neisseria meningitidis;* can be local epidemic; fever, hypotension, altered mental status; petechiae can progress to purpura

Nikolsky's sign, in which normal-appearing skin is denuded when friction is applied. TEN also can be a reaction to drugs, which can be differentiated from *Staphylococcus*-mediated disease on the basis of skin biopsy findings.

Certain streptococci produce toxins that spread rapidly and cause tissue destruction; these organisms are sometimes referred to as *flesh-eating bacteria.* Patients with these skin infections can present with severe local pain and systemic symptoms consisting of chills, fever, headache, nausea, and vomiting.

Vignette Follow-ups

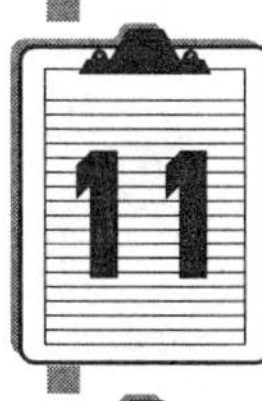

TE undergoes incision and drainage, which leaves a large cavity that requires five bottles of iodoform gauze packing. Blood cultures are sterile, and he is discharged on oral antibiotics and continued wound care.

KR undergoes sinus CT scanning that reveals frontal and maxillary sinusitis. A diagnosis of erysipelas is made, and he is treated with facial ice packs, 1% hydrocortisone lotion applied to his face, and broad-spectrum intravenous antibiotics, with both antistreptococcal and antistaphylococcal activity. Blood cultures are sterile, and his facial erythema and pain slowly resolved as he completed ten days of oral antibiotics for cellulitis and sinusitis. Because of flushing that occurs in association with niacin therapy, this drug is discontinued until the antibacterial therapy is complete.

Vignettes 13, 14, and 15

Janeway lesions and **Osler's nodes:** both are tender, erythematous, small (a few millimeters to 1.5 cm in diameter) cutaneous nodules that occur in association with bacterial endocarditis. Classically, Janeway lesions are nontender and appear on the fingertips, whereas Osler's nodes are tender and form in the finger pads. Additional findings characteristic of bacterial endocarditis include Roth's spots of the fundi, splinter hemorrhages, (dark red streaks under the nails), and petechiae (especially of the conjunctivae and palate).

Raynaud's phenomenon: sequential pallor, pain, cyanosis, and erythema of the distal extremities; caused by arterial vasospasm and often induced by exposure to cold or vibration.

MH is a 38-year-old woman with "joint pains." She was well until approximately 5 months ago, when she noted "shooting pains" in her left shoulder that worsened with activity. Her problem was diagnosed as bursitis and treated with salicylates. About 1 month later, her pain increased and spread to involve both shoulders. She also noted pain and swelling in the small joints of her hands and the metatarsal area of both feet. Although she has been able to do housework and care for her children, the joint pain has prevented her from pursuing other activities. With the exception of these joint complaints, the review of systems does not reveal other problems.

Physical examination reveals a well-nourished woman who moves stiffly and appears to be in mild to moderate discomfort. Her **blood pressure** is 134/80 mm Hg, and her **heart rate** is 76 beats/min. Her **temperature** is normal. **HEENT:** no rash, alopecia, or oral ulceration; thyroid gland is normal to palpation. Funduscopic findings are normal. **Chest:** clear to auscultation. **Cardiac:** normal S_1, physiologically split S_2; no murmurs, gallops, or rubs. **Abdomen:** soft without organomegaly or masses. **Pelvic** exam reveals normal mucosa, and bimanual examination findings are normal. Stool is occult-blood negative. **Extremities:** no edema. **Joint** exam shows her shoulders are painful in all planes during active and passive motion. There is mild swelling of the first through the third MCP joints and the PIP joints of both hands. There is slight swelling and warmth of her right ankle, and her metatarsals are diffusely tender and swollen.

KS is a 45-year-old woman who presents with a 4-month history of painful swelling of her right elbow and both ankles. Her joint complaints began 3 1/2 months ago, when she was seen in clinic for elbow pain. The symptom was attributed to mild trauma, and she was advised to take NSAIDs, as needed. Over the next 3 months, bilateral ankle pain and swelling developed, as well as a painful but not swollen right wrist. She also noted anorexia, weight loss, chills, and sweats. When seen last week, laboratory studies showed a hematocrit of 27% and an ESR of 89 mm/hr. At that time, two blood cultures were drawn, which are now growing *Streptococcus viridans.*

Ms. S had "rheumatic fever" at 6 and 8 years of age. These illnesses lasted approximately 2 weeks and consisted of fever and joint swelling, without rash or chorea. Six years ago, she was hospitalized with atrial fibrillation, requiring electrocardioversion. (Records of that admission are not available.) Since that time, she has been taking digoxin, quinidine, and propranolol. She has been found to be in sinus rhythm at subsequent examinations and is not anticoagulated. Of note is that before her current symptoms arose, Ms. K underwent dental cleaning with scaling, without antibiotic prophylaxis.

Physical examination reveals a well-nourished woman who is cooperative and in no distress. Her **blood pressure** is 130/60 mm Hg; her **heart rate** is 72 beats/min and regular, and she has a **temperature** of 37.0°C orally. **HEENT:** Her pupils are equal, round, and reactive to light; extraocular movements are full; fundi are normal, and no Roth's spots are present. Her neck is supple, without thyromegaly. **Cardiac:** no JVD when sitting at 30 degrees. PMI is in the left fifth intercostal space 2 cm lateral to the midclavicular line; S_1 and S_2 are normal, and she has a grade 3/6 blowing, holosystolic murmur, loudest at the lower left sternal border and radiating to the apex and axilla; no diastolic murmur, S_3, or S_4 are appreciated. **Chest:** clear to auscultation. **Abdomen:** soft, without organomegaly or masses. There is tympany in Traube's space with inspiration (indicating that splenomegaly is not present). **Pelvic** examination findings are normal, and stool is occult-blood negative. **Extremities:** no cyanosis, clubbing, or edema. No Osler's nodes, Janeway lesions, or splinter hemorrhages are present. Joints show no edema, heat, or swelling. **Neurologic** findings are normal. An echocardiogram shows prolapse of the posterior mitral valve leaflet, with thickening of the anterior leaflet and mild left atrial dilatation. Vegetations are not seen.

FN is a 24-year-old man who works in the clinical laboratory. He is in the clinic because of persistent low back pain. He describes a dull low-grade ache and stiffness in his lumbar area; his pain recently increased considerably after he worked in his parents' garden. He denies pain radiation to his legs, and no weakness or sensation changes in his legs are reported. His pain eases when he is flat in bed or standing and increases when he is bending or sitting. He has been taking approximately six aspirins each day for his back stiffness. He also has experienced swelling of his knees over the past few years, which "comes and goes." There is no history of eye complaints, skin rashes, penile lesions, or GI symptoms. He has no family history of arthritis or chronic back pain. His only ongoing medical problem is a long-standing seizure disorder, which is well-controlled with phenytoin.

Physical examination reveals a well-developed, thin man who is standing in the examination room. He does not want to sit in the chair or on the exam table because of his back pain. He stands erect with mild flexion of the dorsal (thoracic) spine. His **blood pressure** is 126/80 mm Hg, with a **heart rate** of 76 beats/min. **HEENT:** normal findings, except for mild gingival hyperplasia. **Chest:** clear to auscultation, but decreased expansion of ribs during inspiration. **Cardiac:** JVP is estimated to be 5 cm H_2O; S_1 and S_2 are normal; no murmur or gallop is heard. **Abdomen:** scaphoid without organomegaly or mass. **Genitourinary** exam: normal. **Joint** exam reveals his back is tender along the lumbar spine, with tenderness also at the sacroiliac joint line. Schober's test is abnormal and reveals only 6 cm of lumbar spine extension. Cervical spine motion is restricted, with inability to extend beyond 180 degrees. Both knees are mildly tender, without erythema, warmth, or effusion.

Vignette Objectives

1. What conditions cause polyarthritis, and what findings help establish the cause?
2. What are the criteria used for establishing the diagnosis of rheumatic fever?

Polyarthritis

Polyarticular arthritis is caused by a broad spectrum of diseases, and there are numerous features that aid in differentiating the causes of oligoarthritis and polyarthritis. These include (1) the pattern of onset, (2) progression, (3) the joints involved, and (4) associated nonarticular manifestations. The causes and common clinical presentation of several types of polyarthritis are summarized in Table 10-13.

Rheumatoid Arthritis

Rheumatoid arthritis affects 1% of adults. It can occur at any age, but onset typically occurs between the ages of 20 to 35 years. Women are affected more than men, and onset can be abrupt or insidious. The disease usually presents with the symmetrical involvement of large and small joints. Although the hands are commonly involved, the DIP joints and thoracic and lumbar regions of the spine usually are spared. Other organ systems can be affected in patients with

Table 10-13. Polyarticular arthritis

Etiology	Findings
Acute viral syndrome (hepatitis B, parvovirus B19)	Diffuse, often symmetrical polyarthralgias; fever and other manifestations of viral illness; usually little evidence of arthritis; resolution in days to weeks
Gonococcal infection (usually one or two joints involved)	Exposure to STDs; prodrome of myalgias, arthralgias, fever, and dermatitis; true synovitis present in only a few joints; generally, only one or two joints involved
Rheumatoid arthritis	Progressive inflammatory, symmetrical polyarthritis; involvement of metacarpophalangeal joints, wrists, knees, ankles, and feet; subcutaneous nodules; see diagnostic criteria in Table 10-14
Acute rheumatic fever	Migratory arthritis, with lower extremity joint involvement most common; new murmur or pericardial rub; typical rash; prior streptococcal infection; see diagnostic criteria in Table 10-16
Spondyloarthropathies (ankylosing spondylitis, Reiter's syndrome, psoriatic arthritis)	Low back pain; oligoarticular in large joints; skin findings; family history; Reiter's syndrome may have preceding STD or diarrheal illness; see diagnostic features in Table 10-15
Systemic lupus erythematosus	Hands and large joints; other features of SLE, which can involve any organ system (see Table 10-17)

rheumatoid arthritis. Manifestations can include pulmonary parenchymal changes, pleural effusions, rheumatoid nodules, splenomegaly, leukopenia, anemia, and vasculitis (Table 10-14).

Spondyloarthropathies

The spondyloarthropathies include ankylosing spondylitis, Reiter's sydrome, and the arthritis associated with psoriasis and inflammatory bowel disease. Each disorder can cause sarcoliitis, arthritis, and enthesitis (inflammation where ligaments insert on the bone). Although ankylosing spondylitis and psoriatic arthritis often involve joints symmetrically, Reiter's syndrome can exhibit an asymmetrical pattern. The features of the two most common disorders, ankylosing spondylitis and Reiter's syndrome, are compared in Table 10-15.

As its name implies, ankylosing spondylitis causes spinal fusion. It is ten times more common in young men than in women. It usually begins with prolonged back pain, leading to loss of lumbar lordosis and spinal flexibility. The hips, shoulders, and knee joints also can be involved. Extraarticular disease is uncommon. The aortic root is involved in approximately 5% of patients, and this can lead to aortic regurgitation or heart block. The eye (iritis) and lung (apical fibrosis) also can be affected.

Reiter's syndrome, like ankylosing spondylitis, is primarily an illness of young men, and often develops after gastrointestinal tract infections. It classically presents as a triad of arthritis of distal joints, urethritis, and conjunctivitis. The characteristic rash is hyperkeratosis of the palms and soles, called *keratoderma blennorrhagicum.*

Psoriasis is associated with several types of joint complaints, and the arthritis usually occurs in those with active skin disease. The skin manifestations of psoriasis are plaques that begin in the scalp, elbows, knees, and sites of skin trauma (Koebner's phenomenon). Pustular forms can involve the palms and soles. In its most characteristic form, psoriatic arthritis occurs as an oligoarthritis that involves the DIP joints (causing "sausage digits"). Other less frequent psoriatic arthritides are more typical of rheumatoid arthritis and Reiter's syndrome.

Table 10-14. Criteria for rheumatoid arthritis*

Swelling in three or more joint areas for at least 6 weeks (progressive inflammatory polyarthritis)
Symmetrical joint involvement
Involvement of hand joints (PIPs and MCPs) and wrists for 6 weeks or longer
More than 1 hour of morning stiffness
Rheumatoid subcutaneous nodules (usually along the extensor surface of the forearm; occur in one-third of patients)
Rheumatoid factor (positive in 70% to 80% of patients)
Radiographically shown erosions in hands or wrist (especially the ulnar styloid) or periarticular osteopenia (due to increased blood flow in bone adjacent to inflamed joint)

*≥four criteria for definite diagnosis. Additional manifestations include weight loss, low-grade fever, ocular scleritis; sicca syndrome (dry eyes); pericarditis and myocarditis; pleuritis with effusion; Felty's syndrome (rheumatoid arthritis + splenomegaly + granulocytopenia); peripheral nerve entrapment syndromes due to synovitis; and cervical myelopathy due to cervical spine involvement.

Table 10-15. Spondyloarthritis

Disorder	History	Physical Examination
Ankylosing spondylitis (Marie-Strümpell arthritis)	Men > women; Caucasian > African-American; usual onset at 15 to 40 years of age; chronic low back pain the initial symptom in 75%; can be family history of the disorder	25% of patients have uveitis; decreased chest expansion (less than 5 cm is abnormal); loss of lumbar flexibility and the normal lordosis[a]; sacroiliac joint tenderness[b]; proximal joint arthritis in 30%; 5% have aortic insufficiency or heart block
Reiter's syndrome (for diagnosis need arthritis plus two of following: GU, eye, or skin involvement)	Onset after episode of infectious diarrhea; men > women; onset in young adults (ages 18 to 40 years); exacerbations and remissions	Urethritis; asymmetrical polyarthritis, tendinitis; conjunctivitis; mucocutaneous lesions, such as oral ulcers; balanitis, keratoderma blennorrhagicum (keratotic desquamating areas over the soles of the feet)

[a]Schober's test measures lumbar mobility: When patient is standing, mark at L-5 level and 10 cm caudal, and remeasure with forward flexion; less than 5 cm additional distance is abnormal.
[b]Patrick's test of the sacroiliac joint is done by positioning lateral malleolus on opposite knee while supine and pushing flexed knee down.

Table 10-16. Criteria for rheumatic fever*

MAJOR MANIFESTATIONS

- Carditis (pericarditis or myocarditis; usually manifested by a new murmur, pericardial rub, or ECG changes showing pericarditis)
- Polyarthritis (migratory, nondeforming, large joint, responds to aspirin therapy)
- Chorea (occurs several weeks after other manifestations)
- Erythema marginatum (transient pink rash with irregular border and pale center)
- Subcutaneous nodules (tender; along joint extensor surfaces, occiput, or palms)

MINOR MANIFESTATIONS

- Arthralgia, fever
- Elevated ESR or C-reactive protein level, prolonged P-R interval on ECG

ANTECEDENT STREPTOCOCCAL INFECTION EVIDENCED BY POSITIVE CULTURE, POSITIVE RAPID STREP TEST, OR RISING/ELEVATED ANTISTREPTOLYSIN-O TITER.

*Diagnosis of rheumatic fever requires evidence of a streptococcal infection + two major or one major and two minor manifestations.

Rheumatic Fever

The criteria for rheumatic fever first were established in 1944 and then updated in 1992 (Table 10-16). Patients with rheumatic fever are at high risk for recurrent disease, and they require long-term antibiotic prophylaxis and follow-up.

Vignette Follow-ups

MH has radiographic and serologic findings characteristic of rheumatoid arthritis. No erosive changes are found on joint radiographs. She initially is treated with high-doses of salicylates, and treatment with antierosive agents is planned.

Ms. S is treated with parenteral antibiotics for 4 weeks. She has no embolic complications and a stable hemodynamic course. No valve replacement is necessary.

FN is believed to have ankylosing spondylitis, and he is treated with high-dose aspirin therapy. Approximately 3 years after his presentation, he has an upper gastrointestinal hemorrhage caused by a gastric ulcer and requires an emergency partial gastrectomy. His disability has progressively worsened over the years, coming to involve his hips and knees, and he has undergone bilateral hip and right knee replacement. Despite his arthritis and spinal deformity, he remains ambulatory and is still working 15 years after the initial presentation.

Vignettes 16 and 17

Cytoid body: round, white lesions of the retina; due to ischemia of the nerve fiber layer; found in 15% of patients with SLE.

BR is a 78-year-old woman admitted to the cardiac care unit with pulmonary edema. She has two major underlying problems: scleroderma and congestive heart failure, complicated by arrhythmias. Her scleroderma has been present for at least 6 years. It has been manifested by Raynaud's phenomenon, pulmonary fibrosis, esophageal atony, and polyarthralgias. Ms. R also has had two myocardial infarctions, one 4 and the other 2 years ago. Since her second infarction, she has been taking digoxin and diuretics. However, the "myocardial infarctions" occurred elsewhere, and records concerning these events are not available. It is not clear from the history whether the patient's congestive heart failure stems from her coronary artery disease, scleroderma involving the heart, or both.

Her admission vital signs are a **blood pressure** of 110/70 mm Hg, without orthostatic change, and a **heart rate** of 88 beats/min, with occasional premature contractions. **Skin:** bound-down, tight-appearing skin over her fingers (sclerodactyly), without ulcerations. **HEENT:** within normal limits; her face does not show evidence of scleroderma, as she has no limitation when opening her mouth and facial wrinkles are present when she makes normal facial expressions. **Chest:** percussion dullness at both bases and "dry" rales to the upper scapula. **Cardiac:** JVP is estimated to be 10 cm H_2O; carotids are 2+ bilaterally, without bruits. Precordial palpation reveals a palpable S_3, a sustained ventricular impulse, a right ventricular heave, and a palpable P_2. A grade 2/6 systolic ejection murmur is heard in the aortic area, and a grade 3/6 holosystolic murmur is audible at the apex, with radiation to the axilla. **Abdomen:** liver is palpable 5 cm below the right costal margin, with a total span of 13 cm; it is nonpulsatile and slightly tender. No mass is present, and stool is occult-blood negative. **Extremities:** 2+ pitting edema to the knees; no cyanosis or ulceration. She had no signs or symptoms of active arthritis. **Neurologic** findings are within normal limits.

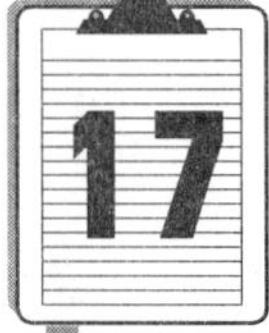

VW is a 15-year-old adolescent with SLE, who has been referred for renal biopsy. The patient was in good health, with normal growth and development, until 4 years ago. At that time, she had an episode of idiopathic thrombocytopenic purpura, which initially responded to steroids. However, she suffered a relapse and required a splenectomy for treatment of her thrombocytopenia. She subsequently did well, until several months ago, when a malar rash developed, followed by the development of arthralgias in both small and large joints. Her SLE serology had become more "positive," and in the last month, her urine (which previously had been normal) was noted to contain protein and red blood cells. She has no history of alopecia, pleuritic pain, oral ulcers, or a heart murmur. Her current medication is four to six aspirins per day.

Her **blood pressure** is 130/80 mm Hg, with a **heart rate** of 80 beats/min. Her **temperature** is normal. **HEENT:** normal scalp; an erythematous rash is present over the malar area; her oropharynx is normal; fundi show normal disks and vessels, without hemorrhages, exudates, or cytoid bodies; her neck is supple, without thyromegaly or adenopathy. **Chest:** clear to auscultation. **Cardiac:** no JVD; PMI is nondisplaced; S_1 and S_2 are normal, and an S_3 is present. **Abdomen:** notable for a splenectomy scar; no tenderness, organomegaly, or mass; stool is occult-blood negative. **Extremities:** fusiform swelling of the PIP joints of both hands. **Neurologic** findings are normal.

Vignette Objectives

1. List the features of SLE.
2. List the manifestations of progressive systemic sclerosis and compare the with those of the CREST (*c*alcinosis, *R*aynaud's phenomenon, *e*sophageal *d*ysmotility, *s*clerodactyly, and *t*elangiectasia) syndrome and mixed connective tissue disease.

Systemic Lupus Erythematosus

SLE affects 1 in 2000 people. It varies widely in its time course and manifestations, but it usually develops among young women, with a female-to-male ratio of 8 : 1, and its initial manifestations often are arthralgias and arthritis. However, any organ system can be involved. Because of its varied manifestations, diagnostic criteria for SLE have been developed (Table 10-17). However, absence of these criteria does not always exclude SLE, in that limited forms of

Table 10-17. Criteria for systemic lupus erythematosus*

Malar rash
Discoid rash (not specific for SLE, and less than 10% of people with discoid lesions have or will have SLE)
Photosensitivity
Oral ulcers
Seizures or psychosis; rarely aseptic meningitis (central nervous system involvement occurs in approximately 25% of patients)
Nonerosive arthritis (arthralgias and arthritis are the most common initial findings; only 10% of patients exhibit deformities due to injury of periarticular structures [Jaccoud's arthropathy])
Pleuritis or pericarditis (a diffuse pneumonitis also occurs, and a myocarditis develops in a small percentage of patients; accelerated atherosclerotic coronary artery disease is a long-term consequence)
Proteinuria or cellular casts (renal disease usually arises within the first 4 years of illness)
Cytopenias (most have mild anemia; 50% have mild lymphopenia [lymphocytes, <1500/mm^3]; can be associated with idiopathic thrombocytopenic purpura; circulating anticoagulants are an additional hematologic abnormality)
Positive antinuclear antibodies (many different antinuclear and anticytoplasmic antibodies have been identified)
Other positive serology (anti-DNA, false-positive VDRL test)

*≥four criteria are need to establish diagnosis. Other findings include cardiac involvement (pericarditis, myocarditis, nonbacterial endocarditis [Libman-Sacks]) and gastrointestinal manifestations (peritonitis and GI tract ischemia resulting in pancreatitis and bowel ischemia).

the disorder can occur. In addition, drug-induced SLE can be caused by many agents (e.g., hydralazine, phenytoin, and quinidine). The manifestations of drug-induced SLE usually include arthritis and serositis, and renal and CNS involvement typically are absent.

Scleroderma and Mixed Connective Tissue Disease

Scleroderma (also called *progressive systemic sclerosis*) is a connective tissue disease of the skin and visceral organs. Its features are presented in Table 10-18. The initial skin finding is edema. Later in the illness, the skin becomes bound down to underlying structures. Limited forms of the illness (Table 10-19) involve the skin but do not affect vital organs (e.g., the heart, lung, and kidney). In addition, there are overlap syndromes, or mixed connective tissue diseases, that can have features of scleroderma, SLE, and polymyositis (Table 10-20). Unlike scleroderma, however, the overlap disorders can respond to immunosuppressive therapy.

Vasculitis

Vasculitis has many manifestations, and it has been classified on the basis of the size of the vessels involved, the type of inflammation, and the organ system, or systems, affected. Other than forms limited to the skin, all the vasculi-

Table 10-18. Features of scleroderma

Symptoms usually present for almost 4 years before diagnosis
History of Raynaud's phenomenon (white, red, and blue discoloration; present in 80% of patients)
Thickening skin (symmetrical involvement of extremities; beginning on fingers; initial edematous phase, followed by induration and thickened taut skin; facial involvement causes loss wrinkles and normal skinfolds and restricts mouth movement; "neck sign" is an indurated anterior-lateral neck seen when the chin is elevated)
Distal digital ulcers
Restrictive lung disease (pulmonary fibrosis usually is asymptomatic)
Myocarditis (approximately half of patients have cardiac involvement)
Myositis
Gastroesophageal reflux (abnormalities can occur throughout the GI tract; reduced bowel motility can cause pseudoobstruction, bacterial overgrowth, and malabsorption)
Hypertension (associated renal disease)
Rapidly progressive glomerulonephritis (combined with marked hypertension can rapidly lead to azotemia)

Table 10-19. Limited scleroderma: CREST

Calcinosis
Raynaud's phenomenon
Esophageal dysmotility
Sclerodactyly
Telangiectasias

tides, are associated with constitutional complaints (e.g., malaise, fever, and weight loss) and symptoms and signs stemming from the involvement of multiple organ systems. The cause of most vasculitides is not known. As in patients with rheumatic arthritis or SLE, most patients respond to immunosuppression therapy consisting of corticosteroids and cytotoxic immunosuppressive drugs. Major features of the vasculitides are given in Table 10-21.

Table 10-20. Features of mixed connective tissue disease*

Affects women >men
Usual onset, 20 to 45 years old
Raynaud's phenomenon
Esophageal dysfunction
Pulmonary fibrosis
Inflammatory myopathy
Polyarthralgias, polyarthritis

*Mixture of features suggestive of SLE, scleroderma, and polymyositis.

Table 10-21. Manifestations of vasculitides

Condition	History	Physical Examination
Temporal arteritis or giant-cell arteritis (granulomatous inflammation of extracranial arteries [large vessel])	Usually Caucasian and >60 years old, headache, jaw claudication, diplopia, amaurosis, proximal myalgias of shoulders and pelvis girdle (polymyalgia rheumatica)	Scalp tenderness, proximal muscle tenderness with polymyalgia rheumatica
Takayasu's arteritis (large-vessel granulomatous vasculitis, primarily of aortic arch and its proximal arteries)	Young women (20 to 30 years old), cerebrovascular accidents	Hypertension, blood pressure differs in upper extremities ("pulseless disease"), bruits, aortic insufficiency
Polyarteritis nodosa (inflammation of small and medium-sized arteries)	History of hepatitis B or drug abuse (especially methamphetamines); fever, weight loss; skin changes; abdominal pain; chest pain; polyarthralgias	Fever, hypertension; palpable purpura; congestive heart failure; hematochezia; mononeuritis multiplex; peripheral neuropathy
Wegener's granulomatosis (granulomatous inflammation of small vessels of the respiratory tract and kidneys)	Onset insidious, often with a delayed diagnosis; affects men > women; fever; upper and lower respiratory tract symptoms (nasal discharge, cough, hemoptysis)	Hypertension; ulcerations and cartilaginous destruction of upper airway; ocular involvement can cause proptosis; serous otitis; pulmonary findings vary with extent of involvement
Hypersensitivity angiitis, which has been replaced by the terms *microscopic polyangiitis* and *cutaneous leukocytoclastic angiitis*	Exposure to foreign protein, drugs, or infection; chronic urticaria	Palpable purpura (especially of legs and feet), urticaria

*Additional vasculitides include Churg-Strauss syndrome (small-vessel vasculitis, eosinophilia, and asthma), Henoch-Schönlein purpura, and cryoglobulinemic vasculitis.

Vignette Follow-ups

Ms. R has a stormy hospital course, complicated by recurrent ventricular arrhythmias, worsening congestive heart failure, and azotemia. An echocardiogram shows regional wall motion abnormalities and poor left ventricular function. During the hospitalization, a new pulmonary infiltrate, fever, and leukocytosis develop. She is thought to have aspirated as the result of her esophageal reflux. She experiences a cardiopulmonary arrest on the 24th hospital day, and per her wishes, she is not resuscitated.

Ms. W has a renal biopsy, and the specimen shows diffuse membranoproliferative glomerulonephritis with marked depositional changes and wire loop hyalinization.

Vignette 18

Trigger point: applying pressure (approximately 4 kg or enough to blanch the examiner's thumbnail) produces pain to a greater degree than when the same amount of pressure is applied to a nontrigger point.

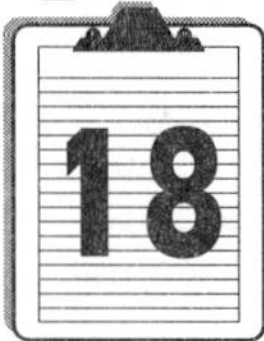

AH is a 36-year-old woman referred because of fatigue and muscle pain. She reports several years of diffuse muscle pain, for which she has seen several physicians. Many blood tests, radiographs, and bone scans have been normal or "negative." She reports that she feels fatigued every day, awakening unrested and feeling like she "had had the air let out." Her only medication is acetaminophen, which she takes two or three times a day for pain. Her past medical history is otherwise noncontributory.

Physical examination reveals a **blood pressure** of 104/78 mm Hg and **heart rate** of 82 beats/min, without orthostatic change. The following components of the physical examination reveals normal findings: **skin** exam, **cardiovascular** exam, **joint** evaluation, and **neurologic** assessment. She has significant bilateral point tenderness at **trigger points** on her trapezius, lateral epicondyles, knee fat pad, and outer buttock. Tenderness also is present over the C-5 and L-5 vertebrae. **Mental status** exam reveals no complaints of depression or anhedonia, and she enjoys her family and home life.

Vignette Objectives

1. What are the most common causes of chronic fatigue among ambulatory patients? How do the history and physical assessment help establish the diagnosis?
2. What are trigger points, and how are they used to diagnose fibromyalgia?

Chronic Fatigue

Fatigue is a common complaint and may affect up to a quarter of adults. It is termed *chronic* when it persists for more than 6 months. The prevalence of different disorders causing fatigue varies with the population studied and potential causes are listed in Table 10-22. Chronic fatigue syndrome is a diagnosis of exclusion in that it can only be diagnosed after other causes (e.g., hypothyroidism, sleep apnea, metabolic myopathy, depression, dementia, and substance abuse) have been ruled out.

Fibromyalgia

Patients with fibromyalgia complain of fatigue and muscle pain and are found to have tender trigger points on physical examination. The disorder is not associated with any abnormal laboratory findings or specific serologic markers. Often these patients are young women, and some clinicians believe affected patients are suffering from depression or a somatization disorder. However, research studies have identified criteria to distinguish a unique group of patients who have fibromyalgia (Table 10-23).

Table 10-22. Causes of chronic fatigue*

Condition	History	Physical examination
Depression	Depressed mood for >2 weeks, appetite or weight change, sleep disorder, anhedonia, guilty ruminations, trouble concentrating, suicidal ideation	Normal (except for mental status)
Somatization disorder	Onset before 30 years of age, "sickly" for years, usually female; complaints in multiple organ systems: vomiting, pain in extremities, dyspnea, amnesia, dysphagia, burning in sexual organs or rectum, dysmenorrhea	Normal, can be scars from prior surgeries
Fibromyalgia (see Table 10-23)	Widespread pain for >3 months	>11 of 18 trigger points tender
Chronic fatigue syndrome	>6 months of fatigue necessitating ≥50% decrease in activity, weakness after exertion, trouble concentrating, myalgias, painful adenopathy, sore throat, chronic headache	Nonexudative, inflamed pharynx, tender cervical or axillary adenopathy, low-grade fever

*Fatigue is a common complaint and can be due to disorders involving any organ system. Initial assessment should exclude problems of the cardiovascular (e.g., congestive heart failure), hematologic (e.g., anemia), and endocrine systems (e.g., hypothyroidism); sleep disorders; and drug abuse.

Table 10-23. Criteria for fibromyalgia

Fatigue, widespread muscle pain for >3 months
Women affected more frequently than men
Diffuse tender points* with ≥11 of 18 points involved
  Occiput (bilateral)
  Upper border trapezius (bilateral)
  Lateral epicondyle (bilateral)
  Origin of supraspinatus muscle (medial to midscapula) (bilateral)
  Second costochondral junction (bilateral)
  Upper outer buttocks (bilateral)
  Greater trochanter (bilateral)
  Fat pad of medial aspect of knee (bilateral)
  Lumbar spine (L-4–S-1)
  Posterior low cervical spine (C-5–C-7)

*Trigger points are assessed with about 4 kg of pressure (which is approximately that needed to blanch the examiner's fingernail). This pressure produces more pain (not just tenderness) at trigger points than at other control sites (such as the forehead and dorsum of the forearm).

Vignette Follow-up

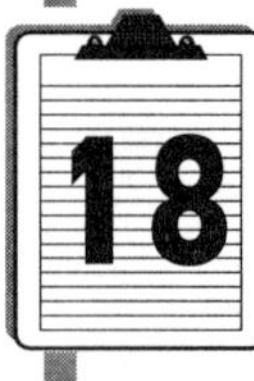

Ms. H is given information about fibromyalgia. She is given a low dose regimen of amitriptyline which she takes at bedtime and which seems to correct the loss of REM sleep that occurs with fibromyalgia. In addition, she begins a low-impact aerobic training program. After 6 months, she continues to have symptoms but does report an approximately 50% reduction in her pain and fatigue.

Objectives Review

1. List the symptoms and signs of anaphylaxis.
2. What are the definitions of and physical examination findings characteristic of urticaria and angioedema?
3. Describe a general approach to defining which structures are causing a joint complaint(s).
4. What is the differential diagnosis for acute monoarticular arthritis, and what history and physical examination findings would relate to these conditions?
5. How do the history and physical examination assist in determining the organism responsible for septic arthritis?
6. Explain how the history and physical examination findings help diagnose the cause of shoulder pain.
7. Describe the physical examination maneuvers used to examine the knee.
8. Explain how the history and physical examination can establish the cause of hip pain.
9. What features of musculoskeletal low back pain indicate the need for radiographs at the initial evaluation?

10. What are characteristics of nerve-root irritation at the L-3, L-4, and S-1 levels?
11. What problems other than musculoskeletal ones cause low back pain?
12. What conditions cause polyarthritis, and what findings help establish the cause?
13. What are the criteria used for establishing the diagnosis of rheumatic fever?
14. List the features of SLE.
15. List the manifestations of progressive systemic sclerosis and compare them with those of the CREST syndrome and mixed connective tissue disease.
16. What are the most common causes of chronic fatigue among ambulatory patients? How do the history and physical assessment help establish the diagnosis?
17. What are trigger points, and how are they used to diagnose fibromyalgia?
18. List terms used to describe skin lesions on the basis of their morphology, location, and configuration.
19. List the features of a pigmented lesion that prompt concern.
20. What are the symptoms and signs of different types of skin infections?

Suggested Reading

Baker DG, Schumacher HR Jr. Acute monoarthritis. *N Engl J Med* 1993;329:1013–20.
This is a brief review from the journal's Current Concepts series; the authors discuss how to differentiate among acute monoarthritis due to infection, crystal-induced and traumatic arthritis, osteoarthritis, and other miscellaneous conditions.

Bennett RM. Fibromyalgia and the facts. Sense or nonsense. *Controv Clin Rheum* 1993; 19:45–58.
The author is an expert on this common, controversial disorder; he reviews potential central and peripheral pathogenic mechanisms.

Bochner BS, Lichtenstein LM. Anaphylaxis. *N Engl J Med* 1991;324:1785–90.
Succinct review article.

Boss GR, Seegmiller JE. Hyperuricemia and gout. *N Engl J Med* 1979;300:1459–68.
This is an extensive and still timely review of gout's pathogenesis, manifestations, and management.

Boumpas DT, Austin HA, Fessler BJ, et al. Systemic lupus erythematosus: emerging concepts. Part 1: renal, neuropsychiatric cardiovascular, pulmonary, and hematologic disease. *Ann Intern Med* 1995;122:940–50.

Boumpas DT, Fessler BJ, Austin HA, et al. Systemic lupus erythematosus: emerging concepts. Part 2: dermatologic and joint disease, the antiphospholipid antibody syndrome, pregnancy and hormonal therapy, morbidity and mortality, and pathogenesis. *Ann Intern Med* 1995;123:42–53.
This two-part review article from the NIH contains a discussion of organ-specific (listed in the articles' titles) manifestations and the status of different managements.

Deyo RA, Rainville J, Kent DL. What can the history and physical examination tell us about low back pain? *JAMA* 1992;268:760–5.
Article from the Rational Clinical Examination series; the authors review the operating characteristics of the history and physical examination for assessing patients with low back pain; they conclude with a summary and recommendations.

Fan PT, Davis JA, Somer T, et al. A clinical approach to systemic vasculitis. *Semin Arthitis Rheum* 1980;9:248–303.
Extensive review of vasculitides, which is organized on the basis of the type and size of vessel involvement; the authors also present information on vasculitis associated with other rheumatic and infectious illnesses.

Fukuda K, Straus SE, Hickie I, et al. The chronic fatigue syndrome: a comprehensive approach to its definition and study. *Ann Intern Med* 1994;121:953–9.
The authors present guidelines for the evaluation of patients with fatigue, discuss the differential diagnosis, and provide an algorithm to assist in patient evaluation.

Gannon T. Dermatologic emergencies. *Postgrad Med* 1994;96:67–81.
Review of pemphigus vulgaris, necrotizing fasciitis, toxic epidermal necrolysis, toxic shock syndrome, and the Stevens-Johnson syndrome; it is illustrated with color photographs of those conditions.

Goldenberg DL, Reed JI. Bacterial arthritis. *N Engl J Med* 1985;312:764–70.
The authors review the pathophysiology of bacterial arthritis, the risk factors for different organisms, distinguishing features of gonococcal and non-gonococcal infections, and the evaluation and management of the disorder.

Good AE. Reiter's disease. *Postgrad Med* 1977;61:153–8.
The author presents the clinical features of Reiter's disease including the joint, skin, ocular, and GU findings.

Goodman, BW, Jr. Temporal arteritis. *Am J Med* 1979;67:839–52.
This is a clear presentation regarding what can be a confusing entity; the relationship of temporal arteritis to polymyalgia rheumatica and the prevalence of different manifestations are reviewed.

Greaves MW. Chronic urticaria. *N Engl J Med* 1995;332:1767–72.
Chronic urticaria differs from the urticaria of acute anaphylaxis; the author discusses the common types of chronic urticaria and presents an algorithm for evaluation and management.

Hoffman GS. Polyarthritis: the differential diagnosis of rheumatoid arthritis. *Semin Arthritis Rheum* 1978;8:115–40.
The author compares features of rheumatoid arthritis with those of other common (e.g., osteoarthritis, spondyloarthritis, and gout) and uncommon (e.g., SLE, mixed connective tissue disease, Lyme disease, and hemochromatosis) causes of polyarthritis.

Hunder GG, Arend WP, Block DA, et al. The American College of Rheumatology 1990 criteria for the classification of vasculitis. *Arthritis Rheum* 1990;33:1065–7.

Hurd ER. Extraarticular manifestations of rheumatoid arthritis. *Semin Arthritis Rheum* 1979;8:151–76.
This is an exhaustive review that includes information about rheumatoid nodules, eye involvement, cardiopulmonary manifestations, Felty's syndrome, and many other extraarticular problems associated with rheumatoid arthritis.

Keat, A. Sexually transmitted arthritis syndromes. *Med Clin North Am* 1990;74:1617–29.
The author reviews the manifestations of Reiter's syndrome, HIV rheumatic syndromes, hepatitis B infection, syphilis, and gonococcal arthritis.

Khan MA. An overview of the clinical spectrum and heterogeneity of spondyloarthropathies. *Rheum Dis Clin North Am* 1992;18:1–10.
Brief review and comparison of these disorders.

Koh HK. Cutaneous melanoma. *N Engl J Med* 1991;325:171–80.
Brief review, which includes 2 pages of color pictures.

Laman SD, Provost TT. Cutaneous manifestations of lupus erythematosus. *Controv Clin Rheum* 1994;20:195–211.

Lupus can have several different dermatologic manifestations, including discoid lesions, malar dermatitis, alopecia, bullous lesions, livedo reticularis, and photosensitivity; the authors succinctly review these topics.

Neustadt DH. Ankylosing spondylitis. *Postgrad Med* 1977;61:124–35.
The authors discuss the manifestations, differential diagnosis, and management of ankylosing spondylitis; the clinical tests for the disorder are illustrated.

Oberlander MA, Shalvoy RM, Hughston JC. The accuracy of the clinical knee examination documented by arthroscopy. *Am J Sports Med* 1993;21:773–8.
If a knee problem is caused by a single disorder, then clinical examination is moderately accurate; chronic and multiple abnormalities are more difficult to accurately diagnose on the basis of the physical examination findings.

Panush RS, Greer JM, Morshedian KK. What is lupus? What is not lupus? *Controv Clin Rheum* 1993;19:223–35.
Lupus has been classified as "classic" and "nonclassic," with the latter sometimes called overlap, subacute, occult, or incomplete lupus; the authors discuss the diagnosis and prognosis in patients with the nonclassic syndromes; they also present an algorithm for categorizing patients' illnesses.

Reisman RE. Insect stings. *N Engl J Med* 1994;321:523–7.
Insect stings are a common patient concern; the author presents information on different insect bites, the types of reactions, the diagnostic evaluation, and treatment.

Report of the Multicenter Criteria Committee. The American College of Rheumatology 1990 criteria for the classification of fibromyalgia. *Arthritis Rheum* 1990;33:160–72.
The sensitivity and specificity of widespread pain and specific tender trigger points as criteria in the diagnosis of fibromyalgia were 88% and 81%, respectively.

Smiley JD. The many faces of scleroderma. *Am J Med Sci* 1992;304:319–33.
The author discusses scleroderma, including the relationship of scleroderma to L-tryptophan—associated eosinophilic fasciitis and the effects of silicone breast implants.

Smith DL, Campbell SM. Painful shoulder syndromes: diagnosis and management. *J Gen Intern Med* 1993;7:327–38.
Shoulder pain is a common problem; the authors describe shoulder anatomy, the distinguishing features of specific shoulder disorders, the utility of imaging studies, and management.

Special writing group of the Committee on Rheumatic Fever, Endocarditis, and Kawasaki Disease of the Council on Cardiovascular Disease in the Young of the American Heart Association. Guidelines for the diagnosis of rheumatic fever. *JAMA* 1992;268: 2069–73.
The original Jones criteria for the diagnosis of rheumatic fever were published in 1944; this article's updated guidelines, including appropriate use of newer laboratory studies in establishing the illness.

Subject Index

D

E

I